Special Issues in Pharmacovigilance in Resource-Limited Countries

Syed Rizwanuddin Ahmad
Editor

Special Issues in Pharmacovigilance in Resource-Limited Countries

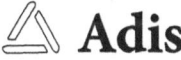 Adis

Editor
Syed Rizwanuddin Ahmad
Adjunct Faculty, Georgetown University School of Medicine
Washington, DC, USA

ISBN 978-981-96-6153-4   ISBN 978-981-96-6154-1   (eBook)
https://doi.org/10.1007/978-981-96-6154-1

This Adis imprint is published by the registered company Springer Nature Singapore Pte Ltd.
The registered company address is: 152 Beach Road, #21-01/04 Gateway East, Singapore 189721, Singapore

If disposing of this product, please recycle the paper.

In loving memory of my deceased parents, Shamsun and Rayaz. "My Lord, have mercy upon them as they brought me up (when I was small) - Quran:17:24." With special thanks to my wife and daughter; my mentors/ teachers and well-wishers.

Foreword

I know Syed since 1991, when I assumed the position of the Coordinator of the Network for Rational Use of Drugs in Pakistan. The UK charity Oxfam established The Network in Pakistan to promote rational use of drugs to continue the work that Syed had initiated in the 1980s as the Coordinator of the consumer advocacy group Health Action International (HAI), Pakistan.

Syed is well qualified to discuss the topic of pharmacovigilance (PV) in developing countries as he is not only trained but also has practical experience in this field at the US FDA and subsequently conducted training and capacity building activities for the staff of National Medicines Regulatory Authorities (NMRA) of several countries.

Since the beginning of times, different systems of medicines have been used to treat diseases but there were no formal system to monitor their safety. The need and the realization to develop a system to monitor the safety of these products came into existence after the thalidomide disaster in the 1960s. Since then, many countries in the Western hemisphere established some form of post-marketing surveillance system to monitor the safety of medicines, which was eventually named PV. In 1968, the PV system got a major boost when the WHO Program for International Drug Monitoring (PIDM) was established following the World Health Assembly's resolution calling for "a systematic collection of information on serious adverse drug reactions during the development and particularly after medicines have been made available for public use."

It took many years for resource-limited countries to establish a system of drug regulation to ensure that all registered medicines on the market meet international quality standards, and are safe and effective. In the last two decades, many countries in the developing world established some form of PV system largely with the technical assistance and financial support of a number of international agencies and development partners.

Traditionally, most clinical trials that lead to development of new medical products are first conducted in the Western world; once these products receive regulatory approval in these countries they may be subsequently approved in resource-limited countries. These trials are largely conducted for diseases that are more common in the Western countries as well. Increasingly, there has been a need to approve drugs and vaccines for infectious diseases such as tuberculosis and malaria that are more common in developing countries. There is not much information about the safety of these products in resource-limited settings where there is a potential for different pattern of adverse outcomes because of genetic makeup and environmental factors. The need for monitoring the safety of medical products post registration is important because of the limitations of clinical trial data such as the small sample size and exclusion of certain population like children, elderly, and pregnant women.

I visited Japan in the early 1990s and became aware of the tragedy with the antidiarrheal drug clioquinol that was associated with thousands of cases of blindness and paralysis. This has been an eye-opener case example for me. On the other hand, despite the availability of clioquinol in Pakistan and many other developing countries for a very long time, we do not know what havoc it has caused. We know about the devastating effects of the drug in Japan because they had an adverse drug reaction (ADR) monitoring system. We will never know how many cases of neurological deficits this drug caused in low resource countries because no such systems existed in these countries.

In recent years, global initiatives to increase access to drugs and vaccines in developing countries by international agencies have been accompanied by efforts to set up PV centers in these countries. However, in many of these countries, PV activities are still either nonexistent or rudimentary. Unfortunately, in low-income countries, PV is being implemented in health systems with poor infrastructure, weak national medicines regulatory authority, unreliable supply and quality of medicines, lack of adequately trained staff, limited training opportunities within the country, lack of awareness and interest of national stakeholders with regard to PV, and limited or no funding for PV activities in the national budget. In general, in resource-limited settings, all these challenges are compounded by the over the counter availability of products from all systems of medicines, which is too often accompanied by aggressive advertising and promotion practices of the industry, and lack of unbiased and reliable information to compliment rational use of these products. This book adequately describes all these issues and more including stories from selected countries and regions. I compliment Syed for undertaking this initiative and hope this work will serve as a useful resource to raise awareness and help develop and strengthen PV systems in resource-limited countries.

Former Minister for Health, Government   Zafar Mirza
of Pakistan, Former Director, Healthcare
System Development, WHO Regional
Office for the Eastern Mediterranean
Islamabad, Pakistan

Preface

In 1989, I attended a drug safety meeting in Minneapolis, Minnesota, USA. This is the same meeting where the International Society of Pharmacoepidemiology (ISPE) was founded. Ever since, I have been a frequent attendee of the ISPE's annual meetings called the International Conference on Pharmacoepidemiology (ICPE). In 2014, I attended ICPE's first annual meeting in Asia that took place in Taiwan. This was my first meeting as a pharmacovigilance[1] consultant after 15 years with the US Food and Drug Administration (FDA), where I was blessed to work with a number of exceptional colleagues.

At the ICPE in Taiwan, I organized a symposium on the topic of "Special Issues in Pharmacovigilance in Resource-limited countries." The objectives of this symposium were to highlight the state of pharmacovigilance in resource-limited countries (RLCs); discuss the challenges being faced by these countries such as lack of fully functional pharmacovigilance systems and infrastructure; lack of resources both financial and personnel expertise; and offer solutions. In this symposium, a number of global funding initiatives such as the Global Fund to Fight AIDS, Tuberculosis and Malaria; the US President's Emergency Plan for AIDS Relief (PEPFAR); and the US Agency for International Development (USAID) that support public health programs for the treatment of HIV/AIDS, malaria, and tuberculosis in RLCs were highlighted. Most of these initiatives support the establishment of a surveillance system to monitor adverse events associated with the use of these medicines. At that ICPE, I met Nitin Joshi, the editor of the journal *Drug Safety*, and he suggested that I consider submitting a book proposal. The idea of this book came from that symposium.

In the early 1980s, when I was a medical student at Dow Medical College (now Dow University) in Karachi, I first became aware of the availability of "banned" drugs in Pakistan and other RLCs. Banned drugs are those that were withdrawn/removed from the market in "developed" countries because of safety reasons but

---

[1] Pharmacovigilance is the science and activities related to detection, assessment, understanding, and prevention of medical products-related adverse effects.

were still marketed and sold by multinational pharmaceutical companies in "developing" countries. My familiarity and interest in the concept of "banned" drugs was facilitated by reading a book "Prescriptions for Death: The Drugging of the Third World" by Milton Silverman, Philip R. Lee, and Mia Lydecker, and by collaboration with several consumer advocacy groups including Health Action International and Consumers International. While I was a medical student, I raised awareness on this subject and campaigned against several drugs including two drugs with serious safety issues.

The first drug was an antidiarrheal hydroxyquinoline/clioquinol (brand name: Entero-Vioform). The use of clioquinol was sometimes associated with what was described as Subacute Myelo-Optic Neuropathy (SMON), a neurological condition accompanied by blindness and paralysis. Over 10,000 cases of SMON were reported in Japan and a few in other countries. As a result clioquinol was banned in Japan and other countries in the 1970s. However, clioquinol continued to be sold in rest of the world for traveler's diarrhea. My campaign to have clioquinol banned in Pakistan was successful and the drug was withdrawn from the market thanks to intervention by the country's Federal Ombudsman.

The second drug for which I advocated for removal was dipyrone/metamizole (brand name: Novalgin). Dipyrone was used as an analgesic (painkiller), antipyretic (fever reducer), and antispasmolytic (muscle relaxant). The use of dipyrone was associated with agranulocytosis, a condition characterized by abnormally low levels of white blood cells called neutrophils that fight infections. This drug was banned in the United States and several other countries in the 1970s.

When I called for the removal of these drugs some medical professionals raised serious questions with regard to my qualification to opine on this topic. These practicing medical doctors stated that they have used both these products for a number of years and have not witnessed any adverse consequences in their patients. My response to them was that the absence of any safety issue is not an evidence of absence of safety problem. I emphasized to them that on the contrary, the situation in Pakistan could be worse because of two main reasons (i) as there was no surveillance system in place to monitor the safety of these products, and (ii) additionally these products were available over the counter without the need for a prescription.

As it is, the full safety profile of a drug is unknown at the time of registration or approval and marketing because of the limitations of clinical trials that are generally conducted in a much smaller population and restricted settings. Until recently, most clinical trials that supported approval of drugs were first conducted in "developed" countries, and these products were later registered in RLCs where the population, disease, and use pattern may be different and as such based on genetics, dietary and environmental factors the adverse outcome profile may be different as well.

As drugs and vaccines become increasingly accessible to people in RLCs, the role of pharmacovigilance systems in these settings have become more critical than ever before. At the same time, more products are being developed for diseases (HIV/AIDS, tuberculosis, malaria, Ebola) that are more prevalent in RLCs, and some of these products are approved under accelerated pathways with limited data on safety.

As such it is all the more important that RLCs develop fully functional and operational PV systems with trained professionals to collect, assess, and evaluate potential safety issues earlier in order to prevent or alleviate drug-associated sufferings and facilitate evidence-based regulatory decisions for patient safety.

COVID-19 pandemic saw a surge in the use of repurposed drugs (finding new use/indications for already approved drugs), accelerated conditional approval of new products with limited safety data, and use of questionable products which were touted as a cure and/or prevention of COVID-19.

During the pandemic it was observed that in general, there was a substantial disparity in the access and roll-out of COVID-19 vaccines between high-income countries (HICs) and RLCs largely because of what has been described as vaccine apartheid. Initially, there was also a major difference in the type and brand of COVID-19 vaccine deployment - non-mRNA COVID-19 vaccines developed in China and Russia were largely used in RLCs compared to mRNA vaccines that were developed and administered in HICs. Several rare but potentially serious adverse events were identified in association with the use of these vaccines in HICs including myocarditis, pericarditis, thrombocytopenia, and clotting disorders. However, perhaps because of less robust PV systems including weak infrastructure; lack of awareness about the existence of surveillance systems (in countries where it existed) resulted in low reporting rates; lack of skilled personnel to evaluate and assess adverse event reports received by the PV centres; low quality reports; practically no new safety signals emerged from the use of these vaccines in RLCs that hadn't already been observed in HICs. This observation is a reaffirmation of the fact that in general, the PV systems in RLCs is rudimentary and needs substantial boost to be fully functional.

This book examines the state of pharmacovigilance system in RLCs; the unique issues and challenges relevant to these settings including medical products safety and product quality problems; the nature of support needed to build pharmacovigilance system capacity in these countries to effective levels; and the challenges being faced and how these are being tackled.

In the final part of the book, we have chapters that describe the global and regional strategies to develop institutional and professional capacity in pharmacovigilance in resource-limited settings. These chapters have been contributed by some government and nongovernmental agencies including representatives of national medicines regulatory agencies and development partners who have programmes in place to advance the PV skill sets of professionals in RLCs to strengthen medical products surveillance systems and improve patient safety (Chaps. 17–25). This is not a comprehensive list but rather a sample of entities who perform activities to improve PV technical capacity and contribute to safe and quality use of medical products. Hopefully, in any future edition, we will strive to showcase activities of other groups including professional societies such as the ISPE and the International Society of Pharmacovigilance (ISoP); and the work of the World Bank, Asian Development Bank, and the United States Pharmacopeia in this space.

I hope this book will be of benefit to all the stakeholders in PV in RLCs, including staff of national centres, national medicines regulatory authorities, pharmaceutical industry, donor agencies, technical assistance providers, and academic centres including pharmacy, nursing, and medical schools.

After all praise and thanks to God, I am grateful to all the contributors of different chapter for their time, and patience during this process. Without their support this book would not have been possible. At Springer, special thanks are due to Rod McNab and to Prasad Gurunadham, for their strong support to bring this project to fruition. Finally, I would like to acknowledge my deceased parents who helped and nurtured me, and provided the best support and guidance during my formative years. It would be amiss if I didn't mention my wife Itrat, and daughter Merium, for their cooperation and understanding throughout the project.

Washington, DC, USA   Syed Rizwanuddin Ahmad

Contents

Chapter 1
Pharmacovigilance in Pakistan: A Neglected Link

Madeeha Malik and Azhar Hussain

1.1 Introduction

"Pharmacovigilance is the functioning of activities in coordinated and interdependent manner focused at improving benefits and reducing harms related to use of medicines by the patients while utilizing services of relevant stakeholders and mobilizing available resources" [1]. A comprehensive medication safety system must be developed and sustained, which calls for in-country capacity building mechanism to reduce gaps in personnel, infrastructure, systems, roles, skills, and tools. For achieving this, it is necessary to specify the roles and responsibilities of the various stakeholders involved such as the pharmaceutical industry, government agencies, public health programmes (PHPs), healthcare facilities, healthcare providers, and expert advisory committees for efficient data collection and reporting [2].

Pakistan's pharmacovigilance and medication safety system is still in its infancy and has significant shortcomings in terms of process, outcome, and structural indicators. The national body responsible for regulating medicines in Pakistan is the Drug Regulatory Authority of Pakistan (DRAP), which was founded in 2012 by an act of parliament. The DRAP is tasked with conducting pharmacovigilance activities to ensure that ethical standards are followed in the promotion and advertising of pharmaceuticals, as per the DRAP Act of 2012. The regulation of import, export, manufacturing, and sale of medicines in Drug Act 1976 bounds the marketing authorization holders (MAH) to regularly monitor and report any safety issues of their products to DRAP [3]. The national pharmacovigilance center (NPC) has been established with a clear mandate under the Directorate of

M. Malik (✉)
Cyntax Health Projects, Islamabad, Pakistan
e-mail: madeehamalik15@gmail.com

A. Hussain
Pharmacy Department, Pak-Austria Fachhochschule: Institute of Applied Sciences and Technology, Haripur, Pakistan

© Springer Nature Singapore Pte Ltd. 2025
S. R. Ahmad (ed.), *Special Issues in Pharmacovigilance in Resource-Limited Countries*, https://doi.org/10.1007/978-981-96-6154-1_1

Pharmacy Services of the DRAP, and the Additional Director of this department has been assigned as the focal person for the NPC. Provincial pharmacovigilance centers have been established in provincial headquarters and in the Islamabad Capital Territory (ICT). The Regional Centre has acquired a proactive approach for effective implementation of pharmacovigilance activities in the ICT and plan to make it a role model for execution in other provinces of Pakistan. The ICT Regional Centre has signed a Memorandum of Understanding with all the hospitals of the ICT for ADR reporting.

Two subregional pharmacovigilance centers have also been notified by Regional Centre. Focal persons have been nominated from all hospitals for ADR data collection and reporting. Moreover, pharmacovigilance committees in all hospitals have been constituted. Academia being an important stakeholder has also been taken on board for the first time for effective implementation of pharmacovigilance system. The Regional Centre has developed a concise road map with clear timelines for achieving the desired outcomes by involving the relevant stakeholders. The strategic plan involves training of all focal persons on ADR reporting and causality assessment. Comprehensive mechanism for reporting of ADRs to Regional Centre has been developed. The ICT Regional Pharmacovigilance Centre will be integrated with the NPC to share good practices all over the country.

Pharmacovigilance Risk Assessment Committee comprised of experts from clinical medicine, pharmacy practice, clinical pharmacology, pharmacoepidemiology, and clinical research has been formed. This committee is responsible to evaluate the risks associated with the use of therapeutic goods, causality assessment, and evaluation of periodic reports. Several meetings of the committee have been conducted, and mechanism to evaluate reports received from healthcare professionals, regional centres, industry, and patients has been devised.

Since 2005, Pakistan's pharmacovigilance centre was an associate member of the WHO/Uppsala Monitoring Centre (UMC) for international drug monitoring [4], and in 2018, it became 134th full member of the programme [5].

Pharmacovigilance guidelines are available in Pakistan, but, detailed Standard Operating Procedures (SOPs) for reporting, evaluation, and collation of ADRs are still missing. The regular publication of safety bulletin/newsletter is considered as a key tool for medicine safety communication but not all the provincial pharmacovigilance centres are publishing such bulletins. The PV centre of Punjab regularly publishes newsletters based on local data and global safety updates [5]. The ADR reporting form has been placed on website; however, the same is not readily and widely available at reporting sites due to which the level of adverse drug reaction reporting is low.

DRAP launched an online reporting portal called "Med Vigilance" on its official website in 2018. Patients, pharmaceutical companies, and healthcare professionals can use this portal to report any adverse drug reactions or adverse events. In November 2020, DRAP launched the Med Safety App for ADR reporting. As per WHO guidelines, pharmacovigilance training should be provided to at least 5% of healthcare workers [1]. In 2018, the pharmacovigilance center conducted training for its staff, focal persons of the provincial centres, and hospital pharmacists in Islamabad. Additional training for the staff of the national PV centre, provincial centres, public health programmes, and the pharmaceutical industry has also been conducted [5]. In November, 2019, Pakistan started using the Vigiflow database to submit reports to the UMC [5]. Overall, efforts to reduce the risk of medicinal products are in their early stages; therefore, specific interventions must be designed to support the legal framework for promoting pharmacovigilance in Pakistan [7].

Med Safety App launched in Pakistan
Drug Regulatory Authority of Pakistan (DRAP) has launched a free mobile application for reporting adverse drug reactions called Med Safety App. This app has been developed by the MHRA—the regulatory agency in the United Kingdom in cooperation with the WHO Uppsala Monitoring Center. The benefits of this app include:

1. Reports can be submitted offline
2. Previously submitted reports can be viewed and updated
3. Reports can be accepted immediately
4. Ability to create a medicines watch list for which alerts can be received

Med Safety App was launched in November 2020. Because of the ease of reporting ADRs, the app has also raised awareness about the pharmacovigilance programme amongst healthcare professionals.

Besides Pakistan, this app has been launched in a few other resource-limited countries including Burkina Faso, Zambia, Armenia, Ghana, Ethiopia, Botswana, Cote d'Ivoire, and Uganda.

1.2 Barriers to Effective Pharmacovigilance

A strong pharmacovigilance and medication safety system is one of the key requirements for effective implementation of the drug regulations. However, many developing countries even lack the most basic pharmacovigilance systems to ensure the safety of pharmaceuticals, and even in those that do, active support from regulators, healthcare professionals, and other relevant stakeholders is missing [8]. Post-marketing surveillance is meant to be an independent discipline under the regulatory authority in order to fulfill a specific role within the regulatory framework. Post-marketing surveillance needs to be kept apart from the processes involved in assessing and approving new medications. The surveillance requires a dedicated source of data, infrastructure, and expertise in order to carry out the necessary tasks; however, for very valid reasons, this system and its resources can be shared with other disciplines [9].

The registered medications in Pakistan are approximately between 76,000 and 88,000, out of which many possess minor therapeutic benefit over others, or are available in multiple different brands with varying prices and quality [10]. Effective market vigilance is mandatory to efficiently combat the major problems of black-marketing and counterfeit medications, which cause fictitious drug shortages. Besides this financing, affordability and availability are also few of the major barrier toward effective pharmacovigilance system, as households are primarily responsible for paying for medications. Clear-cut pricing formula is required. The operational budget allocated to public healthcare facilities is inadequate to guarantee the availability of medications. Procurement information on prices set by the Ministry of Health is not easily accessible. Outdated logistics management systems and low number of qualified personnel result in improper drug storage and poor dispensing [11].

Although Pakistan has extensive regulations regarding the licensing of drug production facilities and registration of drugs, the implementation of these regulations is dubious resulting in poor quality assurance, increased drug expenditure, and irrational prescribing practices. Moreover, lack of baseline data, which can help map prioritized policy concerns, is another missing link. The Central Research Fund, which is managed by the Federal Government in accordance with subrule (14) of rule 19 of the Drugs (Licensing, Registering, and Advertising), Rules, 1976, has not been extensively used for comparative cost analysis or bioequivalency studies. Most of the research in the pharmaceutical area is focused on rational prescribing, while areas including policy, supply side, and financing are significantly neglected. It is necessary to analyze the challenges faced by Pakistan's Essential Medicines Programme for reducing the gap between policy and practice for promoting generics at all levels including policy, supply chain, providers, and consumers [12].

1.3   Punjab Institute of Cardiology Hospital Contaminated Medicine Crisis Case Study

In January 2012, a contaminated medicine crisis occurred at the Punjab Institute of Cardiology (PIC) hospital in Lahore, Punjab, Pakistan, killing over 100 cardiac patients, many of whom were critically ill. The incident involved patients who were being treated at the hospital for cardiac illnesses. Many of these registered cardiac patients in the PIC experienced a sudden decrease in blood platelets and leukocyte count during mid-January, resulting in bleeding from various parts of the body. At first, these signs were thought to be related to the dengue fever outbreak. However, it was soon discovered that the symptoms were limited to the PIC cohort group, suggesting that the cause could be adverse drug reaction. Drug samples were sent to drug testing facilities in France and England for examination. The pharmaceutical companies provided the record of the medications purchased by PIC in December. Six different medications that were suspected of being harmful to heart patients included

Isotab (Isosorbide Nitrate), Lipitor (Atorvastatin Calcium), Cardiovestin (Simvastatin), Alfagril (Clopidogrel), Concort (Amlodipine), and Soloprin (Aspirin). Although, nearly 25,000 patients took similar medications, only one particular batch led to deadly side effects. Approximately 451 patients were affected and 218 patients were admitted to various hospitals for using the aforementioned drugs [13]. Following confirmation of the incident, the distribution of the said medicine to patients was halted, and 70% of the total medicines distributed to 28,000 PIC patients were recovered. The Medicines and Healthcare Products Regulatory Agency (MHRA) in the United Kingdom and the Central Drugs Laboratory in Karachi found that among one of the five suspected drugs, Isotab, was found contaminated. The report also revealed that pyrimethamine, which is used to treat malaria, was present in Isotab leading to toxicity. Pyrimethamine decreased folic acid, which is required for blood synthesis. Heart patients were prescribed Isotab. The contaminant in Isotab was equivalent to ten Fansidar (sulfadoxine/pyrimethamine) tablets, which caused bone marrow suppression, irregular blood production eventually leading to death [14]. As the contaminant was quickly identified, the administration of folic acid as an antidote saved many lives.

Sri Lanka took quick precautionary measures after the incident and banned the import of medicines from Pakistan [15]. Counterfeit medications are usually sold at most of the pharmacies and substandard drugs are supplied to government hospitals and dispensaries, but those who are responsible for this remain unpunished as there is no strong regulatory body in place. The Pakistan Medical Association (PMA) denounced the event and emphasized that the deaths resulting from drug reactions were primarily caused by a failure in quality control during the acquisition of medicines. The PMA also demanded that the federal and provincial governments set up an efficient drug regulatory body to guarantee the safety of medicines in Pakistan [16].

1.4 Adulterated Blood Pressure Control Medicine Crisis Case Study

In July 2018, the European Medicine Agency (EMA) issued a recall of batches of the drug containing valsartan active substance manufactured by Zhejiang Huahai, China. In these batches, the impurity N-nitrosodimethylamine (NDMA) was detected in the raw material. NDMA is classified as a probable carcinogen based on laboratory tests. Consequently, DRAP notified all drug inspectors and health departments that the recall would also apply to all medications containing valsartan produced by the same Chinese company, regardless of whether they were imported or produced locally. Additionally, DRAP directed nine pharmaceutical companies to recall medicines with valsartan raw material. Special instructions were sent to PIC, the largest public health hospital that specializes in heart disease patients. Furthermore, all private hospitals with cardiology departments and healthcare professionals were advised to discontinue the use of valsartan from this source.

Moreover, DRAP informed patients regarding the issue and were advised to take different valsartan medicine (or an alternative treatment) when they go for next prescription. These prompt actions depict that DRAP is taking all possible measures to safeguard people's health.

1.5   Strategies to Improve Pharmacovigilance

An updated ongoing surveillance programme for assessing the impact of policies on medicine availability, price, and affordability must be developed and implemented within the healthcare system. To achieve this goal, pharmaceutical policy and research must be integrated into larger health-system initiatives, reviews, and policy updates. A framework for identifying, regulating, and monitoring standard chronic care therapies must be developed for reducing pricing and increasing availability [17]. Pilot projects on alternative financing mechanisms to supplement the public sector, such as commodity vouchers, general practitioner (GP) contracting, pre-payment schemes, and equity funds, must be considered for increasing drug availability and affordability. The expenditure on households should be reduced through optimal mix of pricing. Consumer health-seeking preferences and involvement in accountability mechanisms must be investigated. The promotion of generics must be addressed at all levels of the healthcare system. It is necessary to deliberate on improving logistics and human resource management in the public sector, as well as mapping the private sector and exploring collaborative working for improved drug access and rational drug use [18]. This necessitates continuous dialogue and interaction among different stakeholders such as the public health sector, pharmacists' and doctors' associations, local governments, industry, researchers, and development partners. Research culture must be promoted along with continuous follow-up mechanism to strengthen evidence-based policies for better pharmacovigilance and medicine safety system [19].

1.6   Conclusion

Effective pharmacovigilance can be accomplished by identifying the obstacles through better systematic collection and accurate documentation of information on substandard drug manufacture and dissemination. This would assist in informing stakeholders about the nature of the problem as well as providing a database against which batches of drugs could be checked. The only way to improve and maintain drug quality is to implement strict regulatory controls. Effective pharmacovigilance programmes must be devised and implemented in true spirit to ensure constant monitoring of the safety of marketed drugs for establishment of a credible and efficient healthcare system.

Conflict of Interest   Dr. Madeeha Malik and Prof. Dr. Azhar Hussain declare that they have no conflict of interest.

References

1. Nwokike J, Eghan K. Pharmacovigilance in Ghana: a systems analysis. Submitted to the US Agency for International Development by the Strengthening Pharmaceutical Systems (SPS) program. Arlington: Management Sciences for Health; 2010.
2. Burke SP, Stratton K, Baciu A. The future of drug safety: promoting and protecting the health of the public. National Academies Press; 2007.
3. Atif M, et al. Pharmaceutical policy in Pakistan. In: Pharmaceutical policy in countries with developing healthcare systems. Springer; 2017. p. 25–44.
4. Jawaid SA. Strengthening drug regulatory authority of Pakistan. Pulse Int. 2013;14(14).
5. Mateen A. From tragedy Pakistan builds vibrant safety system. Uppsala Rep. 2020;82:22–3.
6. Mahmood KT, Tahir F, Haq IU. Pharmacovigilance: a need for best patient care in Pakistan: a review. J Pharm Sci Res. 2011;3(11):1566–84.
7. Wood SM. Postmarketing surveillance: viewpoint from a regulatory authority. Drug Inf J. 1991;25(2):191–5.
8. Rägo L, Santoso B. Drug regulation: history, present and future. In: Drug benefits and risks: international textbook of clinical pharmacology. revised 2nd ed. Ios Press; 2008.
9. Zaidi S, Nishtar N. Access to essential medicines: in Pakistan identifying policy research and concerns. 2011.
10. Zaidi S, Bigdeli M, Aleem N, Rashidian A. Access to essential medicines in Pakistan: policy and health systems research concerns. PLoS One. 2013;8(5):e63515.
11. Hirose A, Hall S, Memon Z, Hussein J. Bridging evidence, policy, and practice to strengthen health systems for improved maternal and newborn health in Pakistan. Health Res Policy Syst. 2015;13(1):S47.
12. Shamim S, Sharib SM, Malhi SM, Muntaha S, Raza H, Ata S, Farooq AS, Hussain M. Adverse drug reactions (ADRS) reporting: awareness and reasons of under-reporting among health care professionals, a challenge for pharmacists. SpringerPlus. 2016;5(1):1778.
13. Babar A, et al. Assessment of active pharmaceutical ingredients in drug registration procedures in Pakistan: implications for the future. Generics Biosimilars Initiat J. 2016;5(4):156–63.
14. Zahid G, Sehrish W. Sri Lanka bans import of Pakistani medicines. Express Tribune, 02 Feb 2012, Pakistan.
15. Imran M, Shafi H, Mahmood Z, Sarwar M, Usman HF, Tahir MA, Ashiq MZ. Fatal intoxications due to administration of isosorbide tablets contaminated with Pyrimethamine. J Forensic Sci. 2016;61(5):1382–5.
16. Gonzalez-Gonzalez C, Lopez-Gonzalez E, Herdeiro MT, et al. Strategies to improve adverse drug reaction reporting: a critical and systematic review. Drug Saf. 2013;36(5):317–28.
17. Fryer KJ, Antony J, Douglas A. Critical success factors of continuous improvement in the public sector: a literature review and some key findings. TQM Mag. 2007;19(5):497–517.
18. Mahmood KT, Amin F, Tahir M, Haq IU. Pharmacovigilance: a need for best patient care in Pakistan: a review. J Pharm Sci Res. 2011;3(11):1566–84.

Chapter 2
Pharmacovigilance Situation in India: Issues and Challenges

Vijay Venkatraman Janarthanan, Vignesh Rajendran, and Ganesan Muniappan

2.1 Introduction: Contemporary Scenario of Indian PV

Pharmacovigilance in India achieved great significance from July 2010 when the new PvPI was launched. The programme gained more impetus when the Indian Pharmacopoeia Commission (IPC) was nominated as the National Coordination Centre (NCC) of PvPI in April 2011. PvPI aims for establishing a unique proactive drug safety ecosystem with an extensive objective to safeguard the health of about 1.5 billion people of India by ensuring that the benefits of a drug outweigh the risks associated with the drug. PvPI performs multiple tasks which include the collection of data, organizing and evaluation of the data, recommending regulatory interventions, and risk communication to HCPs and public [1]. PvPI collaborates with a maximum number of medical colleges and hospitals which function as Adverse Drug Reaction Monitoring Centres (AMCs) that collect suspected Adverse Drug Reaction (ADR) reports and forward them to NCC. PvPI updates information on ADRs that is being reported in India from across all its centres through VigiFlow to the Uppsala Monitoring Centre (UMC) in Sweden, which is WHO's collaborating centre for international drug monitoring [2]. As of November 2022, the total number of AMCs functioning under the PvPI programme was 606 [3]. Also, the Health Ministry had instructed to set up Causality Assessment Committees in all AMCs functioning across the country [4]. The Pharmacy Council of India (PCI) had asked all pharmacy and healthcare institutions across the country to report ADRs to the existing AMCs as part of PvPI. PvPI constantly focuses on skill development and capacity building measures of AMCs to ensure robust functioning of the Pharmacovigilance activities [5, 6]. A representative illustration of the PV System in India is shown in Fig. 2.1.

V. Janarthanan (✉) · V. Rajendran · G. Muniappan
Oviya MedSafe Private Limited, Coimbatore, Tamil Nadu, India
e-mail: vijay.j@oviyamedsafe.com

© Springer Nature Singapore Pte Ltd. 2025
S. R. Ahmad (ed.), *Special Issues in Pharmacovigilance in Resource-Limited Countries*, https://doi.org/10.1007/978-981-96-6154-1_2

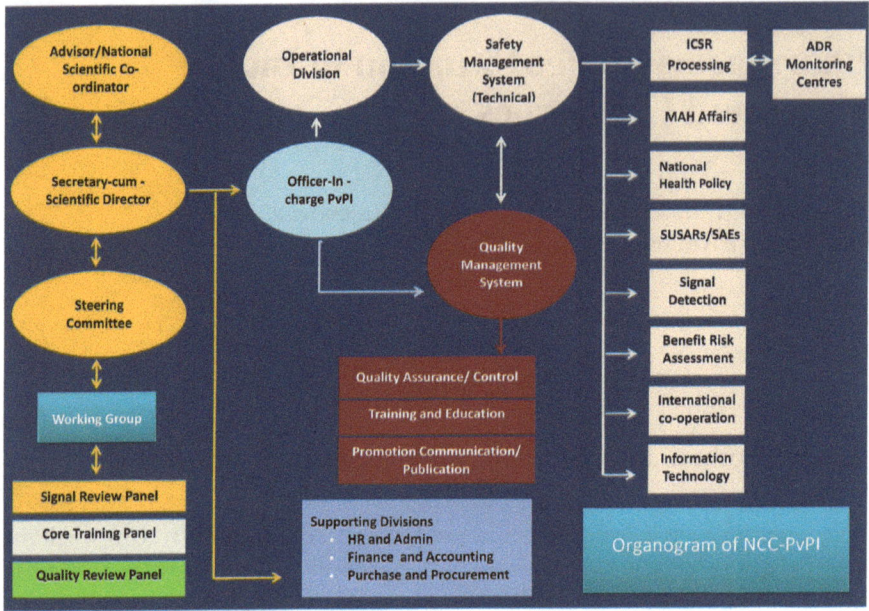

Fig. 2.1 Organogram of PvPI

The initiatives of PvPI encompass several components such as deploying a toll-free hotline, introducing a creative mobile app to streamline ADR reporting, providing ADR forms in various regional languages, and enforcing a requirement for the pharmaceutical industry to submit Individual Case Safety Reports (ICSRs) in XML-E2B (Extensible Markup Language) format. India is the first country to report over 100,000 ICSRs to VigiFlow, UMC's web-based PV system [7]. As of September 2017, over 300,000 ADRs were reported as part of PvPI ever since its inception in 2010 [8, 9]. Further, India ranked 7th (as of April 2015) in terms of its contributions to the international drug safety database (Vigibase) managed by the UMC. The UMC's completeness score assessed for Indian ICSRs was 0.82 out of 1 (as of July 2017) as against the global average of 0.55 accounted on a quarterly basis which elevated India to a position among the highest achievers in the completeness score criterion [10, 11]. The establishment of a benefit-risk assessment cell for drugs included in the risk management plan (RMP) of PvPI marked a significant strategic achievement in enhancing the PvPI initiatives and facilitates the analysis of the benefit-risk ratio of marketed medicines [12]. The presence of pharmacists in every district hospital is now a requirement to oversee ADR monitoring, and this actively contributes to advancing the progress of PvPI. It is worth noting that the March 2016 Gazette notification from India's drug regulatory agency, the Central Drugs Standard Control Organization (CDSCO), spoke of revisions in Schedule Y, which later culminated in the New Drugs and Clinical Trials Rules 2019 that became

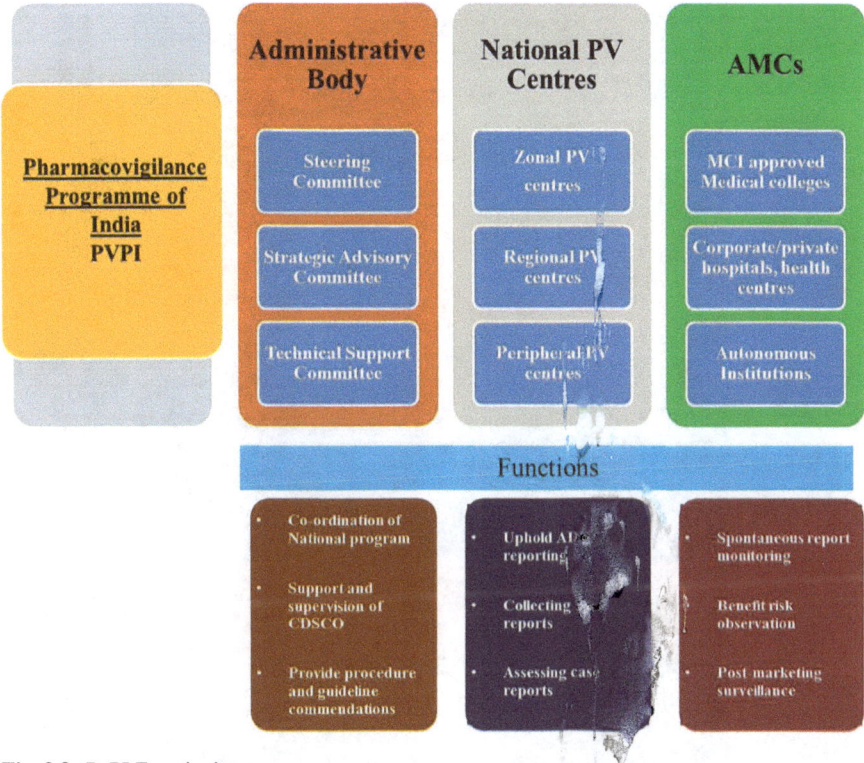

Fig. 2.2 PvPI Functioning system

effective on March 19, 2019. This update imposed a legal obligation on pharmaceutical companies to establish a pharmacovigilance (PV) system staffed with qualified individuals responsible for collecting, processing, and forwarding reports to the licensing authority concerning ADRs associated with the drugs they manufacture or sell. The functioning and achievements of PvPI are shown in Figs. 2.2 and 2.3.

India stands as a prominent player in the pharmaceutical industry in terms of growth. In the last decade, India was projected to become the sixth-largest global market by 2020. Over time, the Indian market has consistently transformed into a key global hub for clinical trials, research, and pharmaceutical development. Compared to the Indian PV system, the growth of PV within the pharmaceutical industry was faster particularly in those companies, which marketed their products in developed countries as they needed a robust PV set-up to ensure compliance to the PV regulations mandated by international regulatory bodies such as US FDA, EMA, etc. The PV outsourcing sector in India has experienced significant growth and expansion over the past 15 years, with the country now having almost 20,000 PV professionals [12]. India's competency range in PV activities has broadened. In spite of these laudable credits, there are some shadow factors that bring in constant challenges in positioning patient safety as a key priority.

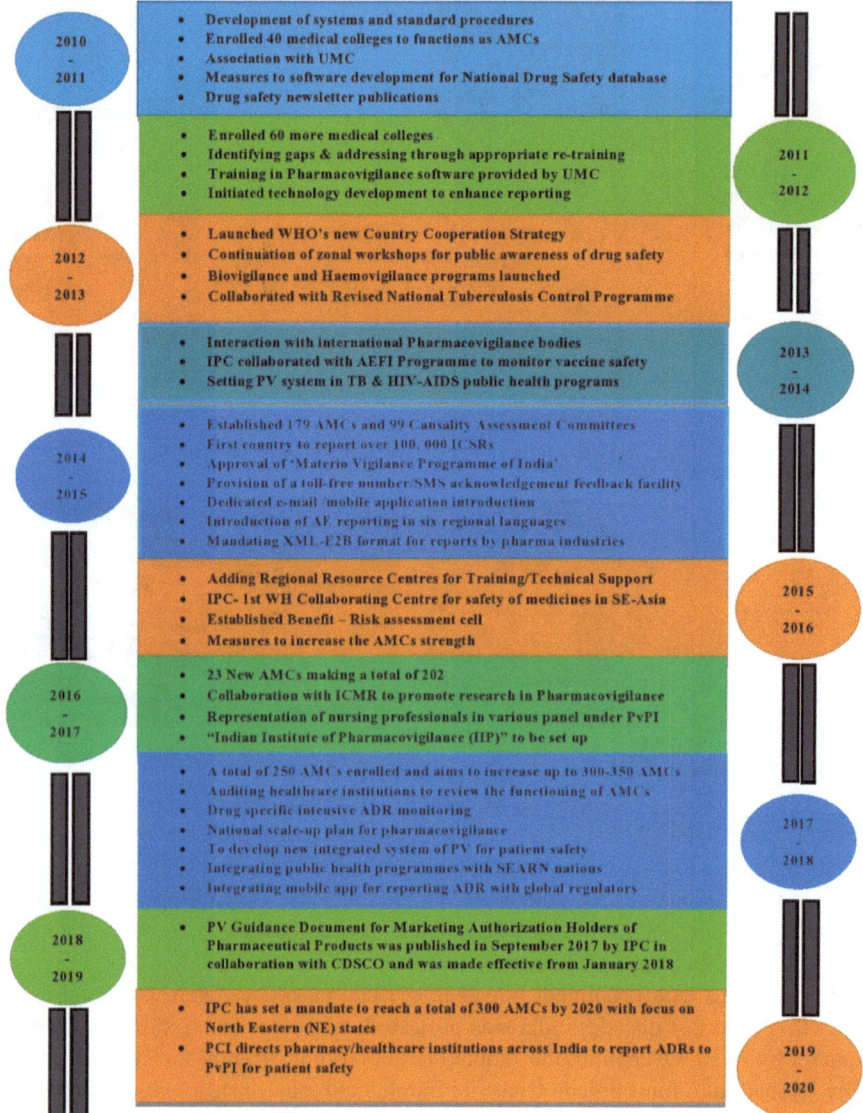

Fig. 2.3 Roadmap of PvPI

2.2 Challenges and Issues

It is indeed a fact that India has achieved quite a lot within a short timeframe in the context of the goals of PvPI, although the country needs to do more to catch up with the developed world. The PV gaps between countries are mainly because of economic, social, cultural, and regulatory differences. In the early years, the income criterion of a nation was a key influence in deciding the involvement of a country in PV activities. For countries under the higher income category, access to medicines was not an issue as the population was limited and PV activities were hence affordable. Earlier in lower- and middle-income countries, the access to life saving medicines was limited by population or by economic issues. These countries considered investing in PV systems as a luxury because to monitor the safety of products, which were not available to most of the population was deemed to be irrelevant [13]. By the continuous efforts of the WHO and some other organizations, the obstructions blocking resource-limited countries from adopting acceptable PV standards were gradually removed.

In a thickly populated country like India which is home to several languages and cultures, it is difficult to expect that a single system of medicine would be accepted by one and all. A part of the Indian population prefers traditional medicines due to their beliefs and by choice, while the other part of the population in remote areas is dependent on traditional medicines due to the lack of essential medicines [13] (See Chap. 13). Moreover, all parts of India cannot be said to have developed comparably. India has a composite healthcare system that involves government-sponsored public healthcare institutions and private hospitals where the cost is borne by patients themselves, by their insurance companies or their employer through corporate healthcare schemes. NGOs also support government/private healthcare initiatives. These are challenges unique to India. Added to these is the menace of counterfeit/spurious medicines. Therefore, implementing a strong PV system amidst these circumstances and overcoming the day-to-day issues is a "Himalayan task." The role of regulatory agencies in monitoring the medicines used in the complex Indian healthcare delivery milieu is still evolving. The monitoring of safety issues due to substandard/spurious/falsely labeled/falsified/counterfeit (SSFFC) medicines has also become a part of PV [13]. A strong PV system is particularly important in resource-limited settings because the absence of or inadequacy in such a system will put the consumers at a higher risk and treating ADRs occurring in such settings will be more expensive. Hence, all efforts need to be put in to safeguard patients from accessing harmful and ineffective medicines.

India although being one of the largest contributors of safety reports is in a need to correlate the ADR data with the population consuming the drug. The unknown ADRs of medicines that occurred previously need to be systematically identified. The Regional Resource Centers for Training and Technical Support (RRCTTS) have a significant impact on raising awareness about PvPI among various stakeholders. Acknowledging the pivotal role of RRCTTs, PvPI has actively considered the expansion of all RRCTTS by implementing necessary measures to enhance infrastructure, technical capabilities, and logistics, as per PvPI guidelines. This expansion will offer consistent training to all AMC(s) teams, foster skill development among PvPI personnel, and bolster the status of the respective AMC [12]. As a promising move to enhance capacity-building measures, PvPI started conducting various training programmes with active industry participation and support. As a requirement of Schedule Y of Drug and Cosmetics Act, 1940, a skill development programme on the Basics and Regulatory Aspects of Pharmacovigilance was started by IPC from January 2017 onwards. The objective of the programme is to sharpen the knowledge and skillset of qualified PV professionals working for better patient safety [14]. In an effort to increase medical community participation in ADR reporting, PvPI has partnered with the Indian Medical Association (IMA), an organization that represents more than 360,000 medical professionals. This collaboration has expanded the scope for private practitioners and corporate hospitals to actively contribute to PvPI, whereas in the past, the programme primarily involved government hospitals, institutions, and colleges [12]. A patient safety monitoring cell equipped with skilled manpower and a dedicated helpline for ADR reporting, and other logistics has been set up at the IMA headquarters in New Delhi. This cell aspires to provide regular training and advocacy to doctors on PV. It is vital to mention that more than 80 corporate hospitals have started coordinating with the AMCs and have started reporting ADRs as part of their pharmacovigilance activities [15].

2.3   ADRs and Regulatory Decisions

2.3.1   Nimesulide Case Study

Nimesulide is a non-steroidal anti-inflammatory drug with analgesic and antipyretic properties indicated for the treatment of acute pain, primary dysmenorrhea, and later advocated as primary anti-pyretic therapy. In India, along with other drugs, nimesulide existed in many tablet forms and multiple fixed dose combinations. Due to the ADRs associated with nimesulide, all European countries and Israel banned the usage of this drug in children. A few countries permitted the use of nimesulide in children above six years of age, and a few other countries refused permission for marketing the drug. In India, seven cases of adverse reactions and five other cases pertaining to child deaths due to nimesulide use were reported. The media reports criticized the government's lack of concern regarding the possible risks associated with the medication and its adverse effects on public health [16].

In order to evaluate the drug's safety and effectiveness when used in children, the government requested inputs from the Indian Medical Association and the Indian Association of Pediatrics. A survey was conducted with physicians and data of 5, 29,792 patients were referred in which 1,70,917 patients were in the age group of 0–1 years, 1,58,528 patients in the age group of 1–5 years, 1,09,589 patients in the age group of 5–12 years, 31,149 patients in the age group 12–30 years, 34,089 patients in the age group of 30–60 years, and 25,520 patients in the age group of above sixty years [16]. Based on the comments of various physicians and available data, IMA declared nimesulide to be safe for use in children. Further it was reported that there was no scientific evidence and causal relationship pertaining to the adverse effects of the drug, and thus, there was no necessity to withdraw the drug from the market or ban its sale. In a study conducted in 2004, it was documented that a 78-year-old man with heart disease was given nimesulide as a treatment for a wrist injury. Subsequently, the patient experienced symptoms such as breathlessness, blue pallor, and restlessness, which rapidly deteriorated and led to his death. On the Naranjo scale, the complications developed after taking nimesulide scored two, indicating the drug could "possibly" have been the cause of cardiac artery insufficiency, a shortage of blood in one or more coronary arteries [17]. These nimesulide-related issues made it clear that India needs a data-driven action.

Later, an appeal was filed in a High Court with an argument, stating that the drug was not marketed for children in any other country in the world except Brazil (children over three years) and Italy (children over six years), whereas in India, the drug was being marketed for new-born [16]. The pharmaceutical companies contended that the suspension of the drug in the mentioned countries seemed to be a precautionary step rather than a definitive conclusion against nimesulide. But in the interim period, a few pharmaceutical companies withdrew some of their nimesulide brands, fixed dose combinations, and tablets for adults from the market [18]. The Drugs Technical Advisory Board (DTAB), which advises the Central and State governments in India on technical matters pertaining to drug regulations, examined the safety-related aspects of the single dose and fixed dose combinations of nimesulide and recommended the use of nimesulide in the form of suspension drops.

Several years following this, experts revealed that nimesulide has a detrimental impact on children's liver and should not be recommended for use. Therefore, the manufacturing, sales, and distribution of nimesulide formulations for use in children below 12 years of age were prohibited under Section 26A of the Drugs and Cosmetics Act 1940. The DTAB considered the use of nimesulide in the population of 12 years and above; and after deliberations they recommended that a box warning should be provided on the label, the package insert, and other promotional literature of formulations containing nimesulide [19, 20]. In spite of the appreciation of the ban, a few experts felt that the ban has come too late and there were disagreements to the ban by a few physicians who suggested to consider Indian clinical conditions rather than foreign standards to test the side-effects of any drug, which are based on foreign genetic make-ups that might not necessarily match Indian conditions [21, 22].There was a case of regulatory decision violation in the usage of nimesulide. The drug has been contraindicated for children of age up to 12 years in India since February 2011. But a case report illustrated that a four-year male child with body weight of 20 kg presented with history of fever for one day with minimal cough. The patient was administered ceftriaxone/cefadroxyl/nimesulide IV, after which the patient developed vesicles and desquamation all over the body including the oral cavity with redness of eyes and puffiness of the eyelids over a period of 4 hours. Causality assessment revealed probable ADR relationship with the suspect drug nimesulide [23].

2.3.2 Pioglitazone Case Study

Pioglitazone is an anti-diabetic drug that has been used globally by 3 million patients for its proven efficacy and is specially valued in the Asian–Indian patients, who have a high level of insulin resistance [24, 25]. The Ministry of Health and Family Welfare

of the Government of India suspended the manufacture and sale of the widely prescribed pioglitazone in the year 2013, citing concerns over adverse effects, particularly bladder cancer [26, 27]. The Indian Pharmaceutical Alliance and a majority of
the medical fraternity considered that the drug regulator's sudden action of suspend-
ing a common and widely used drug appeared to be ill-informed. The action was
criticized, and appropriateness of the decision was under debate as there was no evidence to show that the use of the drug had resulted in adverse drug reactions in India.
Surprisingly, the suspension was not recommended by the DTAB or there has been
no mention of the PvPI reporting suspicious signals for pioglitazone [24]. Later, the
DTAB revoked the suspension and pioglitazone was available with an updated warning for the patients [27]. This episode indicated the need for a regulatory system that
has a predictable, unbiased process based on evidence to suspend or ban a medicine.

2.4   Anti-diabetic Drugs and Pancreatitis

There are various adverse events reported for the first time in India through published literature. A 49-year-old man experienced severe abdominal pain and was
diagnosed with pancreatitis three weeks after initiating vildagliptin to manage his
uncontrolled type 2 diabetes. This seems to be the first documented instance of
acute necrotizing pancreatitis in a patient using vildagliptin in India [28]. There was
another postmarketing case report of liraglutide-induced pancreatitis from India. A
51-year-old patient who had been living with type 2 diabetes for 13 years was given
liraglutide, a medication in the glucagon-like peptide (GLP-1) analogue class
known as Victoza, to manage blood sugar levels and aid in weight reduction.
Approximately eight weeks after starting the GLP-1 analogue, the patient experienced severe abdominal pain, nausea, and vomiting. Laboratory tests and a CT scan
confirmed the presence of pancreatitis, and the patient received treatment for acute
pancreatitis. Liraglutide was discontinued and the symptoms improved [29].

2.5   Pharmacogenomics—Indians Respond Differently
       to Certain Medicines

2.5.1   Carbamazepine

The effective operation of the Signal Review Panel within PvPI is commendable
because it informs CDSCO about the signals it generates, providing CDSCO with
the necessary evidence to request drug manufacturers to modify their labels. The
current focus of PV is primarily on collating and analyzing data related to ADRs.
However, it is anticipated that in the near future, the scope of PV will expand to
encompass pharmacogenomics as an integral part of the scientific aspect of PvPI
[12, 30]. One of the reasons for the need of involving pharmacogenomics in PvPI is

the worrisome incidence of serious ADRs like Stevens-Johnson syndrome (SJS) in India [31]. Reports of ADRs from 100 AMCs across India revealed that the usage of carbamazepine is linked to the occurrence of SJS in a substantial number of patients. SJS is a clinical condition believed to be an allergic response characterized initially by prodromal symptoms like fever, fatigue, and a sore throat. Carbamazepine, available in various brand names, is a commonly prescribed anticonvulsant medication used for managing epilepsy by reducing nerve signals that trigger seizures and pain. It is also utilized for treating conditions such as seizures, nerve pain like trigeminal neuralgia, and diabetic neuropathy, in addition to managing bipolar disorder [32]. PvPI received 119 reports of fatal or life-threatening skin reactions, including SJS and Toxic Epidermal Necrolysis (TEN), which were possibly linked to the use of carbamazepine. These 119 cases were among the 1,887 reported ADRs attributed to carbamazepine in India, as documented in VigiBase up to December 31, 2014. Scientific literature has indicated a heightened correlation between HLA-B 1502 and the development of SJS due to carbamazepine in the Indian population. It was advised to include the statement "It is recommended that patients may be screened for HLA-B 1502 prior to initiating treatment with carbamazepine because it is a known risk factor for carbamazepine induced Stevens Johnson Syndrome. Patients testing positive for the allele should not be treated with carbamazepine unless the benefit clearly outweighs the risk" [7].

A retrospective analysis encompassed 59 instances of SJS reported over a span of four and a half years, spanning from July 2005 to December 2009. Throughout this study period, a total of 1,769 ADRs were documented, with 59 cases specifically related to drug-induced SJS. The prevalence of SJS in this context was approximately 3.33% (with a 95% confidence interval ranging from 2.91% to 4.17%). The age range of individuals afflicted with SJS ranged from 2 months to 85 years, with the median age being 35 years. Among the 59 patients, 15 (approximately 25%) were children or young adults, and nine (around 15%) were over the age of 50. The onset of SJS was observed within a timeframe spanning from 1 to 39 days after the commencement of drug therapy [33]. Within the initial week of treatment, SJS emerged in 36 patients, with an average onset occurring at 10.5 days. For phenytoin, the onset averaged 8.4 days, while for carbamazepine, it was 7.5 days. Among the children included in the research, nearly half of those who developed SJS had previously experienced upper respiratory or nonspecific viral infections. This study revealed a higher incidence of SJS in children with a susceptibility to viral infections, while mortality rates were more elevated among the elderly [33]. With patient safety in mind, the SRP advised CDSCO to instruct all manufacturers to include a clear warning on the drug's label, notifying patients about potential side effects.

2.5.2 Anti-Cancer Medicines

Apart from carbamazepine, PvPI has submitted recommendations to the Centre based on data collected from over 60 AMCs across the country concerning two anti-cancer medications, sunitinib and pazopanib. Sunitinib is prescribed for the treatment of gastrointestinal stromal tumors (GIST) that develop in the stomach, intestine, or esophagus in cases where imatinib treatment was unsuccessful or not possible. It is also used to address advanced renal cell carcinoma (RCC), a type of kidney cancer, as well as pancreatic neuroendocrine tumors (pNET), a specific tumor type originating in the pancreas, particularly in patients with inoperable and worsening tumors. On the other hand, pazopanib is utilized to treat advanced RCC in adults, with its mechanism aimed at slowing down or halting the spread of cancer cells.

In Indian patients with metastatic renal cell carcinoma treated with sunitinib, there have been observed instances of hepatotoxicity, hemorrhage, and cardiovascular events. Moreover, the ICSRs of Indian patients with metastatic renal cell carcinoma undergoing pazopanib hydrochloride therapy have disclosed cases of fatal cardiac dysfunction. These encompass congestive heart failure and ischemic heart diseases, which have resulted in death in approximately 23.40% of patients [7]. Based on the panel's findings, CDSCO has been advised to undertake vigilant monitoring of these two drugs due to numerous instances of ADRs such as pazopanib induced hand-foot syndrome [34] and sunitinib-induced thrombotic microangiopathy [35] reported from the use of these drugs.

2.5.3 Ranitidine

The Signal Review Panel conducted a thorough assessment of ranitidine's utilization and its potential connection to cardiac arrest, relying on Indian case reports featured in various publications. An example from a 2013 literature report highlighted the situation of a 38-year-old female patient who underwent admission for medical termination of pregnancy and laparoscopic tubal ligation at a day care surgery facility [36]. The patient underwent a pre-anesthetic check-up, which showed normal results, including routine tests within normal ranges. An electrocardiogram (ECG) indicated a normal sinus rhythm. Prior to surgery, the patient received an intramuscular injection of 50 mg of ranitidine 45 minutes before the procedure. In the operating room, the patient was administered ondansetron, 4 mg intravenously, given slowly over 30 seconds. However, just 30 seconds after receiving the drug, the patient lost responsiveness to stimuli and stopped breathing, and the ECG displayed a flat line with no detectable peripheral or central pulses. Cardiopulmonary resuscitation (CPR) was initiated. The patient was promptly intubated with a 7.5 mm inner diameter cuffed endotracheal tube. Within two minutes of CPR and the administration of 0.6 mg of atropine, there was a return of spontaneous circulation. The monitor displayed a normal sinus rhythm with a heart rate of 96 beats per minute and a blood pressure of 132/80 mmHg. Subsequently, the patient regained spontaneous breathing within the next two minutes. Upon observation, the patient exhibited adequate spontaneous breathing, maintained oxygen saturation, was conscious, alert, free from neurological deficits, and had stable hemodynamics. The author concluded that it is unclear whether the cardiac arrest in this case was due to a drug combination or ondansetron alone [36]. A 2014 literature report describes an incident where a single intravenous dose of 50 mg ranitidine resulted in sudden cardiac depression, leading to the patient experiencing a sudden cardiac arrest. The patient in question was a 32-year-old female scheduled to undergo a hemithyroidectomy. She received intravenous ranitidine as a preoperative measure. Subsequently, the patient experienced a rapid decline in cardiac function, leading to cardiac arrest. Despite initial resuscitation efforts and intensive care, the patient developed supraventricular tachycardia the day after the initial event and passed away due to cardiorespiratory arrest [37].

A case report from 2015 documented an unusual occurrence involving a 30-year-old male who was admitted for a malunited fracture involving the mandible and zygomatic bones. The patient received oral medications, including cefixime, metronidazole, ondansetron, and ranitidine for three days before the operation, following a normal preoperative workup. The patient had no notable medical history or family history. On the day of the surgery, the patient was administered injectable dexamethasone, cefotaxime, ondansetron, ranitidine, and metronidazole approximately half an hour before the procedure. Within less than five minutes of receiving a rapid bolus injection of ranitidine, the patient experienced a sudden cardiac arrest and received resuscitation from the attending anesthesia team. Subsequently, the patient was transferred to the Intensive Care Unit (ICU) and placed on a ventilator, and maintained stable vital signs for 24 hours following the incident. In all the above reported cases, association of ranitidine with cardiac arrest has been reported. Considering the seriousness, the panel submitted a high-level recommendation to CDSCO, suggesting label change by the manufacturers and concerned Marketing Authorization Holders (MAHs) [38].

2.6 Other Examples

In the PvPI database, there were two ICSRs concerning the anti-rabies vaccine (Rabipur) and erythema multiforme. After a comprehensive assessment of these cases, the Signal Review Panel determined that a significant temporal relationship existed between the administration of the anti-rabies vaccines and the occurrence of erythema multiforme. Given this evidence, the panel has advised the CDSCO to include this warning in the package inserts of the suspected drug available in the domestic market [39]. The panel also confirmed a strong underlying association of hypokalemia and bronchospasm induced by piperacilline and tazobactam and therefore recommended to CDSCO to change the label on the package of a fixed dose combination (FDC) of piperacilline and tazobactam [40]. Table 2.1 shows the drugs, their ADRs, and the Signal Review Panel recommendations [41].

One of the most significant achievements in pharmacovigilance is the timely identification of signals related to potential adverse drug reactions. In the 5th signal review panel meeting held on 9th May 2015 at CDSCO, to promote patient safety, ICSRs of potential signals were evaluated from Indian database. As an outcome,

Table 2.1 Recommendations and actions taken by Indian regulatory authority

Drugs	Adverse Drug Reaction(s)	PvPI Recommendations to CDSCO
Sulfasalazine	Stevens-Johnson Syndrome, Toxic Epidermal Necrolysis	Label change
Meropenem	Hypokalemia	Continued monitoring
Phenytoin	Angioedema, Osteoporosis	Continued monitoring and collection of more reports
Lamotrigine (Phenyltriazines)	Stevens Johnson Syndrome, Toxic Epidermal Necrolysis	Label change
Ceftriaxone (5th gen. cephalosporin)	Stevens Johnson Syndrome	Label change
Betamethasone (corticosteroid)	Photosensitivity reaction	Label change
Azithromycin (macrolides)	Acute Generalized Exanthematous Pustulosis (AGEP)	Label change
Cloxacillin (Penicillin)	Acute Generalized Exanthematous Pustulosis (AGEP)	Label change
Piperacillin and Tazobactum (Penicillin derived)	Hypokalemia, bBronchospasm	Label change
Ranitidine (Antihistamine)	Cardiac arrest	Label change
Anti-Rabies Vaccine	Erythema multiforme	Label change
Surfactant	Pulmonary hemorrhage	Label change
Mannitol	Hypokalemia	Label change
Rota Vaccine	Intussusception	Label change

SJS was considered a potential signal for artemether/lumefantrine which was also suggested by WHO-UMC [42]. In a joint signal detection workshop conducted during 5th –8th October 2015, at IPC-Ghaziabad, the existing signal detection procedure of UMC was replicated to identify potential signals that could be applicable to the Indian context. The ultimate result of the workshop was the review of a total of 168 combinations of drugs and ADRs, with a selection of a few of these combinations being designated as potential signals (Table 2.2) [41]. The list of combinations was compiled using the latest information from VigiBase, the worldwide WHO database of ICSRs, which includes reports of suspected adverse drug reactions. To assess and prioritize these drug-ADR pairs based on the quality of evidence supporting them as genuine adverse effects, the VigiRank algorithm was used. Since this signal detection was reviewed by the signal review panel, the outcomes were considered for appropriate regulatory measures by CDSCO [39]. After discussions during the 15th signal review panel meeting convened on August 21, 2019, at IPC, the panel suggested to PvPI that they inform CDSCO to initiate the essential measures to include "acute kidney injury" in the PIL of proton pump inhibitors [43]. This resulted in CDSCO directing the state drug controllers to instruct

Table 2.2 Signals identified for different drugs

Drug	Signal
Amikacin	Drug hypersensitivity syndrome
Artemisinin derivatives	Stevens Johnson Syndrome
Azithromycin	Acute Generalized Exanthematous Pustulosis (AGEP)
Betamethasone	Photosensitivity
Citicoline	Hallucination
Cloxacillin	AGEP
Phenytoin	Vestibular disorder

manufacturers of proton pump inhibitors like pantoprazole, omeprazole, tanso-prezole, esomeprazole, and rabeprazole to do so. This recommendation was made based on PvPI's review of the ADR reports received for proton pump inhibitor products.

In India, CDSCO approves new drugs to be introduced in the market. Once CDSCO has granted approval, the state regulatory bodies give out licenses for sale and manufacture of drugs. But due to inconsistent enforcement of laws between state and central regulators and based solely on approval from individual state governments, a high number of unapproved FDC products are available over the counter in India. In 2012, an Indian parliamentary committee noted that a high number of manufacturing licenses for FDC products had been granted by state authorities without obtaining prior approval from CDSCO, which contravened regulations. The committee also raised concerns about potential ambiguity regarding the extent of powers delegated to the states, which may have played a role in this situation [44]. Earlier in 2007, CDSCO banned 294 FDCs which had state licenses only, for which the manufacturers of FDCs contested the ban and secured a court-ordered stay [44]. In January 2013, CDSCO sent a letter to all state and union territory drug controllers asking them to order all the drug manufacturers under their jurisdiction to demonstrate the safety and efficacy of their FDCs [45].

In 2014, the Government of India set an expert committee to review the submissions of drug manufacturers [46]. The committee received over 6,220 applications for consideration and found 963 drugs to be irrational, medically inappropriate, ineffective and thereby lacks "therapeutic justification" [47]. Considering the outcome after conducting several product reviews and based on the suggestions from various research papers, in March 2016, the central government banned 349 of the 963 drugs under Rule 26-A stating that they are likely to involve risk to human beings. The therapeutic categories of anti-diabetic drugs, respiratory drugs, analgesics, anti-infective, and gastro-intestinal drugs will be impacted [48]. Many international drug regulatory agencies have voiced apprehensions regarding the quality of medications produced in India [49–51]. The Government of India took necessary measures to regulate manufacturing practices, sales, and distribution of the FDC products. As a result, these combinations did not receive approval for sale in significant pharmaceutical markets, such as the United States, the United Kingdom,

Germany, France, and Japan. At present, there are more than 64,000 different formulations being manufactured and sold through pharmacies across India [52]. The Pharmaceutical Wholesalers Association (PWA) claimed that the ban could affect 7% of domestic drug market resulting in losses of INR 7000 crore (approximately 1.047 billion US$) to pharmaceutical companies [53]. The annual impact of the ban is estimated to be around Rs 3049 crore (approximately 0.46 billion US$) or by 3% of the organized pharma retail market valued at Rs 98,000 crore [54] (approximately 14.67 billion US$). However, the pharmaceutical companies/industry associations questioned the basis of the ban and managed to get a stay of ban through judicial interference [55].

The pharmaceutical industry associations argued that CDSCO should have implemented the ban in a phased manner, giving a cut-off date for stopping production at first and withdrawal in a timeframe. The ban of FDCs by the government was considered as impractical and unacceptable by some pharmaceutical companies as the drugs had been in the market for long, with a few of the combinations having been approved by CDSCO. There was an argument that the drugs were neither spurious nor of substandard quality to be a threat to patient safety. The key arguments [52, 56–59] of the companies against the ban were:

- The sudden ban will cause tremendous void in handling health problems of many patients.
- The ban will force divestment in instant research, which will weaken the research and development capability.
- There will be an impact on the effectiveness of the drugs being developed and may rise the cost of medicines.
- The ban will affect the profitability of industries and will lead small and medium scale companies in financial distress.
- The supply chain will be left with reduced inventories, leading to significant financial losses, particularly for small-scale businesses.
- The products even of non-banned categories are returned along with the banned drugs as these drugs do not hold high sales in the market due to the arrival of newer drugs or other brands.
- The ban caused destruction to contract manufacturing sector.
- This ban will create panic among the patients and confusion among physicians. The patients will have a feeling of insecurity and threat in their mind about the physicians who prescribe these drugs. The physicians may not have any clear idea about the ban and may continue to prescribe the same drugs.
- The retailers are dispensing medicines based on physicians' prescriptions which are in brand names and do not consider the combination of each brand. The drugs that were banned are sold in 3000 brand names, and each pharmacy may have 400–500 brands of these drugs which is too difficult for the retail pharmacists to identify.
- There is inadequate networking between state drugs control departments and CDSCO which have to monitor the millions of pharmacy outlets without adequate of surveillance technology.

- The ban would be a retrograde step and the drug regulatory body has no sufficient mechanism to warrant the drugs' withdrawal from the market. Hence, the government should withdraw the ban on FDC medicines in the interest of all stakeholders.
- India holds the top position globally in the realm of FDCs, and presently, even well-regulated markets are witnessing a gradual increase in the introduction of additional combination products.

The All India Chemists and Distributors Federation (AICDF) pointed out that the ban on FDCs is a beneficial step to the patient community in the country. The AICDF insisted the government to take post-ban steps including monitoring of the market and to ensure that the manufacturers withdraw the banned products from the traders without any financial difficulties. The federation stated that the ban has in no way impacted the traders' business as there were enough alternatives [60]. This ban will give scope for the pharmaceutical industry to develop safer and more effective drugs [52]. A study on the utilization of FDCs, carried out before the FDC ban issued by the Union Health Ministry on March 10, 2016, disclosed that the abundance of FDCs found in the nation's pharmacies encourages their excessive consumption due to a lack of awareness regarding their appropriate and justified usage. A 2015 study suggested that by highlighting the drug withdrawals/bans internationally, the unapproved formulations in India should be banned immediately, conducting an assessment of the benefits and risks for patients when discontinuing or transitioning to alternative medications. A recent study reported that there was a total of 118 systemic antibiotic FDC formulations available for sale in India. Among these, 43 (approximately 36%) had received official regulatory approval, while 75 (around 64%) lacked any documented record of regulatory endorsement. Only four (about 3%) of these formulations were approved for use in the United Kingdom and/or the United States. Nearly half of these formulations (58 out of 118, which is roughly 49%) consisted of a combination of two antimicrobial agents. A significant portion of these dual antimicrobial combinations (43 out of 58, equivalent to approximately 74%) were not authorized for use in India. Many of these combinations posed pharmacological challenges. The 118 FDC formulations resulted in the production of 3307 branded products by 476 pharmaceutical manufacturers, including a dozen multinational firms. Out of these 118 FDC formulations, 53 were produced by multinational corporations. Among these, 20 were not authorized for use in India. Only four of them had received approval for use in both the United Kingdom and the United States [61]. It was strongly felt then that amending drug regulations was necessary to guarantee the safety and efficacy of medications available in the Indian market [46]. In September 2018, the Union Health Ministry banned 328 FDCs because a report submitted to the Supreme Court by the Drugs Technical Advisory Board had deemed all of these drugs as irrational and lacking in efficacy. Though this move could be considered as late, it was lauded as the right decision and as a vital step towards protecting the health of the people from the adverse effects of unnecessary drugs [62],

2.7   The Way Forward

It is imperative for the nation to undergo a significant overhaul in its healthcare sector, prioritizing patient safety to advance PV practices in India. In India, the quantum of self-treatment is considerably high. Regulators should enhance the two-way communication with the primary stakeholders, which include patients and healthcare professionals. Valuable information about medicines should be made available to patients and physicians. Regulatory actions should promote patients to report any new symptoms to their healthcare professionals and inspire healthcare professionals (especially physicians) to submit well-documented reports of suspected ADRs. Patient-generated reports can complement those generated by healthcare professionals and offer valuable insights. However, additional evidence-based strategies are required to enhance physician engagement. Building collaboration between physicians associations and PV experts will bring promising outcomes. The reasons for poor reporting of ADRs include lack of incentives, ignorance, hesitation of reporting serious ADRs, lack of time, and the personal insecurities that refer to the fear of legal liability on the part of physicians, which should be addressed and resolved authentically. The factors required for a proactive futuristic PV system are shown in Fig. 2.4.

Indian regulatory authorities need to guarantee that they collect timely and sufficient information about adverse events in a manner that does not hinder access to essential medications. The awareness to report therapeutic failure should be increased. The pharmacovigilance activities should be incorporated into drug administration programmes by partnering with public health agencies, NGOs, and similar organizations. The communication gap between the regulatory authorities, pharmaceutical companies, and their stakeholders responsible for products safety should be sorted out. Though promising outcomes have been achieved in the past through collaborations, there is a need for sustained partnership between these stakeholders to meet international, national, and local level PV obligations. The roles and responsibilities of the key stakeholders in the pharmacovigilance framework need to be defined. In India, there is a need for medicine-related harm data with strong evidence especially due to the enormous population. The existing literature and reports on medicine-related harm are inadequate, emphasizing the necessity for further extensive research on the issue of harm, including cases stemming from medication errors. It is crucial to reduce the occurrence of false positive results when dealing with the vast amount of electronic data from various sources. The analysis of signals should focus more on preventable problems that can be caused by a drug and then reach out for signals that are novel. Any new sources having the potential to provide drug safety signals should have to be entertained through proper actions. It is essential to obtain comprehensive epidemiological data that actually reflects the use of drugs and treatment outcomes.

By being the 8th WHO collaborative center and as a member of South East Asia Regulatory Network (SEARN), CDSCO-IPC needs to support WHO member countries like Bangladesh, Bhutan, Korea, Indonesia, Maldives, Myanmar, Nepal, Sri

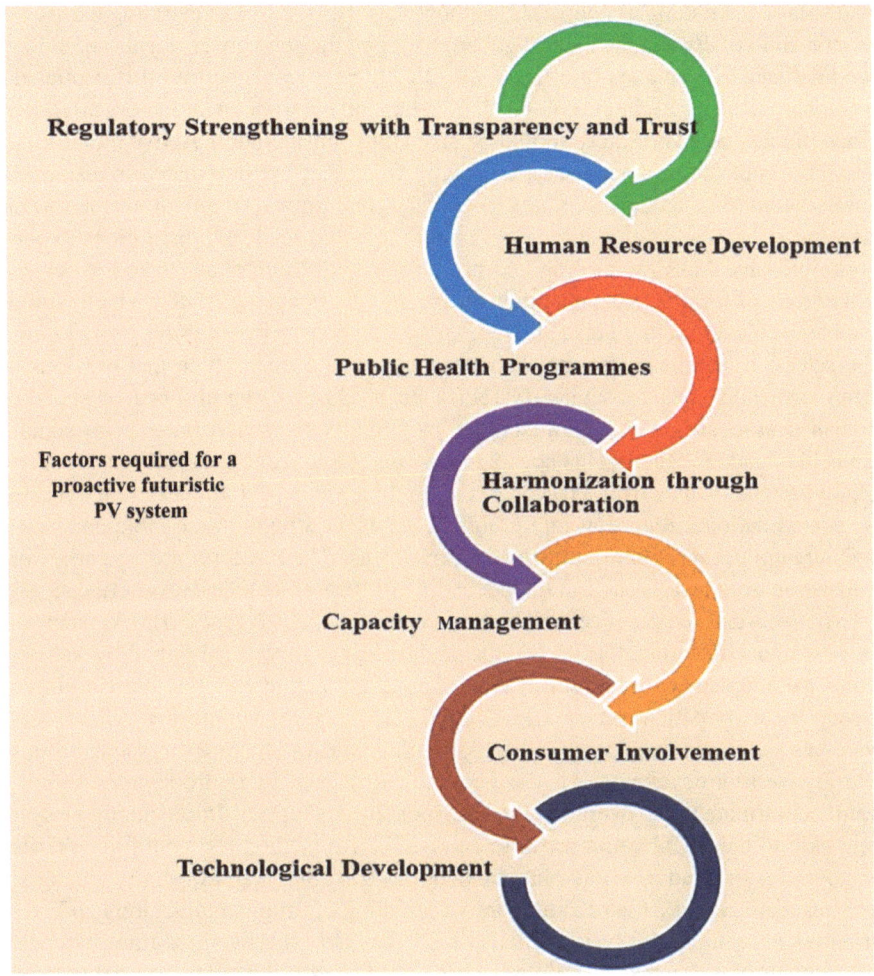

Fig. 2.4 Factors required for a proactive futuristic PV system

Lanka, Thailand, and Timor to build to implement pharmacovigilance programme in their health systems. This will help to develop regulatory collaboration, convergence, and reliance in the South-East Asia region over shared regulatory issues. IPC intends to focus on TB, neglected tropical diseases, vector-borne diseases, HIV-AIDS among other such challenges as part of integrating PV programmes in public health systems for SEARN member countries [63]. IPC also had plans to harmonize PvPI with public health programmes of member countries with UMC's oversight [64].

To predict the harm of drugs premarketing, there is a need for relating post marketing clinical information to premarketing pharmacology and toxicology. For any regulatory decisions taken in India, there is a need for transparency and accountability. Improving these processes will facilitate the public to evaluate and understand the details of approvals, withdrawals, bans, etc. The clouding clarity of responsibility between the central government and the state governments should be well defined. The concept of efficacy and effectiveness must be well differentiated. The pharmacological, immunological, genetic, and environmental factors affecting drug effectiveness and safety should be taken into consideration. Active monitoring of all types of drugs is necessary, especially when they are introduced in resource-limited countries, as they may not have undergone prior testing and evaluation in developed nations. As an initiative, PvPI has identified academic institutions to perform intensive ADR monitoring and has also provided guidelines to follow a specific protocol for prospective studies on specific drugs having ADRs, which would enable the Government to take any regulatory decisions. As part of this programme, the selection was made for the diabetic drug pioglitazone, which had previously been suspended and subsequently reinstated because of the absence of specific Indian data regarding adverse reactions, particularly those associated with conditions like bladder cancer. This specific study on pioglitazone hopefully may generate India specific data over a period of two to three years [65]. India should develop dedicated national reporting rate graphics, establish a public-accessible database, and streamline an online platform for physicians. These efforts are essential for enhancing drug awareness and understanding of their potential adverse effects.

The well-defined practices of the European Medicines Agency (EMA), such as RMPs, signal detection, QPPV, and the paid review of reports submitted by MAHs, could be adopted with the aim of streamlining PV activities while maintaining a strong focus on patient safety. EMA's Medical Literature Monitoring (MLM) service has generated considerable discussion in countries where PV responsibilities are just getting developed. This is because cases from literature sources significantly contribute to the overall volume of spontaneous reports. Implementing a system akin to the MLM could prove to be an effective method for identifying ADRs in countries like India, where pharmacovigilance is emerging, especially when the pharmaceutical market is predominantly consisting of drug manufacturers and distributors who might not have sufficient resources for extensive literature searches. To promote the practice of PV, India has established standardized guidelines for pharmacovigilance in collaboration with the industry. Around 100 pharmaceutical companies joined hands with CDSCO and PvPI to bring up comprehensive guidelines on a level comparable to the established international guidelines [66]. PvPI also appointed a panel of industry experts who submitted their recommendations for the draft PV guidelines. A 15-member committee representing 60 pharmaceutical companies recommended PvPI for setting of pharmacovigilance system at each pharma manufacturing unit which will collect, process, and forward reports to the licensing authority to inform them about ADRs arising from the utilization of the company's drugs within India. The committee also proposed that it should be made compulsory for MAHs and license holders manufacturing products in India to submit risk management plans to ensure drug safety at par with global standards [67]. On September 29, 2017, the Pharmacovigilance Guidance Document for MAHs of Pharmaceutical Products was released by the secretary, ministry of health and family welfare, Government of India. It was developed by the NCC of PvPI, IPC, in collaboration with CDSCO, according to the amendment in the Drugs & Cosmetics Rules, 1945, Schedule Y vide Gazette Notification G.S.R. 287(E) published on March 8, 2016 [68], which was consequently incorporated in the New Drugs and Clinical Trials Rules 2019 that became effective on March 19, 2019. But the compliance to the PV guidance document is yet to see its high point in the country due to lack of strict regulatory action, and it is necessary for the government to take steps to sanctify the PV guidance document as an indisputable regulatory mandate in order to ensure cent percent compliance to it by the industry. As of 2018, around 200 companies have submitted ICSRs to PvPI, and the number has not increased much in 2023 as well. Also, there are expectations from the micro, small, and medium-sized enterprises (MSME) that the guidelines should be feasible for implementation by MSME units as well. Several companies are facing practical difficulties complying with certain provisions of the guidelines as mentioned below [69].

- Every ICSR received by a MAH is required to be sent to the PvPI in XML-E2B format, which necessitates the implementation of an electronic pharmacovigilance database.
- The MAH must assign codes to ADRs using a dictionary, but there is no prescribed dictionary specified. However, it is mandatory to code the indications related to the suspected and concomitant drugs using the most current version of the International Classification of Diseases, which can result in redundancy.
- It remains unclear whether it is necessary to report serious adverse events/ADRs to both the regulatory authority and PvPI, or if reporting to one of them is sufficient.
- The necessity to report serious and unexpected ADRs to the licensing authority, which could be either the CDSCO or one of the state drug licensing authorities, creates ambiguity because it opens up various reporting avenues.
- The drug industry has found it challenging to report PSURs in 30 days in the wake of voluminous data, which could have been at least 60–90 days to report PSURs in line with global practice.
- There is uncertainty regarding whether RMPs are required for products already available in the market or exclusively for products that will be introduced in the future. Furthermore, no specific guidance has been given regarding the format in which a MAH should prepare and submit an RMP.
- Even though the modules on Pharmacovigilance System Master File (PvMF) and PSUR make reference to it, there is no specialized section or module for Signal Detection.

Pharmacovigilance continues to grow with multidimensional challenges, and to overcome these challenges, it is necessary to build a systematic approach with global collaboration for national use, taking advantage of the abundant talent pool available in India.

Disclosure of Conflict of Interest The authors declare that they have no conflict of interest.

References

1. Pharmacovigilance Toolkit. Pharmacovigilance Programme of India (PvPI), 2013. http://ipc.nic.in/writereaddata/linkimages/PDF%20PV%20Toolkit-1898248681.pdf. Accessed 19 Jul 2016.
2. Govt plans to expand PvPI with 50 more AMCs at healthcare institutions across the country http://www.pharmabiz.com/NewsDetails.aspx?aid=107358&sid=1
3. List of ADR Monitoring Centres under Pharmacovigilance Programme of India, 2022. https://ipc.gov.in/mandates/pvpi/pvpi-updates.html Accessed 17 Nov 2022.
4. Health ministry directs AMCs to set up causality assessment committee to detect serious adverse event related to drugs. http://www.pharmabiz.com/NewsDetails.aspx?aid=106822&sid=1
5. IPC launches benefit-risk assessment cell for drugs under PvPI, 2016. http://pharmabiz.com/ArticleDetails.aspx?aid=93612&sid=1 Accessed 19 Jul 2016.
6. Indian drug regulators emphasise on strengthening drug quality on 12th Foundation Day of IPC: Expert http://www.pharmabiz.com/NewsDetails.aspx?aid=120312&sid=2
7. Pharmacovigilance Programme of India Newsletter. 2014;4(10) http://ipc.nic.in/writereaddata/mainlinkFile/File398.pdf. Accessed 19 Jul 2016.
8. PvPI registers 3 lakh adverse drug reactions, as it adds 40 more AMCs. http://www.pharmabiz.com/NewsDetails.aspx?aid=104074&sid=1
9. PCI directs pharmacy, healthcare institutions pan-India to report ADRs in PvPI for patient safety: Expert http://www.pharmabiz.com/NewsDetails.aspx?aid=117515&sid=1
10. Kalaiselvan V, Kumar R, Thota P, Tripathi A, Singh GN. Status of documentation grading and completeness score for Indian individual case safety reports. Indian J Pharmacol. 2015;47(3):325–7.
11. Govt to implement intensive ADR monitoring to report adverse events in specific drugs. http://www.pharmabiz.com/NewsDetails.aspx?aid=103262&sid=1
12. Vijay Venkatraman J, Vignesh R. Pharmacovigilance in India - the past, present and future, 2016. https://www.fpm.org.uk/policypublications/spring_2016_newsletter. Accessed 19 Jul 2016.
13. Olsson S, Pal SN, Dodoo A. Pharmacovigilance in resource-limited countries. Exp Rev Clin Pharmacol. 2015;8(4):449–60.
14. Around 80 corporate hospitals start reporting ADRs as part of PvPI. http://www.pharmabiz.com/NewsDetails.aspx?aid=106640&sid=1
15. India joins hands with SEARN nations for drug safety. http://www.pharmabiz.com/NewsDetails.aspx?aid=108800&sid=21
16. Iyer PK. The science and politics of Nimesulide: retracing the 'Career' of a controversial drug. ISS E-J Indian Soc Soc. 2012;1:1.
17. How India tackles adverse drug reactions - By ignoring data, 2016. http://www.mid-day.com/articles/how-india-tackles-adverse-drug-reactions%2D%2D-by-ignoring data/16941177. Accessed 11 Jul 2016.
18. Health ministry bans Nimesulide and 2 other drugs, 2011. http://www.hindustantimes.com/health-and-fitness/health-ministry-bans-nimesulide-and-2-other-drugs/story-c5RZYL8fI7uplYRGEnlcZO.html. Accessed 19 Jul 2016.
19. DCGI issues directive to state drug controllers to ensure 'Box Warning' on nimesulide, 2012. http://pharmabiz.com/NewsDetails.aspx?aid=68683&sid=1. Accessed 19 Jul 2016.
20. Pharmacovigilance Programme of India Newsletter. 2012:2. http://ipc.nic.in/showfile.asp?lid=547&EncHid= Accessed 19 Jul 2016.
21. Sharma S. Health ministry bans Nimesulide and 2 other drugs, 2011. http://www.hindustantimes.com/health-and-fitness/health-ministry-bans-nimesulide-and-2-other-drugs/story-c5RZYL8fI7uplYRGEnlcZO.html. Accessed 26 Aug 2016.
22. Doctors dispute government fiat against Nimesulide, 2012. http://timesofindia.indiatimes.com/city/patna/Doctors-dispute-government-fiat-against-Nimesulide/articleshow/13143275.cms. Accessed 19 Jul 2016.

23. Newsletter: Pharmacovigilance Programme of India (PvPI). 2012:2(1) http://ipc.nic.in/showfile.asp?lid=546&EncHid=. Accessed 19 Jul 2016.
24. Hashmi A. Pioglitazone suspension and its aftermath: a wake up call for the Indian drug regulatory authorities. J Pharmacol Pharmacother. 2013;4(4):227–9.
25. Health ministry bans two drugs Analgin and Pioglitazone; industry protests, 2013. http://articles.economictimes.indiatimes.com/2013-06-27/news/40233626_1_drug-pioglitazone-rosiglitazone-drug-controller-general. Accessed 20 Jul 2016.
26. Govt bans popular diabetes drug and analgin, 2013. http://timesofindia.indiatimes.com/india/Govt-bans-popular-diabetes-drug-and analgin/articleshow/20789831.cms. Accessed 20 Jul 2016.
27. Pioglitazone Back on Market in India. Medscape Medical News, 2013. http://www.medscape.com/viewarticle/808990. Accessed 10 Aug 2016.
28. Kunjathaya P, Ramaswami PK, Krishnamurthy AN, Bhat N. Acute necrotizing pancreatitis associated with Vildagliptin. JOP J Pancreas (Online). 2013;14(1):81–4.
29. Jeyaraj S, Shetty AS, Kumar CRR, Nanditha A, Krishnamoorthy S, Raghavan A, Raghavan K, Ramachandran A. Liraglutide-induced acute pancreatitis. J Assoc Physicians India. 2014;62(1):64–6.
30. Pharmacogenomics to address ADRs specific to vulnerable populations under PvPI, 2016. http://pharmabiz.com/ArticleDetails.aspx?aid=92820&sid=1. Accessed 19 Aug 2016.
31. Government plans to fund projects in pharmacogenomics to expand scope of PvPI, 2016. http://pharmabiz.com/PrintArticle.aspx?aid=95137&sid=1. Accessed 19 Aug 2016.
32. IPC recommends caution on 3 lifesaving drugs in market to CDSCO based on ADRs, 2015. http://www.pharmabiz.com/NewsDetails.aspx?aid=89566&sid=1. Accessed 20 Aug 2016.
33. Patel PP, Gandhi AM, Desai CK, Desai MK, Dikshit RK. An analysis of drug induced Stevens-Johnson syndrome. Indian J Med Res. 2012;136(6):1051–3.
34. Sundriyal D, Kumar N. Pazopanib induced hand-foot syndrome. Oxf Med Case Rep. 2015;2015(2):206–7.
35. Noronha V, Punatar S, Joshi A. Rushi V Desphande and Kumar PrabhashSunitinib-induced thrombotic microangiopathy. J Cancer Therap Res. 2016;12(1):6–11. https://doi.org/10.4103/0973-1482.172575.
36. Vinit K. Srivastava, Parineeta Jaisawal, Sanjay Agrawal and Diwakar Kumar. Cardiac arrest associated with ranitidine and ondansetron combination in day care gynecologic surgery. J Anaesthesiol Clin Pharmacol. 2013;29(4):563–4.
37. Mahajan R, Nagaraj TM, Kumar P, Patil S, Moyin R. A rare case report: single intravenous dose of ranitidine leading to cardiac arrest. Int J Pharm Bio Sci. 2014;5(1):(b) 1043–45.
38. Upadhyay KJ, Parmar SJ, Parikh RP, Gauswami PK, Dadhaniya N, Surela A. Intravenous ranitidine: rapid bolus can lead to cardiac arrest. J Pharmacol Pharmacother. 2015;6:100.
39. Pharmacovigilance Programme of India Newsletter. 2015;5(13) http://ipc.nic.in/writeread-data/mainlinkFile/File499.pdf. Accessed 20 Jul 2016.
40. Pharmacovigilance Programme of India Newsletter. 2016;6(14):12. http://ipc.nic.in/writeread-data/mainlinkFile/File534.pdf. Accessed 20 Jul 2016.
41. Pharmacovigilance Programme of India (PvPI) Performance Report 2015-16. http://ipc.nic.in/showfile.asp?lid=675&EncHid=. Accessed 30 Jun 2017.
42. Pharmacovigilance Programme of India Newsletter. 2015;5(12) http://ipc.nic.in/writeread-data/mainlinkFile/File453.pdf. Accessed 20 Jul 2016.
43. DCGI directs cos of proton pump inhibitors to list kidney injury as ADR in package insert: Expert http://www.pharmabiz.com/NewsDetails.aspx?aid=119232&sid=1
44. Singh GN. Approval of the safety and efficacy of fixed dose combinations (FDCs) permitted for manufacture for sale in the country without due approval from the office of DCG(I)—regarding. (2013Jul5).http://www.cdsco.nic.in/writereaddata/Approval_of_the_safety_and%20efficacy_FDC.pdf. Accessed 21 Jul 2016.
45. McGettigan P, Roderick P, Mahajan R, Kadam A, Pollock AM. Use of Fixed Dose Combination (FDC) drugs in India: central regulatory approval and sales of FDCs containing

Non-Steroidal Anti-Inflammatory Drugs (NSAIDs), metformin, or psychotropic drugs. PLoS Med. 2015;12(5) https://doi.org/10.1371/journal.pmed.1001826.

46. The FDC Drugs Ban Will and Must Go to the Supreme Court, 2016. http://www.caravanmagazine.in/vantage/fdc-drugs-ban-supreme-court. Accessed 21 Jul 2016.

47. DCGI may ban 619 more FDCs based on review of expert panel report, 2016. http://www.pharmabiz.com/NewsDetails.aspx?aid=94168&sid=1. Accessed 21 Jul 2016.

48. Harris G. Medicines made in India set off safety worries. New York Times, 2014. http://www.nytimes.com/2014/02/15/world/asia/medicines-made-in-india-set-off-safety-worries.html. Accessed 26 Aug 2016.

49. European Medicines Agency. GVK Biosciences: European Medicines Agency confirms recommendation to suspend medicines over flawed studies, 2015, Jan 23. http://www.ema.europa.eu/ema/index.jsp?curl=pages/medicines/human/referrals/GVK_Biosciences/human_referral_000382.jsp&mid=WC0b01ac05805c516f. Accessed 26 Aug 2016.

50. Porecha M. Vietnam shows the door to 45 Indian pharma companies. DNA (Diligent Media Corporation); 2014. http://www.dnaindia.com/mumbai/report-vietnam-shows-the-door-to-45-indian-pharma-companies-1980761. Accessed 26 Aug 2016

51. Banning FDCs a right move by govt as it help to reduce unwanted intake of medicines: experts, 2016. http://www.pharmabiz.com/NewsDetails.aspx?aid=94062&sid=1. Accessed 20 Jul 2016.

52. Confusion prevails amongst retailers over sale of banned FDCs as Delhi HC granted stay to several cos, 2016. http://pharmabiz.com/ArticleDetails.aspx?aid=94603&sid=1. Accessed 20 Jul 2016.

53. Overnight ban on FDC drugs will cripple domestic market growth: PWA, 2016. http://pharmabiz.com/ArticleDetails.aspx?aid=94081&sid=1. Accessed 10 Aug 2016.

54. Drug ban: Pharma market to see immediate loss of Rs 1k cr, 2016. http://timesofindia.indiatimes.com/business/india-business/Drug-ban-Pharma-market-to-see-immediate-loss-of-Rs-1k-cr/articleshow/51418326.cms.

55. Sudden ban of FDCs to impact more on patient-community rather than industry: TN IDMA, 2016. http://www.pharmabiz.com/NewsDetails.aspx?aid=94082&sid=1. Accessed 20 Jul 2016.

56. Dr BR Jagashetty. Regulatory authority should have given at least 15-30 days timeframe to recall 344 FDCs, 2016. http://www.pharmabiz.com/NewsDetails.aspx?aid=94039&sid=1

57. FDCs of cos with no data submitted to DCGI to prove safety, efficacy banned, 2016. http://www.pharmabiz.com/NewsDetails.aspx?aid=94537&sid=1. Accessed 10 Aug 2016.

58. Taking advantage of FDC ban, traders in Kerala return even non-banned drugs resulting in big loss to companies, 2016. http://www.pharmabiz.com/NewsDetails.aspx?aid=94726&sid=1. Accessed 10 Aug 2016.

59. AICDF hails FDC ban, urges govt to force industry to take back banned drugs from traders, 2016. http://www.pharmabiz.com/NewsDetails.aspx?aid=94707&sid=1. Accessed 10 Aug 2016.

60. Study on use of FDCs reveals lack of awareness of use helps promote its overuse, 2016. http://www.pharmabiz.com/NewsDetails.aspx?aid=94486&sid=1. Accessed 10 Aug 2016.

61. McGettigan P, Roderick P, Kadam A, Pollock A. Threats to global antimicrobial resistance control: centrally approved and unapproved antibiotic formulations sold in India. Br J Clin Pharmacol. Published Online: February 5. 2018; https://doi.org/10.1111/bcp.13503.

62. Ban on 328 FDC drugs to cost Rs. 2,500 crore for pharma companies: expert http://www.pharmabiz.com/NewsDetails.aspx?aid=111307&sid=1

63. IPC to focus on TB, tropical diseases as part of integrating PV programmes in public health systems for SEARN nations. http://www.pharmabiz.com/NewsDetails.aspx?aid=107642&sid=1

64. IPC to discuss plans with UMC to harmonise PvPI with public health programmes of member countries. http://www.pharmabiz.com/NewsDetails.aspx?aid=108928&sid=1

65. Health ministry comes out with suspected ADR form and medicine side-effect reporting form for intensive ADR monitoring. http://www.pharmabiz.com/NewsDetails. aspx?aid=109473&sid=1
66. 100 pharma cos join hands with CDSCO, PvPI to frame guidelines for good PvP practices. http://www.pharmabiz.com/NewsDetails.aspx?aid=99045&sid=1. Accessed on 07 Jul 2017.
67. Pharma industry waiting for CDSCO's revised post marketing surveillance guidelines. http:// www.pharmabiz.com/NewsDetails.aspx?aid=101465&sid=1. Accessed on 07 Jul 2017.
68. Vijay Venkatraman J. New pharmacovigilance obligations for MAHs in India. DIA Global Forum. https://globalforum.diaglobal.org/issue/january-2018/ new-pharmacovigilance-obligations-for-mahs-in-india/
69. Pharmacovigilance guidance document should be made part of D&C Act to ensure 100% compliance of drug industry: Expert http://www.pharmabiz.com/NewsDetails. aspx?aid=109565&sid=1

Chapter 3
Challenges and Opportunities for Pharmacovigilance Development in the Arab World

Danya M. Qato

3.1 Introduction

This chapter explores the challenges and opportunities for pharmacovigilance development in the Arab world. An overview of the current state of public health and pharmacovigilance policies in the region is also discussed. Typically, the Arab world is defined as the 22 member countries of the Arab League of States. While bound loosely by some shared linguistic, religious, and cultural traits, countries of the region are heterogeneous with respect to demographic and ethnic composition, economic development, health systems organization and capacity, sociopolitical context, health status of the population, exposure to war and political violence, and political stability. Some researchers have argued that this diversity is too great to allow for meaningful prescriptive analysis and that any broad generalizations are misleading [1]. As an alternative strategy, they recommend considering more meaningful disaggregated groups among the countries to inform the construction of effective interventions and to more rigorously engage the particular challenges to health policy development. As level of economic development is often the primary determinant for advancing a health system, this approach classifies countries based on economic strength.

In this chapter, I will address the countries collectively for comparative purposes and to keep in line with previous literature while acknowledging the unique environments that characterize each country or group of countries based on shared political environments and economic capacities. Thus, this chapter will address challenges and opportunities for pharmacovigilance development in the following countries in the Arab world: one group defined by comparatively well-developed public health services with limited resources (middle-income countries: Algeria, Egypt, Iraq, Jordan, Lebanon, Libya, Morocco, and Tunisia) and the other group

D. M. Qato (✉)
University of Maryland, Baltimore, MD, USA
e-mail: danyaqato@gmail.com

© Springer Nature Singapore Pte Ltd. 2025
S. R. Ahmad (ed.), *Special Issues in Pharmacovigilance in Resource-Limited Countries*, https://doi.org/10.1007/978-981-96-6154-1_3

defined by protracted political instability, lack of resources for healthcare, and poor population health outcomes [Mauritania, Comoros, occupied Palestinian territories, Syria (officially known as the Syrian Arab Republic), Djibouti, Somalia, Sudan, South Sudan and Yemen]. Except in general terms, countries commonly referred to as the Gulf countries, will not be addressed here as they are not considered resource-limited countries but rather are high-income countries. These countries are Bahrain, Kuwait, Oman, Qatar, Saudi Arabia, and the United Arab Emirates.

Importantly, the political transitions and ruptures that occurred from the late 2000s and onwards have ushered in a new era of politics and socioeconomic development. The repercussions to public health systems of these events are ongoing and yet to be defined or fully examined [2]. To varying degrees, what is known is that the political uprisings have exposed the vulnerabilities of the health systems in the region, especially in Libya and Syria. Syria until recently was in the throes of a humanitarian crisis with no signs of abating, and as a result there has been massive population displacement from the country. Some estimates hold the number displaced at half the population [3], resulting in what aid agencies have called, "the worst refugee crisis since World War II" [4]. The short- and long-term public health ramifications of such violence, damage and destruction to healthcare infrastructure, and population transfer —including that of health professionals [5]—are unclear. The experiences in Iraq and occupied Palestine provide illuminating if not devastating examples of the negative implications of conflict and war on population health and national healthcare infrastructure. In light of the fact that there is a paucity of comprehensive up-to-date reliable data, this chapter (except where noted) focuses on the state of pharmaceutical policies and health systems prior to the political schisms that have overtaken the region.

More recently, the COVID-19 global pandemic has played a critical role in shaping the priorities of healthcare systems in the Arab world. The COVID-19 pandemic exacted multiple population-level health and economic shocks to the region, which will likely be long-standing [6]. With respect to pharmacovigilance, there was a diversity of reported experiences by national pharmacovigilance centres with respect to preparedness and ability to perform necessary functions during the pandemic. A recent report suggested that digital infrastructure was a key area for improvement for pharmacovigilance centers in the region [7].

Importantly, while I refer to the collection of healthcare activities undertaken by each country as a healthcare "system," that characterization may be generous. Inasmuch as "systems" connote the systematized and organized functioning of health practitioners, resources, and institutions that together deliver healthcare services for a population and realize a comprehensive vision for public health, and given that many of the countries' health systems are fragmented and underfunded, such a characterization is "deliberately futuristic" [8].

3.2 Health and Pharmaceuticals in the Arab World

While great progress has been made in increasing life expectancy and reducing mortality from communicable diseases and injuries in the Arab world over the past twenty years, profound inter- and intra-country inequalities in population health outcomes still exist. In the sixteen countries addressed in this chapter, there is marked diversity reflected in differential performance on health status metrics and health systems financing and development. Life expectancy ranges from 51.2 and 57.9 years in Somalia and Djibouti to 72.6 and 75.0 years in Lebanon and Libya, respectively. Maternal mortality ratio, per 100,000 live births, ranges from 1295.4 and 962.8 in Mauritania and Somalia, respectively, to 76.4 per 100,000 live births in Lebanon. Under-5 mortality (or deaths per 1000 live births) ranges from 9.3 in Lebanon to 180 in Somalia [2]. The epidemiological transition of the Arab world is increasingly resembling that of Western nations, with a growing prevalence of non-communicable diseases, including cardiovascular disease, obesity, mental health disorders, motor vehicle injuries, and disability and trauma due to state and interpersonal or self-inflicted violence [9]. It remains unclear if any of the gains in recent decades have been lost due to recent political dynamics, especially in Libya, Syria, Algeria, Egypt, South Sudan, and Sudan.

Pharmaceuticals and medical devices have played a central role in the increased life expectancy across the globe, and in the Arab world, as elsewhere, they continue to be the primary modes of treatment for chronic and acute health conditions. Total international spending on prescription medicines was forecasted to surpass the US$1.2 trillion threshold by 2017 [10] and in the Arab world is expected to surpass US $60 billion by 2025 [11], with Saudi Arabia and Egypt accounting for 40% of the total [12]. According to 2012 data, Arab governments spent 10–40% of total health expenditures on pharmaceuticals and consumables [8]. The World Health Organization (WHO), Eastern Mediterranean Regional Office (which encompasses most countries in the Arab League in addition to Afghanistan, Iran, and Pakistan), estimates that in 2015, average pharmaceutical expenditure per capita in the region was US$57 [13]. In 2013, per capita spending on pharmaceuticals was lowest in Yemen at US$5.3 compared to Lebanon, the highest spender outside the Gulf countries, at US$261.9 followed by Jordan at US$122.5 [14].

Pharmaceutical industry capacity has also developed in the past three decades and varies widely as a function of population size, investments, and extent of the market penetration of multinational pharmaceutical companies. It is estimated that approximately 250 pharmaceutical manufacturers operate in the Arab world [15]. The Egyptian pharmaceutical industry is the largest and as of 2013 has 130 licensed pharmaceutical manufacturers [16, 17], covering 30% of the pharmaceuticals supply in the Middle East and North Africa market, second only to Jordan. Jordan is the leading exporter of pharmaceuticals in the Arab world, registering sales of US $1.4 billion USD in 2020 [18]. Other countries with strong local manufacturing capacity include Syria with 45 companies, Morocco 35, Jordan 18, Lebanon 9, Palestine 7, and Algeria 5 [8]. There is little research and development into novel drug therapies in the region, and the majority of pharmaceuticals produced are either generics or licensed branded products. Due to the absence of local manufacturing facilities, Somalia, Qatar, and Libya import all of their required pharmaceuticals [12].

3.3   Current State of Pharmacovigilance in the Arab World

In the Arab world, national pharmacovigilance programmes are still in their nascent phase, if extant at all. Just as there is significant heterogeneity with respect to health systems development, local pharmaceutical manufacturing capacity, and financing, there is also diversity in terms of the stage of development of pharmacovigilance and drug safety programmes and policies. In one of the few reports on pharmacovigilance in the Middle East region, researchers noted that among ten national bodies responsible for drug safety that were interviewed, only six described a formal drug safety programme at the national level [19]. As of October 2022, more current review of the literature and online information from national governments suggests that Palestine is the only Arab League country that has no formal pharmacovigilance programme or regulation. These populations are thus living in a public health environment with a weak safety net in place to protect them from unsafe medications that enter the market—either because they are counterfeit, of poor manufacturing quality, because they are being prescribed and/or used inappropriately, or because emerging evidence suggests new unanticipated adverse effects. More promisingly, of 18 Arab countries responding to a 2015 survey,[1] 16 or 88% noted the presence of a standard adverse drug reaction (ADR) reporting form at the national level [20].

For those countries that do have a pharmacovigilance programme in place, efforts are often fragmented, weak, and unable to protect the public adequately, with leaders struggling to effectively formulate their pharmacovigilance policies and programs amidst a complex and ever-shifting political, economic, and health systems terrain. Countries that have comparatively stronger pharmacovigilance systems and drug regulation, for example, Morocco and Egypt, rely singularly on ADR reporting as the central tool of their drug safety armamentarium. This is not surprising, because reliance on passive modes of reporting is the least costly and burdensome for a national healthcare system that is yet to build sufficient health information technology capacity and establish comprehensive electronic healthcare and pharmaceutical claims databases. For the functioning of their drug safety programme, these systems are thus relying primarily on the goodwill of the industry, the public, and

---

[1] A descriptive cross-sectional study utilizing online survey instrument was conducted by the author between May and September 2015 to describe the current state of pharmacovigilance systems in Arab and Eastern Mediterranean countries. Of 21 Arab countries invited to participate in the survey, only respondents from Bahrain, Somalia and Syria did not respond. Although Mauritania is a member of the Arab League, it was not represented in the survey because a reliable focal point from this country could not be identified. South Sudan is not represented in the survey.

their providers [21], some of whom are unaware of the existence of such pro-grammes, have suspicions about the privacy of submitted reports, or fear litigation resulting from reporting medication problems [22]. As elsewhere, underreporting and incomplete reporting of ADRs is pervasive in Arab countries [23]. Quality of reporting, measured by the vigiGrade completeness score where a perfect score is 1 and a score greater than 0.8 is considered well-documented [22], also varies and ranges from 0.2 in Oman to 0.7 in Egypt in 2015 (personal communication with Uppsala Monitoring Centre). To add to the problem, the majority of information relied on by Arab countries related to drug safety still arises from Western countries, such as the United States [24]. While data from these countries are helpful for local or national regulatory bodies to make drug safety decisions regarding approval and possibly removal of a drug from the market, information may not be relevant or generalizable given the distinct pharmaceutical markets and the diversity of popula-tions with unique traditions, diets, and sociopolitical environments in each country.

To assist governments in pursuing their own nationally based pharmacovigilance systems, the WHO offers different support programmes and educational materials, including general guidelines to help identify the particular challenges to monitoring the safety of drugs effectively and approaches for overcoming them [25]. As of December 2024, 17 (Algeria, Egypt, Iraq, Jordan, Kuwait, Lebanon, Libya, Mauritania, Morocco, Oman, Saudi Arabia, South Sudan, Sudan, Syria, Tunisia, United Arab Emirates, and Yemen) of the 22 countries in the Arab region are full members of the WHO Programme on International Drug Monitoring, while five are associate members (Bahrain, Comoros, Djibouti, Qatar, and Somalia) [26]. However, given a context of weak political will and poor financing, generic guide-lines and formulas applied bluntly without regard to unique population needs and composition do little to change the political economy of drug regulation. This is especially true in health systems where public health policies have been politically undervalued and historically deprioritized.

3.4 Current Efforts at Promoting Pharmacovigilance in the Arab World

Due to the absence of a common Arabic language describing adverse drug events in particular and pharmacovigilance programme components more generally, efforts to harmonize Arabic terminology for pharmacovigilance were undertaken among members of the Arab and Eastern Mediterranean region in a series of meetings that began in 2013. At the culmination of the final meeting, in Rabat, Morocco, in September 2014, countries agreed on 20 common Arabic terms using an iterative Delphi consensus process, and that terminology was formally published in the jour-nal *Drug Safety* [27]. The ultimate aim of this endeavor is to facilitate intellectual contributions to the field of pharmacovigilance from the region and to support com-munication and collaboration cross-nationally.

Simultaneous to these efforts, the Common Arab Guidelines in Pharmacovigilance began to be developed and became effective, though not legally binding, in July of 2015. Under the institutional umbrella and support from the Arab League of States, the guidelines were conceptually and operationally led by leadership from Egypt, Saudi Arabia, Jordan, Oman—Arab States with relatively stronger pharmacovigilance strategies—and the United Arab Emirates, Qatar, Kuwait, Bahrain [28]. Pharmaceutical companies and regulators in the region were invited to comment on the proposed guidelines [29]. Though the broad distinctions of the region are taken into account, the Arab guidelines borrow heavily from European risk management and European Good Vigilance Practice and, for this reason, have been criticized for not adequately addressing the complexity and heterogeneity of unique contexts within which each country in the Arab region finds itself [personal communication with PV leadership in several Arab countries]. Furthermore, because of the overwhelming scope of the guidelines (the document spans 523 pages and includes 16 modules) [30], critics have noted the difficulty in encouraging buy-in from policymakers who are hesitant to take on such full-scale projects with little funding and even less promise of success.

To mobilize for collaboration and enhance unified efforts at improving drug safety in the region, the Arab and Eastern Mediterranean Pharmacovigilance Network (AEMPN) online platform was launched in March of 2016 [31]. The AEMPN is a burgeoning online network of healthcare professionals and policymakers actively working towards developing and advancing pharmacovigilance in their countries and regionally. According to the founders, the platform is also intended as a tool for real-time knowledge dissemination and resource pooling.

3.5   Challenges to Pharmacovigilance Development in the Arab World

Inasmuch as each Arab country is enmeshed in a unique set of sociopolitical and economic conditions, the matrix of challenges to the creation and development of a pharmacovigilance programme in each context can vary considerably. In the same 2015 survey mentioned previously, leaders of pharmacovigilance programmes and pharmaceutical policy in the Arab world were asked about the greatest challenges to pharmacovigilance development in their country (Table 3.1). Not surprisingly, the primary challenges to development of a pharmacovigilance system, as relayed by the country respondents, were lack of funding and inadequately trained staff able to undertake rigorous pharmacovigilance work. Other challenges noted by respondents include the following: low prioritization of pharmacovigilance in public health policy development; weak political commitment and leadership; lack of resources and capacity (trained staff, funding, physical and technical facilities); lack

Table 3.1 Challenges to pharmacovigilance development, as reported by Pharmacovigilance Leadership in Select Arab Countries, 2015 Survey[a]

Algeria	Require greater reporting by all national and international companies Mandated reporting Involvement in studies conducted by our centre if needed
Djibouti	Developing better collaboration with pharmacists and local pharmaceutical industry
Iraq	Lack of human resources Collaboration from some health institutions
Jordan	Lack of political commitment in the country regarding patient safety. Low priority of pharmacovigilance Lack of human resources Lack of information technology resources Lack of training(s) in pharmacovigilance Lack of international communication and coordination
Libya	Financial problems (lack of facilities, dedicated specialized personnel, training personnel, hardware, software etc.)
Morocco	Building capacity Financial and technical assistance
Palestine	How to start is the most important challenge
Sudan	The primary challenges are financial: To support our activities To attend annual pharmacovigilance meetings worldwide To attend pharmacovigilance training courses
Tunisia	Lack of human resources Lack of public awareness Lack of reporting
Yemen	Lack of capacity building opportunities for pharmacovigilance entity staff Low knowledge of clinical staff and public on medicine safety and adverse drug reactions Low interest of research institutions on medicines Lack of research facilities Low interest of donors Illegal importation and diversity of medicine in the local market

[a]Qato [20]

of coordination, communication, and collaboration with other pharmacovigilance leaders, nationally, regionally, and internationally; lack of coordination with local and international pharmaceutical manufacturers; low interest of donors; inability to access high quality training resources; poor enforcement of policies and illegal importation of pharmaceuticals into the market; and low reporting and underreporting of ADRs. Inadequate follow-up and education of health professionals, reflected in the underreporting of ADRs, was also noted.

In this chapter, I will explore these common challenges in depth while emphasizing that they do not apply to each country in equal measure.

3.6 Funding

The Arab region constitutes 5% of the world population [8] but spends less than 1% of global health expenditures [32]. Total estimated government spending on health in the Arab world is between US$72 and $80 billion [33, 34]. Levels of economic development and incomes vary widely, as does per capita spending on health, calculated as the sum of public and private health expenditures as a ratio of total population. In 2013, Syria spent US$43 per capita on healthcare—down from US$97 in 2011—while Comoros spent US$51 and Somalia spent US$8. In contrast, Lebanon spent US$664 per capita, the highest rate outside of the Gulf countries [35].

Healthcare funding is derived from a variety of sources including household out-of-pocket payments, health insurance via private or public mechanisms, personal and corporate taxes, and external sources. External funding is primarily channeled through international development aid from nongovernmental organizations and donor countries [32]. The percentage of total healthcare costs covered by out-of-pocket contributions is greatest in the low-income countries of Mauritania, Comoros, Palestine, Syria, Djibouti, Somalia, South Sudan, Sudan, and Yemen. These conditions reflect the greater vulnerability of the poor to catastrophic health changes that may thrust them into greater impoverishment. The maxim that "poverty magnifies the need for health care while shrinking the capacity to finance it" holds true for lower income groups in the Arab world [36].

Health systems development requires significant investment, and in order for a pharmacovigilance programme to be established and enhanced, initial and sustained financial support and commitment is necessary. Such a commitment entails the allocation of significant structural resources. The following are considered by the WHO to be the minimum resource requirements for establishment of a pharmacovigilance center: a dedicated workspace to undertake pharmacovigilance activities; access to quality computers and data analysis software; access to current drug safety literature; funding for training opportunities for pharmacovigilance staff and other personnel; and at least one full-time staff member devoted to working on the creation and organizing of programme activities [37]. Financial resources are also necessary for the creation of a functional and sustainable organizational plan, national guidelines for pharmacovigilance and medicine safety monitoring, and educational materials.

In the Arab countries addressed in this chapter, public health programmes are woefully underfunded. Even in countries with more robust financing schemes, pharmacovigilance is simply not a priority. The scarcity of funding is often due to the dual obstacles of insufficient financing earmarked for public health programming and a weak national economy. The inexorable rise in healthcare costs across the board further compounds the problem, putting pressure on governments to prioritize the allocation of already-strained resources to meet the acute (and primarily curative) healthcare needs of the population. In the often-tenuous political climate within which health ministers in the Arab world must make budget decisions, allocating funding for public health programmes, which by nature require long-term investment and payoff in the distant future, may be difficult to justify. At a personal level, motivations are oftentimes tepid because the long-term nature of public health investments suggests that any health policy benefits will only come to fruition after an employee leaves their position. This uncertainty entrenches the historical inertia and fear of change that prevents the advancement of innovative projects, programmes, and policies [38].

Additionally, misuse of scarce funding is prevalent in the region. Because of a combination of poor management, inefficiency, corruption, and policy imperatives created without the support of sound cost-effectiveness analysis—due in part to the absence of trained health economists able to undertake such analyses [32]—even generous investments made into public health may never bear substantive fruit and may in fact increase costs and put the population at risk. Furthermore, it is no secret that "Health authorities often have a vested interest in the commercial, unregulated deals they are supposed to regulate" [39]. The poorly regulated healthcare and pharmaceutical markets, rife with counterfeit, repackaged, and expired medications, may also serve the profit-making interests of health authorities and public managers [39], who may receive substantial kickbacks for certain procurements or particular political (in)decisions [8].

3.7 Policy Prioritization and Legal Frameworks

In the absence of critical buy-in and support from policy makers, it is unlikely pharmacovigilance development will make it on the policy agenda and receive the funding and support to evolve in the form of codified and enforced rules and regulations. The difficulties in building momentum among leadership in the Arab world are manifold, and especially in crisis or shifting contexts, working towards a long-term goal of institutional development and capacity building is a formidable challenge. Most prominently, there is a lack of education and communication among the public, health professionals, and policymakers, about the significant role a strong pharmacovigilance system plays in improving public health. Insufficient evidence at the local and/or national level to estimate the burden of adverse drug related events on population health is an additional obstacle to effectively communicate this pivotal role. The scarcity of databases and underfunding of rigorous intersectoral research [40] is status quo in the Arab world, and without empirical evidence, it is difficult to prove to policymakers the positive impact a pharmacovigilance programme will have on population health. The interest and incentive to take on this topic, either as a national priority or even at all, is therefore weak.

Moreover, even in cases where pharmacovigilance may have political support, persistent political conflict may subsume efforts at uptake and prioritization of pharmacovigilance, as resources are perpetually siphoned off to focus on exigent health situations and complex emergencies. For instance, in the Palestinian context, leadership within the Pharmaceutical Information Department of the General Directorate of Pharmacy continue to face an uphill battle as they attempt the seemingly Sisyphean task of developing a pharmacovigilance system. While the Ministry of

Health is focused on the proximate health crises resulting from the occupation—including poor access to healthcare, violence, and inconsistent funding streams—pharmacy leadership is requesting a commitment to a project that may take years to fully realize with little guarantee of success. Especially in dynamic political and economic contexts, leaders are often unwilling take on these risks.

Third, in several countries, there is a high turnover of health ministers and managers working within the government [8]. By the time the Ministry of Health may be convinced to tackle a project related to pharmacovigilance, a new minister may step in, and the policy building and lobbying process begins anew. The impact of this latter phenomenon cannot be overemphasized, as it leads to duplicative efforts that are time consuming and costly. Due to a perceived failure of the project by incoming officials, future efforts are also negatively impacted. The exhaustive emotional and professional toll of these recurring failed policy pushes on those who mobilize for them can be formidable.

3.8   Patient and Provider Engagement

The central beneficiary in any pharmacovigilance narrative is the patient—the ultimate consumer of pharmaceutical products. The healthcare practitioner, as the primary mediator of the linkage between patients and their pharmaceutical care, is a pivotal supporting figure in this narrative. While the aim of future drug safety surveillance programmes is to rely on integrated electronic databases, reliance on voluntary reports remains the mainstay and can serve to flag any potential problems before they appear in the data. Underreporting of adverse drug events by both patients and healthcare providers has long been noted as a barrier to the efficient and timely functioning of pharmacovigilance activities. As many countries still rely on voluntary submission of reports as the central pillar of their pharmacovigilance system, the hurdle associated with costs of the distribution and completion of the forms, for patients and for the health system, can be substantial. Combined with inherent bureaucratic delays in delivering a case report from the local to the national office, costs and time associated with adherence to this strict protocol [22] may be enough to discourage reporting.

Even in countries where there are a greater number of incoming reports, the poor quality and incompleteness of these submitted reports renders them insufficiently usable and even in some instances entirely unusable. The lack of sustained and targeted public outreach efforts by pharmacovigilance programmes and personnel on the imperative of reporting adverse effects; and the absence of drug safety and pharmacovigilance principles in medical and pharmacy curricula has facilitated this predicament. Further, a lack of access to current up-to-date drug safety information in the Arab world forces practitioners to rely on tertiary sources for drug information. While important, these sources do not reflect current drug safety evidence that emerges post-marketing. With improved access to the Internet, this problem is steadily diminishing, yet given that the vast majority of quality journals remain accessible only to subscribers, the issue is still important since poor access to current literature and research effectively puts practitioners outside the purview of "modern" medicine.

It warrants noting that compared to private sector employment, public sector salaries in the Arab world are often comparatively lower. Therefore, it is difficult to motivate public sector health providers to participate in a pharmacovigilance programme or submit reports, when there is no mechanism for compensation or even, minimally, acknowledgment and follow-up. In other developing countries, this disparity in compensation leads to the professional migration of pharmacovigilance professionals towards the private sector. A high staff turnover then results in the deterioration or even discontinuation of pharmacovigilance programmes [22]. While greater educational efforts to motivate healthcare providers are necessary, education alone is not sufficient to encourage active involvement in the pharmacovigilance process.

3.9 Political Will and Leadership

"Leadership is central to healthcare systems reform" [41] is a tired cliché, but especially for Arab health systems with low resources and an inadequate number of highly trained staff, this assertion rings forcefully true. Historically, it has been a select group of enthusiastic healthcare providers that have laid the groundwork necessary for the inception and development of strong pharmacovigilance systems in the Arab world. These leaders, practicing in the public or private sector, have served to catalyze reform and build around them a group of core supporters that worked collectively to advocate for pharmacovigilance efforts and mobilized around cultivating political will towards policy change. Examples can be gleaned from Egypt, Morocco, and Tunis, and more recently in the efforts undertaken by staff at health ministries in Qatar, Palestine, and Lebanon. In some cases, staff have worked without compensation, patiently mobilizing for a national pharmacovigilance system as a second vocation, in addition to their official full-time responsibilities. The ability to take on additional duties above and beyond the job requirements is not typical and thus the ability for those working within severely resource constrained health systems to pursue additional projects is often not possible. To be sure, inasmuch as pharmacovigilance is a comprehensive health systems programme, enthusiasm alone was and is not sufficient to manage the complexities and challenges inherent in this expansive enterprising work. The regulatory, economic, and political tools of the state need(ed) to be engaged in order to build a sustainable pharmacovigilance system [22].

By nature, constructing effective public health programmes, especially one as wide-ranging as pharmacovigilance, is a deeply interdisciplinary process. Not unlike other parts of the world, policymaking in the Arab region is a highly bureaucratic space with clearly demarcated professional turf. Collaboration across different sectors and departments is a profound and sensitive challenge, with clear lines of engagement that are difficult to navigate when trying to build the collaborative relationships necessary for the construction of effective and evidence-based public health programmes. Diplomatic, patient, and experienced leadership is required to engage these overlapping spaces while promoting collegial and collaborative exchange.

3.10   Trained Professionals and Training Opportunities

Foundational to the development of effective and robust health systems are trained health professionals able to spearhead and implement the procedures and policies necessary for institution building and policy promulgation. In several countries, there is a dearth of trained professionals able to fill these roles. This is especially true in the lowest income countries of Comoros, Djibouti, Mauritania, occupied Palestine, Somalia, South Sudan, Sudan, and Yemen. One reason for the lack of qualified trained professionals is human capital flight or the "brain drain" phenomenon, wherein researchers and clinicians leave their home countries in order to pursue higher training and do not return due to a lack of opportunities. The inability for training opportunities to be brought into the country further compounds the problem. In politically and financially fragile health systems, this latter problem in part explains the stasis in the development of pharmacovigilance. For example, in Palestine, efforts to obtain an entry permit for a director of pharmacovigilance in a neighboring country to conduct training activities were delayed for over two years because of political reasons. This is emblematic of a wider problem related to travel and security assurances for expert consultants able to conduct training in countries severely disrupted by occupation, conflict, and war.

3.11   Donor Interest and Dependence on Donor Funding

In countries reliant on international aid and development funding for support, there are persistent challenges to securing a funding stream that is predictable, reliable, and sustainable [42]. Official development assistance and health aid are notoriously unpredictable, dynamic, short-term, and prone to political, economic, and socially motivated shifts that may not always reflect the needs of the population. In 2013, the largest recipients of international donor aid (among countries covered by this chapter) were Egypt (US$5.5 billion), Syria (US$3.6 billion), and the occupied Palestinian territories (US$2.6 billion) [43].

Much has been written about, indeed entire disciplines have been devoted to, the problem that long-term international aid dependence has had on thwarting the development of robust and self-reliant indigenous institutions [44] and health reform programmes. Among the legacies of aid is that donors may not invest in local experts and may rely on external contractors to consult on health reform projects.

These consultants are not accountable to the long-term success (or failure) of programmes they have consulted on and may not reside in the country, rendering their expertise effectively inaccessible to policymakers as the programme matures. This lack of accountability produces an unfortunate cycle of incompetence and failure that further entrenches the status quo and prevents the evolution of the healthcare system. Gottret and Schieber summarize the breadth of the serious problems attendant development assistance and health aid in particular and write that these problems include "Lack of predictability, increased focus on specific diseases or interventions, large numbers of new actors and donors, lack of responsiveness and flexibility to crises, and donors' lack of accountability for the absence of results and progress" [36]. In addition, the volatility of aid is especially damaging as "commitments are made for short maturities (three years at best)." All of these factors hamper the ability of any government to plan strategically and commit funding to long-term public health projects.

In a qualitative study aimed at examining pharmaceutical systems in severely disrupted countries, key informants noted that "there is a distinct lack of coordination between donors and the ministry, and it is unclear where the accountability lies for meeting goals" [45]. The problem of fragmented care is linked to waste and mismanagement at the national level, as duplicative costly efforts are undertaken by multiple organizations with little to no accountability mechanisms in place to measure impact. The volatility of aid and lack of accountability of aid agencies push Ministries of Health further into the "poverty trap" cycle, where curative medical treatment is by necessity privileged over public health programmes as existent resources are rarely sufficient to meet the demands of both missions [46].

3.12 Improving Governance

The Universal Declaration of Human Rights outlines the right of all people to the highest attainable standard of health, which includes the right to access essential medicines. The WHO estimates that upwards of 100 million people in the Arab region lack regular access to essential medicines [47]. In order for a state to fulfill its core duties towards its citizens, it must maintain a functioning healthcare system that ensures health products are accessible, safe, and effective. In countries with limited financial and human resource capacity, this assurance is extremely difficult, particularly so in states of chronic conflict without good governance. Good governance is the "participatory, transparent, accountable and efficient exercise of economic, political and administrative authority to manage a countries affairs at all levels" [48]. Because health systems are part and parcel of larger political frameworks and undertaking their reform does not happen in a vacuum, it is naïve to assume that decisions at the health policy level are immune from the political circumstances of the population. A major challenge for pharmacovigilance leadership in health ministries in the Arab world aiming to build comprehensive health programs is therefore the inability to effectively and sustainably enforce policies and laws in a perpetually contentious, perhaps antidemocratic, environment. This weak regulatory environment is prone to nepotism and corruption. As a result, importation and distribution of poor quality and counterfeit drugs flourishes. The proliferation of these poor-quality medications leads to health tragedies and scares (provoked by media), which in turn promote distrust and cynicism by the public towards the health system more broadly. Furthermore, even if it is required legally to have a prescription to purchase medications, enforcement of pharmacy legislation is often poor, so patients are able to purchase most pharmaceutical products without a prescription or oversight from a health provider. The lack of oversight of pharmaceutical systems has profound implications for public health. Growing evidence suggests that high risk prescribing practices are not outliers, but rather the norm [49]. This has had a devastating impact on health systems by leading to "treatment failure, drug resistance, loss of confidence in the health system, and increased morbidity and mortality" [50].

The pharmaceutical industry has capitalized on this lax regulatory environment by engaging in what are considered by international standards as unethical and aggressive promotional and educational activities [8, 51]. In Somalia, researchers noted that "The opaque nature of the pharmaceutical system could in fact be deliberate to facilitate illegal business. The ease and impunity with which counterfeit, expired or repackaged medicines can enter into a large market has obvious appeal to criminal networks" [45]. The pharmaceutical industry exploits and indeed financially thrives in this regulatory vacuum, "as attested by the proliferation of import-export dealers and selling outlets [that serve as] conduits through which medicines transit unchecked and unrecorded to supply neighboring countries-undermining their attempts at regulated import, and quality control" [39]. The lack of an accountability structure, an insufficiently trained health professional workforce, and inadequate access to emerging scientific evidence and literature have enabled these unchecked pharmaceutical industry practices to continue unabated [8].

3.13   Weak Health Information and Data Systems

With rare exceptions (primarily the Gulf countries and Egypt), health information systems and disease surveillance in most Arab countries is weak or nonexistent [52, 53]. Basic vital statistics, disease burden, and death registries may not be available to policy makers. Greater efforts at incorporating technology and health information systems in the health sector are being made but in most cases, are fragmented and yet to be fully operationalized. Governmental efforts to answer health services-related questions are often hindered by scarce and restricted access to current data. These barriers compel policymakers to rely on inaccurate estimates when planning health care programmes, and such reliance inevitably, "shift(s) decision making in the health care field from the realm of health policy to that of politics" [54].

3.14 Opportunities

In order to advance pharmacovigilance systems in the Arab world and build opportunities for change, focus should be directed to the following tasks: promoting educational efforts aimed at patients, the public, health providers, and policymakers; centering the public narrative by incorporating patients into the initial and development phases of the construction of pharmaceutical policies; greater funding for public health efforts writ large; more efficient and streamlined use of health information technologies; greater collaborations nationally, regionally, and internationally across the private and public sector; maximizing the benefits of current capacity and infrastructure through consolidation nationally and regionally; combating corruption and crafting policies to ensure accountability and transparency in health policy construction and promulgation; and ultimately developing sustainable methods for funding pharmacovigilance activities in the long term. All of these efforts will need to be tailored to the specific capacities and resources available in each context, especially with respect to the political and economic environment.

3.15 Increased Educational Opportunities

In the Arab world, the greatest opportunity for the realization of a strong and robust pharmacovigilance programme will be investment in improving cultures of reporting by the public and the healthcare professional community. Consensus building requires networking and collaboration between public and private actors and greater outreach and educational efforts that are harmonized nationwide. To increase public awareness, countries can partner with the media and the pharmaceutical industry (local and international) to produce culturally sensitive multimedia and print campaigns. For health providers, educational efforts should begin at the undergraduate and graduate university level. Embedding principles of drug safety and pharmacovigilance early in the educational curricula of pharmacists, nurses, and physicians will build support and momentum among healthcare providers, who will be central to the successful implementation of future pharmacovigilance programmes. Incorporating pharmacovigilance training into continuing education programmes at professional conferences and framing adverse drug event reporting as one of professional and civic responsibility are also worthwhile endeavors to push forward a culture of reporting.

When it comes to developing educational tools, policymakers do not have to reinvent the wheel and can capitalize on available outside resources. In 2013, the WHO established the WHO Collaborating Centre for Pharmacovigilance in Education and Patient Reporting, charged with assisting countries in integrating pharmacovigilance in the curricula of health training programmes [55]. Materials and support from the WHO Centre can be adopted and tailored to the particular needs of healthcare provider groups in the country.

The "brain drain," or the emigration of highly trained or qualified people from their native country, has long hampered efforts at maintaining indigenous knowledge creation and ensuring a pipeline of local researchers deeply knowledgeable about context and culture. Fortunately, there has more recently been, "a reverse trend, spurred by a flat job market and low economic growth in the West, and the rise of opportunities in the Internet technology and other sectors in the region" [56]. This greater exchange of highly trained nationals returning to native countries will promote development efforts so long as the collaborative energy is recognized and encouraged. These repatriates also bring with them professional networks that can facilitate national and international collaborations.

Recognition for promoting pharmacovigilance can come in many forms. One method can be greater remuneration more broadly for public sector professionals working in the public health field. Increased salaries can help redress the problem of high turnover of healthcare professionals practicing in the public sector that ultimately fragments efforts at expanding and developing pharmacovigilance programmes [22].

3.16   Improved (Use of) Health Information Technology

To justify the creation and long-term development and funding of a pharmacovigilance programme, policymakers need evidence. Evidence of the public health burden of unsafe pharmaceuticals requires sound and rigorous research methodologies and data collection processes. Owing to a lack of integrated health information technologies and to a lack of funding for research related-activities, this requisite local evidence is lacking. As a precursor to the efficient and cost-effective mobilization of resources for pharmacovigilance development, more and better data is needed to: 1) allow researchers to quantify the public health status of the population; 2) measure the impact of public health interventions; and 3) enable governments to plan, prioritize, and exploit available local, national, regional, and international resources.

Greater use of emerging technologies to enable the construction of reliable databases for evidence holds promise as a critical tool for building a robust pharmacovigilance system [57]. Given that the past five years has seen unprecedented growth in the use of Internet technology in the Arab world, the option of vigorously promoting adverse drug event reporting online has largely been unexplored and could be better harnessed as a mechanism to facilitate data solicitation, collection, and consolidation. Information technology can be utilized to support evidence-based decision making and enhance the ability of pharmacovigilance authorities to expeditiously communicate safety risks to the public and health professionals. Enabling patients and healthcare providers to input adverse drug reaction reports confidentially via the Internet can serve as a complementary strategy to hard copy submission of case reports and may be more user-friendly and cost-effective in the long term. Data derived from online sources allows regulators to streamline access and consolidate information, circumventing the burdensome steps of collecting, sorting, and analyzing hard copy reports.

With the increased regional emphasis on incorporating information technology in the health sector, measures to proactively build in integrated data consolidation (through, for example, standardized data entry fields) across countries in the Arab world should be explored in earnest. Making such data sources publicly available can help foster innovative and critical health services research, and "the availability of these datasets on a regional basis will also allow exploring comparable regional variations for benchmarking" [54].

Membership in the WHO Programme for International Drug Monitoring, the global clearinghouse for individual case safety reports (ICSRs) from around the world, allows countries access to international pharmacovigilance data that can be utilized for local purposes. The utility of this internationally sourced data is primarily a function of the makeup of the local pharmaceutical market. Because of shared manufacturers and suppliers, consolidation and aggregation of adverse drug event data at the regional level may be most beneficial to facilitate timely and relevant detection of adverse drug events. Furthermore, given the prevalence of self-medication, population level surveys may be necessary to capture the full scope of adverse drug events in the population.

3.17 Collaboration and Cooperation

Ministries of Health must regain their important role in fostering transparent relationships between the pharmaceutical industry, the public, and health practitioners that ensure decisions in prescribing are evidence-based. Such a strategy will serve to further the goal of privileging public health over commercial interests and thus improve the performance and functioning of the health system and advance the health of the nation by promoting accountability among all relevant actors and institutions. Greater research collaborations between academia and public and private partners, in particular the pharmaceutical industry, should be encouraged. At a minimum, partners from within the pharmaceutical industry may have critical expertise, especially related to medicine supply chains and manufacturing. The insights from the industry can help regulators and researchers create and implement effective pharmacovigilance strategies [58]. Careful consideration of the role private industry can play in establishing and supporting pharmacovigilance systems should be explored in each context and should be tailored to avoid conflicts of interest. This latter concern is especially complicated given the poor accountability structures in place at the political and commercial level.

3.18 Patient-Centeredness

The primary end user of pharmaceuticals is the patient. As such, the cornerstone of any effort to promote pharmacovigilance must privilege patient safety and health [59]. As it currently stands, voluntary reports are the main tool for pharmacovigilance programmes; hence, encouragement of quality patient and provider reporting should continue, as the more complete the case report the more useful it is to providing critical and timely information. With greater use of social media and the emergence of popular struggles mobilizing for and demanding governmental transparency, accountability, and reform, the ingredients for nurturing patient and provider cultures of engagement are ever more present yet not fully realized. Regulatory agencies and pharmacovigilance systems should "redouble their efforts to strengthen bidirectional communication with their most important stakeholders, patients and healthcare practitioners" [59]. In the context of low-resource settings, and given the prevalent problem of underreporting that has dogged pharmacovigilance systems globally, it behooves national health agencies to ensure case reporting mechanisms are as low-cost and user-friendly as possible. As noted by the WHO, "Many factors influence the choice of reporting means for a specific country. Receiving reports over the telephone or through local pharmacies might be the best solution for some countries, especially those where literacy rates are not high, while in other countries this option might be considered too resource demanding compared to an electronic reporting form sent over the Internet" [60].

3.19 Consolidation of Funding and Resources

Increased global emphasis on pharmacovigilance and health data infrastructure and technologies provides a fruitful avenue by which Arab countries can leapfrog developed countries experiences in order to expeditiously and cost-effectively suit their local needs and aims. Especially in low-resource settings, efforts to capitalize on this emerging global movement can save governments' time and money. Building initiatives aimed at creating alliances regionally and internationally to consolidate and complement local health data resources and capacity is one avenue that should be exploited. The ability for leadership to proactively network and collaborate with other national, regional, and international partners will be critical to building these alliances.

While efforts should be undertaken to develop viable long-term funding solutions for pharmacovigilance programmes, countries reliant on development aid may need to continue to rely on such aid in the interim. Efforts "to increase the maturity of resources, decrease volatility, and improve harmonization" are necessary, and "It is particularly important for donors not to second guess recipient countries' preferences, but rather to fund gaps in country programmes" [36]. Thus, the onus to maximize the efficiency of funding lies on both the donor institution or country and on the recipient country.

Greater cooperation and pooling of resources, policies, and programmes among Arab countries in the region should be improved. These unified efforts, including of resources and experiences of people and non-governmental organizations, can help bridge health disparities in the region [61].

3.20 Improved Governance with Better Evidence

In light of the ongoing political, economic, and social transformations engulfing the region, a central consideration that emerges as health ministries are encouraged by their populace to adopt a human rights framework in the reconstruction of the health system is how best to operationalize this paradigm. In the initial stages of health reform where unfettered commercial interests may take advantage of ambiguous, newly drafted regulations, it is crucial to set policies that are informed by the medical evidence and uphold standards of accountability and transparency at all levels of the healthcare system. The pharmaceutical sector must be one of the focal points of such efforts [62]. Although the promotion of rational drug use and utilization have been on public health agendas for at least the past two decades vis-à-vis programmes such as the WHO Programme on Essential Drugs; insufficient progress has been made because of weak oversight of the industry and the lack of clear and enforceable pharmacy practice laws.

Discouraging self-medication and encouraging shared decision making with physicians and other experienced health care providers, through requiring prescriptions for medicines, will also improve prospects for appropriate drug use and enable more efficient monitoring of pharmaceutical use at the population level. This requires harmonized efforts between the public health sector, government, and across markets—both informal and formal [45]. Where laws are already in place mandating prescriptions for pharmaceuticals, they should be coupled with better enforcement mechanisms.

3.21 Conclusion

Given the increased use of pharmaceuticals and rising healthcare costs globally, there is a greater focus at the national, regional, and international level on the imperative for the development and nurturing of pharmacovigilance as a core component of public health systems. This global push, led principally by global non-governmental organizations, is a welcome change to the previously singular focus on access (rather than access and safety) to medicines and fosters a positive environment for embarking on the journey towards the creation and development of a pharmacovigilance system. In October 2012, health ministers in the Arab world agreed on five key priority areas for the advancement of health, including the strengthening of health systems [63], which necessarily includes pharmacovigilance as a core component. Despite the obstacles policymakers face, they should remain focused on enabling and constructing a sustainable pharmacovigilance system that will improve pharmaceutical quality and pharmaceutical use and ultimately nurture improved health nationally and regionally.

Conflict of Interest Dr. Qato declares no conflicts of interest.

Funding This study was supported in part by a grant from the Arab Council for the Social Sciences and the Swedish International Development Agency.

References

1. Blair I. The 'Arab World' is not a useful concept when addressing challenges to public health, public health education, and research in the Middle East. Front Public Health. 2014;2:30.
2. Batniji R, et al. Governance and health in the Arab world. Lancet. 2014;383:343–55.
3. Almost Half of Syria's population has been uprooted - The Atlantic; http://www.theatlantic.com/international/archive/2014/08/half-of-syrias-population-is-displaced/379407/. Accessed 15 Aug 2020.
4. United Nations High Commissioner for Refugees, "EU says world facing worst refugee crisis since WWII", 16 Aug 2015; http://www.unhcr.org/cgi-bin/texis/vtx/refdaily?pass=52fc6fbd5&id=55d17e7b5. Accessed 15 Aug 2020.
5. Coutts A, et al. The Arab spring and health: two years on. Int J Health Serv. 2013;43:49–60.
6. United Nations Policy Brief: The Impact of COVID-19 on the Arab Region an opportunity to build back better; July 2020. https://www.un.org/sites/un2.un.org/files/sg_policy_brief_covid-19_and_arab_states_english_version_july_2020.pdf. Accessed 1 Oct 2022.
7. Al-Zubiedi SA, Younus M, Al-Khalidi S, Ekilo M, Alshammari TM. Pharmacovigilance regulatory actions by national pharmacovigilance centers in Arab countries following COVID-19 pandemic. Expert Opin Drug Saf. 2022;18:1–10. https://doi.org/10.1080/14740338.2022.2108398. Epub ahead of print. PMID: 35915555.
8. Jabbour S. Public health in the Arab World: at a crossroads. J Public Health Policy. 2013;34:356–60.
9. Mokdad AH, et al. The state of health in the Arab world, 1990–2010: an analysis of the burden of diseases, injuries, and risk factors. Lancet. 2014;383:309–20.
10. IMS, The Global Use of Medicines: Outlook through 2017.; http://www.imshealth.com/en/thought-leadership/ims-institute/reports/global-use-of-medicines-outlook-through-2017. Accessed 1 Feb 2016.
11. Rise & Growth of Pharma Distributors in the Middle East; PharmaSolutions; March 2, 2022. https://www.pharmasolutions-int.com/rise-growth-of-pharma-distributors-in-the-middle-east/. Accessed 1 Oct 2022.
12. Kandil O. The pharmaceutical industry in the Arab world: challenges, controversies, and future outlook. Drug Discov Today. 2004;9:543–5.
13. WHO EMRO | Essential medicines and pharmaceutical policies; http://www.emro.who.int/entity/essential-medicines/index.html. Accessed 10 Jan 2021.
14. Abdollahias A. Pharmaceutical market and health system in the Middle Eastern and Central Asian countries: time for innovations and changes in policies and actions. Arch Med Sci. 2011;7(3):365–7.
15. Ayoub R. Pharmaceuticals in Jordan Sectoral Report. http://www.awraq.com/uploads/research/51d41ed210403895b5ecc1d665b191433f4ee02a.pdf. Accessed 1 Feb 2016.

16. WHO, Egypt Pharmaceutical Country Profile 2011.; http://www.who.int/medicines/areas/coordination/Egypt_PSCPNarrativeQuestionnaire_27112011.pdf. Accessed 1 Feb 2016.
17. The Report: Egypt 2013. Oxford Business Group, 2013.
18. Jordan's Pharmaceutical Exports Reach 1BN; Jordan Times, 2021 Dec 8.; https://www.jordantimes.com/news/local/jordans-pharmaceutical-exports-reach-jd1b-%E2%80%94-japm. Accessed 1 Oct 2022.
19. Wilbur K. Pharmacovigilance in the Middle East: a survey of 13 Arabic-speaking countries. Drug Saf. 2013;36:25–30.
20. Qato DM. Current state of pharmacovigilance in the Arab and Eastern Mediterranean region: results of a 2015 survey. Int J Pharm Pract. 2018;26:210–21.
21. Olsson S, Pal SN, Stergachis A, Couper M. Pharmacovigilance activities in 55 low- and middle-income countries: a questionnaire-based analysis. Drug Saf. 2010;33:689–703.
22. Olsson S, Pal SN, Dodoo A. Pharmacovigilance in resource-limited countries. Expert Rev Clin Pharmacol. 2015;8:449–60.
23. Alsaleh FM, Alzaid SW, Abahussain EA, Bayoud T, Lemay J. Knowledge, attitude and practices of pharmacovigilance and adverse drug reaction reporting among pharmacists working in secondary and tertiary governmental hospitals in Kuwait. Saudi Pharm J. 2016;25:830.
24. Ferner RE, Aronson JK. National differences in publishing papers on adverse drug reactions. Br J Clin Pharmacol. 2005;59:108–11.
25. WHO, supporting pharmacovigilance in developing countries: the systems perspective; http://apps.who.int/medicinedocs/documents/s18813en/s18813en.pdf. Accessed 1 Feb 2016.
26. Uppsala Monitoring Centre; https://who-umc.org/about-the-who-programme-for-international-drug-monitoring/member-countries/. Accessed Dec 2024.
27. Bham B. The first Eastern Mediterranean region/Arab countries meeting of pharmacovigilance. Drugs - Real World Outcomes. 2015;2:111–5.
28. Al-Essa RK, Al-Rubaie M, Walker S, Salek S. Pharmaceutical regulatory environment: challenges and opportunities in the Gulf Region, 2015. http://search.ebscohost.com/login.aspx?direct=true&scope=site&db=nlebk&db=nlabk&AN=990730. Accessed 1 Feb 2016.
29. Common Arab guidelines on good vigilance practice; http://www.lexology.com/library/detail.aspx?g=9a96c38d-c3b0-4588-ad02-199a1ddeb5bb. Accessed 1 Feb 2016.
30. Guideline on Good Pharmacovigilance Practices (GVP) for Arab Countries; http://www.jfda.jo/Download/JPC/TheGoodPharmacovigilancePracticev2.pdf. Accessed 1 Feb 2016.
31. Arab & Eastern Mediterranean Pharmacovigilance Network. Available at: http://www.arabemrpvnetwork.org/. Accessed 21 April 2016.
32. Jabbour S, Yamout R, editors. Public health in the Arab world. Cambridge: Cambridge University Press; 2012.
33. Up to $40 billion of Arab world's spending on health care wasted | The National; http://www.thenational.ae/business/economy/up-to-40-billion-of-arab-worlds-spending-on-health-care-wasted. Accessed 1 Feb 2016.
34. WHO Global Health Expenditure Atlas; http://apps.who.int/nha/atlasfinal.pdf. Accessed 1 Feb 2016.
35. World Bank Health expenditure per capita (current US$); http://data.worldbank.org/indicator/SH.XPD.PCAP?order=wbapi_data_value_2013+wbapi_data_value+wbapi_data_value-last&sort=asc. Accessed 1 Feb 2016.
36. Gottret PE, Schieber G. Health financing revisited: a practitioner's guide. World Bank; 2006.
37. WHO safety monitoring medicinal products: guidelines for setting up and running a Pharmacovigilance Centre; http://www.who.int/medicines/areas/quality_safety/safety_efficacy/EMP_ConsumerReporting_web_v2.pdf. Accessed 1 Feb 2016.
38. Merrill JC. The road to health care reform: designing a system that works. Plenum Press; 1994.
39. Hill PS, Pavignani E, Michael M, Murru M, Beesley ME. The 'empty void' is a crowded space: health service provision at the margins of fragile and conflict affected states. Confl Heal. 2014;8:20.
40. Makhoul J, El-Barbir F. Obstacles to health in the Arab world. BMJ. 2006;333:859.

41. Becker's Hospital Review, Leadership is Central to Healthcare System Reform; http://www.beckershospitalreview.com/hospital-management-administration/leadership-is-central-to-healthcare-system-reform.html. Accessed 1 Feb 2016.
42. Bräutigam D. Aid Dependence and Governance; http://www.swisstph.ch/fileadmin/user_upload/Pdfs/swap/swap404.pdf. Accessed 1 Feb 1 2016.
43. World Bank, Net official development assistance and official aid received (current US$); http://data.worldbank.org/indicator/DT.ODA.ALLD.CD/countries?display=map. Accessed 1 Feb 2016.
44. Van de Walle N. Overcoming stagnation in aid-dependent countries. Center for Global Development; 2005.
45. Kohler JC, et al. An examination of pharmaceutical systems in severely disrupted countries. BMC Int Health Hum Rights. 2012;12:34.
46. Ooms G, Stuckler D, Basu S, McKee M. Financing the millennium development goals for health and beyond: sustaining the 'Big Push'. Glob Health. 2010;6:17.
47. Medicine prices and access to medicines in the Eastern Mediterranean Region. Technical discussion at the fifty-forth session of the Regional Committee for the Eastern Mediterranean. Agenda item 5(a). Cairo, World Health Organization Regional Office for the Eastern Mediterranean, 2007; http://applications.emro.who.int/docs/EM_RC54_Tech_Disc_1_en.pdf?ua=1. Accessed 1 Feb 2016.
48. United Nations Development Programme. Fighting corruption in the health sector: methods, tools, and good practices; http://www.undp.org/content/dam/undp/library/Democratic%20Governance/IP/Anticorruption%20Methods%20and%20Tools%20in%20Health%20Lo%20Res%20final.pdf. Accessed 1 Feb 2016.
49. Khatib R, Daoud A, Abu-Rmeileh NME, Mataria A, McCaig D. Medicine utilisation review in selected non-governmental organisations primary healthcare clinics in the West Bank in Palestine. Pharmacoepidemiol Drug Saf. 2008;17:1123–30.
50. Newton PN, Green MD, Fernández FM. Impact of poor-quality medicines in the 'developing' world. Trends Pharmacol Sci. 2010;31:99–101.
51. Petryna A. Global pharmaceuticals: ethics, markets, practices. Duke University Press; 2006.
52. WHO Regional Office for the Eastern Mediterranean. Health systems priorities in the Eastern Mediterranean Region: challenges and strategic directions; http://web.worldbank.org/archive/website01055/WEB/IMAGES/HEALTHSY.PDF. Accessed 1 Feb 2016.
53. WHO, Country Health Information Systems; http://www.who.int/healthmetrics/news/chis_report.pdf. Accessed 1 Feb 2016.
54. Saleh SS, Alameddine MS, El-Jardali F. The case for developing publicly-accessible datasets for health services research in the Middle East and North Africa (MENA) region. BMC Health Serv Res. 2009;9:197.
55. WHO Collaborating Centre for Pharmacovigilance in Education and Patient Reporting; http://www.lareb.nl/whocc?lang=en-GB. Accessed 1 Feb 2016.
56. Salih C. "Middle East 'Brain Drain' Reverses" - Al-Monitor: the Pulse of the Middle East; http://www.al-monitor.com/pulse/originals/2012/al-monitor/reversebraindrain.html#. Accessed 15 Aug 2020.
57. Lu Z. Information technology in pharmacovigilance: benefits, challenges, and future directions from industry perspectives. Drug Healthc Patient Saf. 2009;1:35–45.
58. Bill and Melinda Gates Foundation, A Report of the Safety and Surveillance Working Group; https://docs.gatesfoundation.org/documents/SSWG%20Final%20Report%2011%2019%2013_designed.pdf. Accessed 15 Aug 2020.
59. Dal Pan GJ. Ongoing challenges in pharmacovigilance. Drug Saf. 2014;37:1–8.
60. WHO safety monitoring of medicinal products: reporting system for the general public; http://www.who.int/medicines/areas/quality_safety/safety_efficacy/EMP_ConsumerReporting_web_v2.pdf. Accessed 15 Aug 2020.
61. Jabbour S. Health and development in the Arab world: which way forward? BMJ. 2003;326:1141–3.

62. Waterston T. Child health and the Arab spring. J Trop Pediatr. 2011;57:239–40.
63. Alwan A. Responding to priority health challenges in the Arab world. Lancet. 2014;383:284–6.

Danya M. Qato is an Associate Professor at the University of Maryland Baltimore School of Pharmacy and School of Medicine where she teaches epidemiology and health policy. She is a former United States Fulbright Scholar and a pharmacist and epidemiologist with over 20 years of experience in public health and pharmacy practice. She holds a PhD in Health Services Research from the Brown University School of Public Health, a Master of Public Health from the Harvard University School of Public Health, and a PharmD from the University of Illinois at Chicago.

Chapter 4
What Should Be the Focus of Pharmacovigilance in the Pacific Island Countries?

John McEwen, Amanda L. C. Sanburg, Agnes Mathias, and Lasse S. Vestergaard

4.1 Challenges for Pharmacovigilance in the Pacific Island Countries

4.1.1 Introduction

Both the Global Fund to Fight AIDS, Tuberculosis and Malaria (Global Fund) and the World Health Organization (WHO) have programmes supporting national and international pharmacovigilance (PV) activities. We have previously published a Current Opinion paper titled 'Pacific Island Pharmacovigilance: The Need for a Different Approach' [1]. In this current chapter, we provide where available updated information and comment. Ten of the 14 Pacific Islands Countries (PICs) are recipients of Global Fund support [2]. However, most PICs do not yet meet the Global Fund and WHO minimum requirements for a functioning PV system [3].

Of the 14 independent PICs, only four (Fiji, Papua New Guinea, Solomon Islands, and Vanuatu) have populations greater than 300,000, while the mean of the other ten PICs is approximately 67,700 persons (Table 4.1) [4]. Enrollment rates in primary school have improved, for example, it had reached 91.7% in Vanuatu in 2018, while the enrollment rate in secondary school was only 42.4% and only 23%

J. McEwen (✉)
Deakin, ACT, Australia
e-mail: mcewenj253@yahoo.com

A. L. C. Sanburg
East Deep Creek, QLD, Australia

A. Mathias
Ministry of Health, Port Vila, Vanuatu

L. S. Vestergaard
Infectious Disease Epidemiology and Prevention, Statens Serum Institut,
Copenhagen, Denmark

© Springer Nature Singapore Pte Ltd. 2025
S. R. Ahmad (ed.), *Special Issues in Pharmacovigilance in Resource-Limited Countries*, https://doi.org/10.1007/978-981-96-6154-1_4

Table 4.1 Independent Pacific Island countries and populations

Country	Population (2023)
Cook Islands	17,000
Federated States of Micronesia	114,000
Fiji	930,000
Kiribati	131,000
Nauru	13,000
Niue	2000
Palau	18,000
Papua New Guinea	10,143,000
Republic of Marshall Islands	42,000
Samoa	222,000
Solomon Islands	724,000
Tonga	107,000
Tuvalu	11,000
Vanuatu	327,000

Source: World Statistics Pocket Book 2023 edition [4]

continued school until Year 13 [5]. Consequently, there are very limited numbers of local doctors and pharmacists. A reflection of the small populations is limited infrastructure, which is further challenged by a geographical setting comprised of many small islands in many of the countries. In all but urban centres, access to a letter box may involve many hours walk or boat travel, greatly impeding postal-based reporting systems. Internet connectivity and mobile phone networks are often unstable, if available at all. The economies of all these countries are dependent on foreign aid, including support for government health services. While there are some private medical services and pharmacies in these countries, the majority of their peoples obtain prescription medicines from public hospitals, health centres, nurse-operated rural clinics and aid posts with volunteer health workers.

The 14 independent PICs do not include New Caledonia or the French Overseas Territories of French Polynesia and Wallis and Fortuna. The medicines in these countries are mostly imported from France and pharmacy is practiced according to French law.

Almost all medicines in the PICs, including prescription medicines, are imported. We estimate that no more than five PICs have active programmes currently for authorization or licensing of medicines. Otherwise, there is virtually no regulatory control over imports so medicines are imported from all over the world with only basic requests for evidence of quality from national authorities. The health service priorities are such that PICs have little or no customs controls or internal inspectorates to ensure compliance with current legislation. Inspections of shops, supermarkets, public and private pharmacies (there are small numbers of private pharmacies in most PICs), medical facilities and veterinary practices are largely unknown. In at least one PIC (Vanuatu), the sale of medicines by private pharmacies to customers in other countries via the Internet is permitted by law, and several pharmacies are actively involved in this practice.

Some coordinated control programmes targeting specific diseases such as malaria in some of the PICs include supply of a specific medicine of known quality. Also in some PICs, there have been recent programmes promoting Antimicrobial Stewardship [6] consistent with WHO Western Pacific Region (WPR) recommendations [7]. Such activities increase the focus on the availability of essential medicines of appropriate quality.

Overall, in the PICs, there is very little monitoring of the quality and effects of the general supply of medicines, most of which are included in national Essential Medicines Lists (EMLs). In addition to the main channels through agents and wholesalers, some medicines enter some PICs in the supplies of aid organizations sponsoring visiting or permanent clinics, often in the more remote areas. Many of these items are not on the national EML. For example, compound tablets containing diclofenac sodium 15 mg, chlorpheniramine maleate 2.5 mg and ox bile 15 mg labelled with Chinese characters found their way into the pharmacy of a PIC public hospital. In some PICs, various products, some of dubious medical value, are the subject of 'quackery'—promoters and agents try to profit through inappropriate health claims for the products. Promotion is often direct to would-be consumers.

The WPR includes 37 countries and stretches over a vast area from China in the North and West to the Pacific Islands and French Polynesia in the East. The Region includes a mixture of low-income, middle-income and high-income countries, with a target of at least 80% of WPR countries having 'medicines policy and implementation mechanism in place' by 2016 [8]. Having such a policy and mechanism in place is possible to attain in high-income countries but is difficult to apply directly to the PICs which are in the low- and middle-income groups.

We estimate that currently ten independent PICs have developed National Medicines Policy documents. Once prepared and adopted, it is a challenge for the smaller PICs to monitor their implementation and regularly update their content. In Vanuatu, it is intended that the impact of the National Medicines Policy (2015–2020) will be assessed against defined indicators with regular reporting of outcomes to appropriate committees and personnel.

The Regional Framework for Action on Access to Essential Medicines in the Western Pacific (2011–2016) [8] promoted 'strengthening of the performance of drug and therapeutic committees or their equivalent in health care centres, especially in hospitals'. The Framework also proposed as an indicator of progress that 'a national programme or committee (involving government, civil society and professional bodies) exists to monitor and promote rational use of medicines' in 100% of WPR countries. While such arrangements may be achievable in high-income countries and in the larger PICs, the existence of a single functioning National Drugs and Therapeutics Committee (NDTC) should be the preferred approach in the smaller PICs. A role for Drug and Therapeutics Committees in monitoring and analysing medicine quality problems has been proposed previously [9]. Given the workload pressures on doctors and pharmacists who might be NDTC members, there is a strong need for support and strengthening of these committees.

'Pharmacovigilance' (PV) is not a word known to many health care workers in the PICs [10]. There is a need for training of health workers at all levels and for community awareness about the basics of PV and the risks of not having PV.

To date, issues of maintenance of supply of essential medicines and difficulties in operational aspects of supply chains have taken precedence over pharmacovigilance activities. We have, for example, observed that the Vanuatu pharmaceutical sector is affected by several constraints: (i) lack of a quality assurance system for pharmaceutical goods, (ii) difficulty in logistics distribution due to the geographical setting, (iii) inadequate reporting and health information systems, (iv) inadequate organization and supervision and (v) insufficient human and financial resources [11]. These constraints are quite similar across all the PICs to varying degrees. Indeed, there are very few staff in the PICs primarily committed even part-time to PV activities as would be found in larger developed countries.

Some prescription products have been pre-qualified by WHO, but the quality of others may be less certain. Package insert information for health professionals, if available, is of variable quality and sometimes in a foreign language and patient information leaflets are largely unknown. The range of available prescription medicines in each country is largely based on national EMLs. Fiscal restraints limit the introduction of new medicines. Conventional pharmacovigilance may detect unusual or uniquely high incidences of adverse events in these populations and also prescribing practices leading to Adverse Drug Reactions (ADRs). However, much more pressing issues are about the quality of a product—arising as an obvious physical defect (e.g. crumbling tablets) or as a clinical suspicion that a medicine is not effective—and the growing risk of counterfeit medicines [12]. When a substandard product is identified, it is important that information about it is shared regionally. With the exception of a laboratory established in Papua New Guinea, no regulatory agencies in the PICs have comprehensive medicine testing facilities.

Rather than emphasizing pharmacovigilance with a focus on ADRs, we argue that an alternative approach is required and have proposed an initiative in which WHO, the Global Fund and development partners would adopt, as a priority over a number of years, the implementation of an adequately resourced programme clearly described as being for the reporting of 'Problems with Medicines'. Such a programme would not exclude reporting of ADRs and medication errors but would rebalance the emphasis towards more pressing problems to do with provenance, quality and efficacy of currently used medicines.

4.1.2 Current Pharmacovigilance in Pacific Island Countries

In brief, there is little or no functioning pharmacovigilance in place in most PICs. A 'Problems with Medicines' reporting form has been developed in Vanuatu by a volunteer Australian pharmacist with help from the WHO Collaborating Centre for International Drug Monitoring at the Uppsala Monitoring Centre (UMC) in Sweden [13]. It nonetheless awaits resources for more permanent implementation.

Globally, the WHO Programme for International Drug Monitoring ('WHO Programme') is central to international co-operation and development of pharmacovigilance. A key element is the UMC [14]. Full members of the WHO Programme (180 full member countries and 22 associate member countries as of May 2025) are expected to submit Individual Case Safety Reports (ICSRs) of ADRs to the UMC at least every quarter and preferably more frequently [15]. WHO requires prospective members:

- To have in place a system for the collection of ICSRs
- To have the necessary funding of a national centre authorized by the competent national health authority to ensure continuity of operations
- To have access to appropriate staffing and technical facilities

Initially a successful applicant country will become an Associate Member country with progression to full membership dependent upon, amongst other things, submission to the UMC of at least 20 ICSRs. These must be collected in the applicant's national pharmacovigilance programme and be confirmed by the UMC for compatibility of those reports with their requirements [16]. Of all PICs, only Fiji, Papua New Guinea and Cook Islands have applied for membership of the WHO Programme. Fiji has been a full member since 1999 and Papua New Guinea became a full member in March 2018. Cook Islands is currently an associate member [17].

The Global Fund pays for medicines used in many low-income and middle-income countries to treat HIV, tuberculosis and malaria [2]. A joint Global Fund and WHO document sets out the 'Minimum requirements for a functioning PV system' [3].

They are:

1. A national pharmacovigilance centre with designated staff (at least one full time), stable basic funding, clear mandates, well-defined structures and roles and collaboration with the WHO Programme for International Drug Monitoring.
2. The existence of a national spontaneous reporting system with a national individual case safety report form, i.e. an ADR reporting form
3. A national database or system for collating and managing ADR reports
4. A national ADR or pharmacovigilance advisory committee able to provide technical assistance on causality assessment, risk assessment, risk management, case investigation and, where necessary, crisis management including crisis communication
5. A clear communication strategy for routine communication and crisis communication

The Global Fund in 2012 indicated that 'Countries have a clear opportunity to conduct pharmacovigilance strengthening activities, drawing on budgeted requests for financial support from the Global Fund' [18]. The Global Fund's Technical Review Panel has more recently (2015) stressed the need for more attention to establishing and supporting PV systems [19], and in 2017 that applicants for funding should include technical support for pharmacovigilance in their funding requests [20]. As at 2025, notwithstanding Global Fund allocations to ten Pacific Island Countries none of those countries (apart from Papua New Guinea and Fiji) yet has a National Centre for the safety monitoring of medicines and/or vaccines designated and recognized by its Ministry of Health (or equivalent). It may be hoped that Global Fund support will further promote pharmacovigilance in the Pacific Island Countries with small populations.

In our Current Opinion paper, we suggested that it may be an unrealistic proposition that any but the largest of the PICs could justify that there should be national ADR or pharmacovigilance advisory committees, especially as many of the PICs do not yet have a National Medicines Policy or a functioning Drugs and Therapeutics Committee [1]. Concerning the conjoint PV Minimum Requirements document, the WHO Advisory Committee on Safety of Medicinal Products indicated in 2016 the need for a revised document [21]. That document should consider special needs of smaller countries, and provide broad guidance on the implementation of the requirements together with references to any existing guidelines.

We have presented an alternative proposal [1]. Based in one of the countries with a mid-range population, spread over numerous islands (such as Solomon Islands or Vanuatu), we proposed that the initial programme, externally funded, would provide opportunities to involve and train personnel ranging from aid post attendants to hospital staff and explore the use of the resources of more established countries to facilitate testing of suspect products and causality assessment of suspected adverse reactions. Possibilities for later extension to other PICs should be explored. The following principles were proposed:

- Management of the Problems with Medicines reporting programme should be part of the duties of a full time pharmacist.
- There should be active liaison between the Problems with Medicines reporting programme and the NDTC, which should perform at least some of the roles of a National Pharmacovigilance Committee.
- Both the programme and the NDTC should have ready and prompt access to specialist advice about medicine quality and clinical safety and assistance with causality assessment.
- The programme should have ready and prompt access to testing of suspect products by accredited laboratories. Results of testing should be shared with other PICs, enabling efficiencies in product testing programmes.
- A key objective is the development of requisite skills and capacity in qualified citizens.

To these, we now add:

- Regional sharing of 'Problems with Medicines' information where relevant.

4.1.3 Learning from Other Countries

Our proposal does not exclude the PICs drawing on experience in other countries. Pharmacists employed by national authorities should be supported to attend pharmacovigilance training offered by the UMC. In time, the use of modern technology such as mobile phones, as occurs in Kenya [22] and Nigeria [23], may have a place, but to date problems have been encountered when mobile phone systems have been used in other health projects in PICs, such as inadequate phone coverage. In 2019, a WHO-convened meeting of PICs was briefed about the Caribbean Regulatory System (See Chap. 6) [24].

4.1.4 Recent developments

A Pacific Medicines Testing Programme providing testing by the Australian Therapeutic Goods Administration Laboratories at no cost to participating PICs was initiated in 2018 [25]. There are 13 countries participating in the Programme. In the financial year 2023–2024, 21.9% of 32 samples failed testing. In February 2024, the TGA hosted the Training Course in Medicines Regulation-Detect, Respond, and Prevent, which focused on enhancing regional regulatory capabilities. This course trained 26 delegates from the participating countries and 2 WHO observers, and covered both regulatory and laboratory-based aspects of identifying and managing substandard medicines (See Chap. 21) [26]. Also a Pacific regional website (www.medqualityassurance.org) was developed in 2017 to aid with regional information sharing of test results as well as visual inspection reports. In 2017, 12 PICs had enrolled in this information platform. It appears however to not be supported currently.

4.1.5 Conclusion

Small independent countries deserve no less than other nations the protections provided by pharmacovigilance. Given the current challenges in ensuring proper PV capacity in many settings, support for an alternative solution is needed. International requirements have their virtues but on occasions, one size does not fit all. Hopefully, the conjoint PV Minimum Requirements document is being adapted to better cater for low-income countries with very small populations. The primary focus of Pacific Island pharmacovigilance should be on monitoring the quality of medicines and sharing that information regionally.

Declaration of interest John McEwen is a former pharmacovigilance consultant, Ministry of Health, Vanuatu. Amanda Sanburg is the former Principal Pharmacist, Ministry of Health, Vanuatu. Agnes Mathias was Principal Pharmacist (2014–2022), Ministry of Health, Vanuatu. Lasse Vestergaard is Senior Medical Officer, Infectious Disease Epidemiology and Prevention, Statens Serum Institute, Copenhagen, Denmark. He was a Medical Officer (2008–2012), WHO, Vanuatu and was a member (2020–2024) of the Global Fund's Technical Review Panel.

References

1. McEwen J, Vestergaard LS, Sanburg ALC. Pacific Island Pharmacovigilance: the Need for a Different Approach. Drug Saf. 2016; https://doi.org/10.1007/s40264-016-0439-4.
2. Anon. The Global Fund. Funding Model allocations 2014–2016. www.theglobalfund.org/en/fundingmodel_2020-2022 allocations_table_en(1). Accessed 27 June 2020.
3. Anon. The Global Fund and World Health Organization. Minimum requirements for a functional Pharmacovigilance System. www.who.int/medicines/areas/quality_safety/safety_efficacy/PV_Minimum_Requirements_2010_2.pdf. Accessed 27 June 2020.
4. Department of Economic and Social Affairs Statistics Division. World Statistics Pocket Book 2023 edition. Series V, No 47. New York: United Nations; 2023. https://unstats.un.org/UNSDWebsite/Publications/StatisticalPocketbook/. Accessed 12 Oct 2023
5. Anon. Republic of Vanuatu. Ministry of Education and Training. Annual Statistical Digest Report 2016–2018. https://moet.gov.vu/docs/statistics/2016-2018%20MoET%20Annual%20Statistical%20Digest%20-%20ENG%20version_2019.pdf. Accessed 27 June 2020.
6. Anon. Antimicrobial resistance in the Pacific: How Pacific nations are working to address drug-resistant pathogens. 23 November 2022 https://www.who.int/westernpacific/newsroom/feature-stories/item/antimicrobial-resistance-in-the-pacific--how-pacific-nations-are-working-to-address-drug-resistant-pathogens. Accessed 30 April 2025.
7. Anon. Framework for Accelerating Action to Fight Antimicrobial Resistance in the Western Pacific Region. https://www.who.int/publications/i/item/9789290619284. Accessed 30 April 2025.
8. The regional framework for action on access to essential medicines in the Western Pacific (2011–2016). World Health Organization 2012. http://www.wpro.who.int/publications/emt_framework_for_action_lite2.pdf?ua=1. Accessed 27 June 2020.
9. Holloway K, Green T, editors. Drug and therapeutics committees a practical guide. Geneva: World Health Organization; 2003. p. 56.
10. Escalante S, McEwen J. National policies for safety of medicines in the Asia-Pacific region. WHO South-East Asia J Public Health. 2013;2:118–20.
11. Brown A, Gilbert B. The Vanuatu medical supply system-documenting opportunities and challenges to meet the Millenium Development Goals. South Med Rev. 2012;5(1):14–21.
12. Hetzel MW, Page-Sharp M, Bala N, et al. Quality of Antimalarial drugs and Antibiotics in Papua New Guinea: A survey of the Health Facility Supply Chain. PLoS One. 2014;9(5):1–10.
13. Hagstrom A. Asia Pacific Training. Uppsala Rep. 2015;69:17.
14. Olsson S. UMC Redesignation. Uppsala Rep. 2013;62:114.
15. Anon. Uppsala Monitoring Centre. Being a member of the WHO Programme for international drug monitoring. www.who-umc.org/media/1434/being-a-member.pdf. Accessed 22 June 2020.
16. Anon. Joining the WHO Programme for international drug monitoring. https://www.who.int/medicines/areas/quality_safety/safety_efficacy/Joining_the_WHO_Programme.pdf?ua=1. Accessed 22 June 2020.
17. Anon. Members of the WHO Programme for International Drug Monitoring. https://who-umc.org/about-the-who-programme-for-international-drug-monitoring/member-countries/ Accessed 30 April 2025.

18. Xueref S. The Global Fund to fight AIDS, TB and Malaria: an opportunity to strengthen pharmacovigilance systems in beneficiary countries. WHO Pharm Newslett. 2012;5:15–7.
19. Anon. Report of the TRP on concept notes submitted in the third and fourth windows of the funding model. February 2015. Archive of Technical Review Panel Reports. https://www.theglobalfund.org/en/technical-review-panel/reports/ Accessed 30 April 2025.
20. Anon. The technical review panel's observations on the 2017-2019 allocation cycle. https://archive.theglobalfund.org/technical-review-panel/. Accessed 18 Oct 2023.
21. Anon. Report from the thirteenth meeting of the WHO Advisory Committee on Safety of Medicinal Products (ACSoMP) 21-22 June 2016. WHO Pharmaceuticals Newsletter. 2016;4:25.
22. Pandit J, Kusu N. Electronic reporting launched in Kenya. Uppsala Rep. 2013;62:11.
23. Jajere F. Rapid consumer reports. Uppsala Rep. 2014;65:16.
24. Anon. Pacific Island meeting on subregional regulatory systems for medicines 28 February-1 March 2019.WHO regional Office for Western Pacific. July 2019. Accessed 27 June 2020.
25. Anon. The Pacific Medicines Testing Programme. https://www.tga.gov.au/safety/product-testing-and-investigations/laboratories-branch-international-affiliations#pmtp.
26. Anon. Therapeutic Goods Administration.Performance Report 2023-24 https://www.tga.gov.au/resources/publication/publications/therapeutic-goods-administration-performance-report-2023-24. Accessed 30 April 2025.

Chapter 5
Pharmacovigilance and Public Health in Latin America Countries

Mónica Tarapués and Mariano Madurga

5.1 Introduction

The safe use of medicines is one of the most important steps in the management of patients with any disease. This takes a high relevance when we talk about diseases considered public health problems, especially in countries with low or middle income. Due to the limited budget assigned to national health programmes, this must be used in the best possible way. For that reason, it is appropriate that pharmacovigilance is introduced in public health programmes [1].

In Latin America, there are several diseases that are considered public health problems because of its high social and financial burden, such as tuberculosis, malaria, HIV, as well as some non-communicable diseases. The approaches to tackle these diseases have changed over time, with changes in the law or in the internal structure of the health ministries under which these initiatives are controlled [2].

In the past, some countries had one unique national health program for each disease, managed in a vertical process and with no relationship with other health departments. Roughly ten years ago, these national health programs were restructured into "strategies," with the objective to function as one integrated program. Some national strategies, especially those regarding pharmacotherapy, focus on access to quality medicines. Pharmacovigilance would fit perfectly within that framework, and if successfully incorporated, it can have a huge impact on the overall public health system—not the least in terms of health spending.

M. Tarapués (✉)
International Society of Pharmacovigilance, Quito, Ecuador
e-mail: monica@tarapues.com

M. Madurga
Pharmacovigilance, Majadahonda, Madrid, Spain

© Springer Nature Singapore Pte Ltd. 2025
S. R. Ahmad (ed.), *Special Issues in Pharmacovigilance in Resource-Limited Countries*, https://doi.org/10.1007/978-981-96-6154-1_5

Besides spontaneous reporting, there are other specific safety monitoring methods that can adapt into public health programs, such as cohort-event monitoring (CEM) or targeted spontaneous reporting. The latter has more advantages in our context, especially because it is less costly—however, its success depends upon the training of individual healthcare professionals [3, 4].

5.2   National Immunization Plan

One example of an integrative model is in the program called "national immunization plan"; this includes the management of vaccines for the prevention of several diseases. For decades, this program has been the most successful and admired program in the region, but with the use of new vaccines, this program needed an integrative model with vaccine surveillance and pharmacovigilance centres for causality assessment. The national immunization plan and the national pharmacovigilance centre show an exceptional interaction in the case of Colombia, Uruguay, Chile, and Peru [5–7]. In fact, Chile together with International Institute of Vaccines (IVI) is working in an electronic standardized format that allows to harmonize the adverse events following immunization (AEFI; in Spanish: ESAVI, Eventos Supuestamente Atribuibles a la Vacunación o Inmunización) suspected from vaccines. This pilot project was presented in the last global meeting of IVI. Their objective is to create one single form in the region that serves as a bridge to the global pharmacovigilance database of the program for international drug monitoring (PIDM) of the World Health Organization (WHO): Vigibase® [8].

5.3   National Tuberculosis Programme

Other Latin American countries already work hard to connect safety monitoring activities to other health initiatives. In Peru, for example, the national pharmacovigilance centre has implemented the cohort-event monitoring (CEM) method in order to follow up all patients in the national program of tuberculosis. For their national program for tuberculosis in Peru, they have also developed an adverse drug reaction reporting form to overcome the problem of underreporting [9]. Additionally, in the region, there is a project, coordinated by the Pan-American Health Organization (PAHO), to tackle the antimicrobial-resistant tuberculosis; the main goal is integrating pharmacovigilance activities into public health strategies regarding tuberculosis.

This regional project, called FAVIA-TB, started in 2017, with the participation of Paraguay, Colombia, Peru, El Salvador, Panama, and Honduras [10]. The project has the support of the health authorities of the included countries. Its objective is to follow the patients especially those who suffer from Multi-Drug-Resistant (MDR) TB, in order to identify potential problems related to medicines earlier. It is important to bear in mind that WHO has released guidelines regarding safety monitoring of second-line drugs, bedaquiline and delamanid [11, 12]. The goal of FAVIA-TB is to improve the surveillance of these and other second-line anti-tuberculosis drugs in the region. For example, in Paraguay, which has more experience in FAVIA-TB project, one objective is to standardize the definition of some adverse drug reactions (ADR), such as hematological toxicity, hepatotoxicity among others, and its incorporation as part of the clinical record. However, the incorporation of these terms in an electronic database is still a challenge, as well the direct connection with the national pharmacovigilance centre and international database. This project has just one year of implementation; for that reason, there is no data available yet [13].

5.4 Surveillance of Hepatitis C Drugs

In the region, some countries have experience in the surveillance of Hepatitis C drugs. In the case of Argentina, there is a strong and beneficial relationship between the regulatory agency of Argentina, ANMAT (Administración Nacional de Medicamentos, Alimentos y Tecnología Médica), as part of Health Ministry and the pharmaceutical industry with the support of PAHO. This program started in 2015, after the postmarketing authorization of sofosbuvir in the country. An online form of the National Pharmacovigilance program was utilized, and another questionnaire was created for patients in order to overcome the underreporting by health professionals. This is the first experience in a Latin America country to evaluate and follow up 1152 patients with Hepatitis C on sofosbuvir with ribavirin. The adverse reactions reported were 245 from health professionals and 528 from patients. The most common adverse reaction reported by health professionals was anemia. In the causality assessment, this was mostly associated with rivabirin. In the reports from patients, fatigue was commonly reported; among these reports, only three cases of serious adverse events were reported. This work supported the concept of surveillance in public health. However, so far no safety signal has been identified through this project [14].

5.5 Surveillance of Antimalarial Drugs

Another important project is the surveillance of the antimalarial therapy, namely, primaquine, in the region where there is a widespread use of this drug. However, primaquine has hemolytic toxicity especially in those who are deficient in glucose-6-phosphate dehydrogenase (G6PD). In Latin American countries, there is no screening of G6PD deficiency because of its low prevalence. However, some patients can be resistant to the treatment and relapse with the standard therapy, and for those patients, there is a new drug under study called tafenoquine. But in order to use tafenoquine and monitor those with primaquine, it is important to follow these patients during their treatment. In the Latin American region, PAHO is reinforcing

the surveillance of antimalarial drugs. However, this project is not fully implemented yet, although some countries such as Brazil, Colombia, Ecuador, Peru, and
Venezuela have expressed interest [15, 16].

These successful examples should be reinforced in the region because it is necessary to achieve this integrative model and make all the efforts to bring the theoretical
concept to practical work across the whole region.

Nevertheless, in many countries, the integrative model is not completely applied
yet. There are several reasons for this, from lack of political interest to a deficiency
of technological support. There is a general lack of knowledge of how medicines
safety systems work. Nor is it fully understood that the patients are the start and
end-point of this work and how it fits into the objective of national health. For that
reason, joint work between pharmacovigilance centres and public health programmes with other healthcare sectors is necessary and should be mandatory.

In addition, there is a need to work on educating professionals in the field. Most
people think that including pharmacovigilance is synonymous of a heavier workload, and changing this perception should be the main goal.

Pharmacovigilance is vital for the safety of patients. There are other successful
experiences in Africa, such as South Africa, that offer a good example of how safety
monitoring activities can be included even with limited resources [17]. In our region,
as well as in other parts of the world, patient populations with a high disease burden
deserve the best possible healthcare, and pharmacovigilance could help to achieve
that goal.

References

1. Olsson S, Pal SN, Dodoo A. Pharmacovigilance in resource-limited countries. Expert Rev Clin
   Pharmacol. 2015;8(4):449–60.
2. Shabir B, Embrey Martha JM. Apoyo a la Farmacovigilancia en los países en vías de desar-
   rollo. La perspectiva de sistemas [Internet]. Strength Pharma System. 2009; Available from:
   http://apps.who.int/medicinedocs/documents/s21530es/s21530es.pdf
3. Pal SN, Duncombe C, Falzon D, Olsson S. WHO strategy for collecting safety data in public
   health s: complementing spontaneous reporting systems. Drug Saf. 2013;36:75–81.
4. Rachlis B, Karwa R, Chema C, Pastakia S, Olsson S, Wools-Kaloustian K, et al. Targeted
   spontaneous reporting: assessing opportunities to conduct routine pharmacovigilance for antiretroviral treatment on an international scale. Drug Saf. 2016;39(10):959–76.
5. Instituto Nacional de Vigilancia de Medicamentos y Alimentos. INVIMA. In 2018 [cited 2018
   Nov 12]. Available from: https://www.invima.gov.co/farmacovigilancia-invima.html
6. Vigilancia de ESAVI | Ministerio de Salud Publica – Republica Oriental del Uruguay [Internet].
   [cited 2018 Nov 26]. Available from: http://www.msp.gub.uy/publicación/vigilancia-de-esavi
7. Juan Roldán QF. Farmacovigilancia: Datos sobre el estado actual de esta disciplina en Chile.
   Rev Médica Clínica Las Condes. 2016;27(5):585–93.
8. International Vaccine Institute. Global vaccine safety initiative fifth meeting secretariat report
   [Internet]. 2016 [cited 2018 Nov 26]. Available from: http://www.who.int/about/licesing/copy-
   right_form/en/index.html
9. DIGEMID. Boletín de farmacovigilancia y tecnovigilancia. Bol Farm y Tecnovigilancia.
   2015;9(1):1–6.

10. Alarcon E. Perspectivas del Programa Regional de Tuberculosis MDR XDR. In: Memories of the XIV International congress of Pharmacovigilance [Internet]. 2018 [cited 2018 Nov 12]. Available from: https://www.invima.gov.co/images/pdf/farmacovigilancia_alertas/eventos/IV-ENCUENTRO-NACIONAL/MEMORIAS/2-3-Perspectivas-del-Programa-Regional-de-Tuberculosis-MDR-XDR.pdf

11. World Health Organization WHO | Interim guidance on the use of bedaquiline to treat MDR-TB [Internet]. WHO. World Health Organization; 2013 [cited 2018 Nov 26]. Available from: https://www.who.int/tb/challenges/mdr/bedaquiline/en/

12. Word Health Organization WHO | WHO position statement on the use of delamanid for multidrug-resistant tuberculosis [Internet]. WHO. World health Organization; 2018 [cited 2018 Nov 26]. Available from: http://www.who.int/tb/publications/2018/Position_Paper_Delamanid/en/

13. Ojeda C. Proyecto FAVIA-TB Experiencia Paraguay. In: Memories of the XIV International congress of Pharmacovigilance [Internet]. [cited 2018 Nov 26]. Available from: https://www.invima.gov.co/images/pdf/farmacovigilancia_alertas/eventos/IV-ENCUENTRO-NACIONAL/MEMORIAS/2-5-Comentarios-de-pais-con-miras-a-la-implementacion-del-proyecto-FAVIA.pdf

14. Carranza J, Vidiella G. Pharmacovigilancia public health programs: the experience in interaction with the programanational of viral hepatitis (in Spanish). [Internet]. 1st ed. In: Papale RM, Schiaffino S, García MG, editors. Manual de Buenas Prácticas de Farmacovigilancia Edición America Latina. Buenos Aires: Ediciones Farmacológicas; 2018. p. 623–32. Available from: https://isoponline.org/wp-content/uploads/2018/10/FVG_II_digital_con-Hipervinculos.pdf?fbclid=IwAR3r_pXMsuw3f5Ta_roDHHxvvMAIgdTbaSH2cR0TxbTeoDdON1L-HEx4Qm0s.

15. Malaria Policy Advisory Committee Meeting. Point-of-care G6PD testing to support safe use of primaquine for the treatment of vivax malaria [Internet]. 2015 [cited 2018 Nov 26]. Available from: http://www.who.int/malaria/mpac/mpac-march2015-erg-g6pd.pdf?ua=1

16. Ade MP. Perspectivas del Programa Regional de Malaria. In: Memories of the XIV International congress of Pharmacovigilance [Internet]. [cited 2018 Nov 26]. Available from: https://www.invima.gov.co/images/pdf/farmacovigilancia_alertas/eventos/IV-ENCUENTRO-NACIONAL/MEMORIAS/2-4-Perspectivas-del-Programa-Regional-de-Malaria.pdf

17. Isah AO, Pal SN, Olsson S, Dodoo A, Bencheikh RS. Specific features of medicines safety and pharmacovigilance in Africa. Ther Adv Drug Saf. 2012;3(1):25–34.

Chapter 6
Caribbean Network for Pharmacovigilance: Sharing Resources for Regional Vigilance

Rian Marie Extavour and Joy St John

6.1 Background

The Caribbean Regulatory System (CRS) was established in 2016 through an agreement between the Caribbean Public Health Agency (CARPHA) and the Pan American Health Organization/World Health Organization (PAHO/WHO), with funding support from the Gates Foundation [1]. This arose out of findings about regulatory challenges and key functions that were not performed by the 15 countries of the Caribbean Community (CARICOM) and other CARPHA Member States, including systems for pharmacovigilance of medicines and vaccines used in the subregion. In 2013, CARICOM Ministers of Health approved the Caribbean Pharmaceutical Policy that outlined the development of a subregional regulatory framework and stronger collaboration for the regulation of pharmaceuticals, with a focus on access to quality, safe, and effective medicines [2]. Because of these efforts, the CRS started its operations to support two key regulatory functions, which are recommended for small developing states with limited resources: (i) market authorization/market registration and (ii) pharmacovigilance and post-market surveillance [3].

In late 2017, the CRS launched the regional network for pharmacovigilance and post-market surveillance (called VigiCarib), which is managed by the CRS team: programme manager, a technical officer, and an administrator. CARPHA Member States were invited to nominate national regulatory focal points and/or national pharmacovigilance officers to comprise the network. To date, there are focal points for 20 CARPHA Member States who are included (Table 6.1). A representative of the Pharmaceutical Procurement Service of the Organisation of Eastern Caribbean States and advisors of PAHO/WHO are also part of the network. Based on the limited capacity noted among CARPHA Member States, support for subregional

R. M. Extavour (✉) · J. S. John
Caribbean Public Health Agency, Newtown, Trinidad and Tobago
e-mail: rextavour@hotmail.com; extavori@carpha.org

© Springer Nature Singapore Pte Ltd. 2025
S. R. Ahmad (ed.), *Special Issues in Pharmacovigilance in Resource-Limited Countries*, https://doi.org/10.1007/978-981-96-6154-1_6

vigilance that is provided by the CRS includes hosting of electronic reporting tools, promotion of vigilance, education and training of regulatory personnel and health professionals, and information sharing among regulators, inspectors, and pharmacovigilance officers.

6.2 Subregional Vigilance

Pharmacovigilance in CARPHA Member States varies based on the available capacity of the individual country. Of the listed Member States in Table 6.1, three have identified dedicated officers for pharmacovigilance (Barbados, Jamaica, St Vincent and the Grenadines), while other Member States assign pharmacovigilance activities to technical officers and/or inspectors, who may have other routine

Table 6.1 CARPHA member states included in CRS-VigiCarib network

Country	Total population, as of July 1, 2021 (thousands)	Male population (thousands)	Percent	Female population (thousands)	Percent
Anguilla	16	8	49	8	51
Antigua and Barbuda	93	45	48	49	52
Bahamas	408	195	48	213	52
Barbados	281	135	48	146	52
Bermuda	64	31	48	33	52
Belize	400	201	50	199	50
British Virgin Islands	31	15	48	16	52
Cayman Islands	68	34	50	34	50
Dominica	72	36	50	36	50
Grenada	125	62	50	62	50
Guyana	805	394	49	411	51
Haiti	11,448	5673	50	5775	50
Jamaica	2828	1403	50	1425	50
Montserrat	4	2	53	2	47
Saint Kitts and Nevis	48	23	48	25	52
Saint Lucia	180	89	50	91	50
Saint Vincent and the Grenadines	104	53	51	51	49
Suriname	613	305	50	308	50
Trinidad and Tobago	1526	753	49	773	51
Turks and Caicos Islands	45	23	50	22	50

Source: United Nations, Department of Economic and Social Affairs, Population Division [4]

regulatory functions. The most common pharmacovigilance activity conducted is spontaneous reporting of suspected adverse drug reactions (ADRs) and detection of substandard and/or falsified products. While some countries, like Barbados, have implemented electronic reporting systems, some continue to use paper-based systems for spontaneous reporting. Given that subregional (Caribbean) pharmacovigilance is primarily reliant on the activities at the national level, which may be limited in countries without dedicated staff or infrastructure, the CRS provides support to Member States by facilitating spontaneous reporting from health professionals and market authorization holders. This is done via the collection of individual case reports of suspected adverse drug reactions (ADRs), adverse events following immunization (AEFIs), also called "events supposedly attributable to vaccination or immunization" (ESAVIs), and reports of substandard and/or falsified medical products. Collection of case reports is primarily via online reporting forms, which have enabled market authorization holders, health professionals in private practice, and the public to submit reports to national authorities where a national reporting form is not publicly available or easily accessible. For CARICOM countries that are members of the World Health Organization (WHO) Programme for International Drug Monitoring but lack personnel to enter reports into the global database at the Uppsala Monitoring Centre, the CRS assists in this area as well. Since the establishment of the VigiCarib network, case reporting of incidents via the CRS has increased in Bahamas, Belize, British Virgin Islands, Cayman Islands, Dominica, St Vincent and the Grenadines, and Trinidad and Tobago. In all, 585 case reports have been shared via the VigiCarib network since its inception, consisting of suspected adverse drug reactions (380–65%), substandard/falsified medical products (120–20.5%), and adverse events following immunization (85–14.5%).

6.3   Role in COVID-19 Vaccine Safety Monitoring

With the use of vaccines against COVID-19 disease among CARPHA Member States, the importance of vigilance of these novel vaccine technologies was highlighted. The CRS modified its reporting form to enable the collection of AEFIs involving COVID-19 vaccines and supplemented these with a social media campaign and training workshops for health professionals to develop awareness and competence for reporting of AEFIs. In May 2021, the CRS hosted a webinar to sensitize health professionals, academics, and regulatory authorities of the lifelong nature of pharmacovigilance of COVID-19 vaccines, from non-clinical studies, to human trials, to post-market surveillance of vaccine safety.

   To date, the VigiCarib reporting system has facilitated the collection of AEFI case reports, which were transmitted to the respective Member States for investigation and follow-up as needed. Along with reports in the global database, the CRS has reported on 1625 spontaneous case reports of AEFIs involving COVID-19 vaccines as of July 15, 2023, from four Member States. These reports were mostly for expected, non-serious events, where most of the vaccine recipients were female

(73.8%) and under 65 years (85%). The predominance of female vaccinees may be reflective of a difference in reporting behavior compared to males, given that the sex distribution among CARPHA Member States is generally balanced (on average 51% are female (Table 6.1)). Three hundred and fourteen reports (19.3%) were classified as serious, but these include coincidental reports that require further investigation and causality assessment to remove non-attributable cases. Considering the number of doses of COVID-19 vaccines administered among the reporting countries, the CRS noted a reporting rate of 61 events per 100,000 doses over the period. However, with the decline in vaccinations against COVID-19 across the Caribbean, the number of AEFI reports has also declined. Nevertheless, individual Member States reported that national activities and sharing of VigiCarib News have helped increase collaborations with managers of the national Expanded Programmes for Immunization and increased collection of reports of AEFIs involving other vaccines.

6.4 Supporting Post-market Surveillance

Market surveillance of the quality of medicines in the Caribbean are supported by two CARPHA units: the Caribbean Regulatory System (CRS) and the Medicines Quality Control and Surveillance Department (MQCSD, formerly the Caribbean Drug Testing Laboratory). The MQCSD conducts quality control testing of medicines and coordinates a subregional risk-based post-market surveillance programme where predetermined medicines are sampled by the national regulatory authorities and sent to the MQCSD for testing. The CRS shares the findings of post-market surveillance activities through sharing of information on incidents detected in the CARPHA Member States, irrespective of the method of detection, for example, visual or physical inspection, laboratory testing, or reports of treatment failure. Incidents may involve substandard, falsified, or unregistered medical products, including devices. Hence, the CRS-VigiCarib network enables increased vigilance as Member States can identify medicines and other medical products that may be on their markets that would warrant closer monitoring, public awareness campaigns, and/or education of health professionals. During the COVID-19 pandemic, the CRS shared reports on various medicines used to treat COVID-19 that were found to be substandard through testing by MQCSD (e.g., dexamethasone tablets) or falsified (e.g., tocilizumab). In addition, the CRS includes alerts or incidents in the region of the Americas and by the WHO Rapid Alert system in its monthly newsletter for medicines, vaccines, or devices that are substandard or falsified. One example of an incident shared with CARPHA Member States that led to a global alert for 8240 falsified HIV test kits, which were detected in a CARPHA Member State (Guyana) in 2020 [5]. There is a need for ongoing monitoring of substandard, falsified, and unregistered medical products particularly where there may be deviations from good storage and distribution practices, lack of legal provisions, prevalence of unauthorized imports, and/or a lack of capacity for the national authorities to assess or test the quality of medical products directly. These create severe vulnerabilities among affected Member States and highlight the importance of information sharing in the subregion.

6.5 VigiCarib News

To ensure that national reporting systems are not working in isolation, the CRS issues a monthly newsletter to regulatory focal points, pharmacovigilance officers, Chief Medical Officers, and other partners including PAHO networks for pharmacovigilance. This newsletter provides periodic updates on the case reports received by the VigiCarib network and by the global database (VigiBase) from CARPHA Member States. However, the limitations of spontaneous reporting are well noted, where further investigation and analyses at the national level are needed before the cases can be attributed to the suspected medicine or vaccine. These intermediate steps continue to be a challenge to countries with limited resources, staffing, and/or information systems. A public version of the newsletter is periodically posted on the CRS-VigiCarib website [1] at: https://carpha.org/What-We-Do/CRS/VigiCarib.

In addition to the newsletter issued by the CRS, CARPHA developed a page for COVID-19 vaccine information [6], which provided answers to frequently asked questions, material for the use of vaccines common to the Caribbean, and a link to the Vaccine Update supplement prepared by the CRS during the pandemic.

6.6 Future Scope

With the growing awareness for the need for strengthening of pharmacovigilance in the Caribbean, the CRS intends to continue expanding its scope to support Caribbean pharmacovigilance, particularly to strengthen detection, reporting, investigation, and assessment of safety and quality reports at the national level. The area of pharmaceutical inspections is of growing interest, specifically the harmonization of standards for inspections, and the sharing of information to identify vulnerabilities or non-compliance. This aspect will be key for the regulation of pharmaceutical distribution and manufacturing facilities to enable Member States to be confident in the quality of manufacturing, storage, and distribution and to better investigate issues related to poor quality medicines that are reported. In addition, towards capacity building, the CRS continue hosting training workshops on topics such as report handling for case safety reports, training of health professionals for detection of substandard and/or falsified products, and training of pharmaceutical inspectors.

6.7 Conclusion

The key elements for pharmacovigilance by CARPHA Member States include legal provisions, sustainable financing, development of capacity, and information systems, but some Member States face challenges to these that reduce their ability to fully implement systems for national, subregional, and global pharmacovigilance. The VigiCarib network of the CRS offers some important efficiencies that may support the Member States' processes and help to create awareness and promote pharmacovigilance through the VigiCarib network, its systems of reporting, communication tools, and educational resources for CARPHA Member States.

Acknowledgements The Caribbean Regulatory System is a unit of the Caribbean Public Health Agency. Its operations are funded via a grant from the Gates Foundation, and the Pan American Health Organization.

References

1. Caribbean Regulatory System [online]. Available at: http://carpha.org/What-We-Do/Laboratory-Services-and-Networks/CRS. Caribbean Public Health Agency, Port of Spain; 2020.
2. Pan American Health Organization. Caribbean Pharmaceutical Policy. Available at: https://iris.paho.org/handle/10665.2/28437. PAHO/WHO, Washington: PAHO; 2013.
3. Preston C, Freitas Dias M, Peña J, Pombo ML, Porrás A. Addressing the challenges of regulatory systems strengthening in small states. BMJ Glob Health. 2020;5:e001912. https://doi.org/10.1136/bmjgh-2019-001912.
4. United Nations, Department of Economic and Social Affairs, Population Division. World population prospects 2022, Online Edition. Available at: https://population.un.org/wpp/. New York; 2022.
5. WHO Global Surveillance and Monitoring System for Substandard and Falsified Medical Products. Medical Product Alert N°2/2020: falsified HIV rapid diagnostic tests. Available at: https://www.who.int/news/item/27-03-2020-medical-product-alert-n-2-2020. Geneva: World Health Organization; 2020, Updated 1 April 2020.
6. Caribbean Public Health Agency. COVID-19 Vaccine Information [online]. Available at: https://www.carpha.org/What-We-Do/Public-Health/Novel-Coronavirus/COVID-19-Vaccine-Information. Caribbean Public Health Agency, Port of Spain; 2021.

Chapter 7
The State of Pharmacovigilance in Brazil

Marcelo Vogler de Moraes and Yannie Silveira Gonçalves

7.1 Introduction

As it happened in most countries, Brazil was hit by the thalidomide tragedy in the 1960s; however, it was only in the 1980s that researchers started discussing the need to implement pharmacovigilance in a concrete way to warn the population and healthcare professionals about the risk related to the use of medicines.

In the 1990s, Drug Information Centres were created in some states of the country, and the accumulated knowledge in pharmacovigilance pointed to the need to develop a National Pharmacovigilance System (NPS). However, pharmacovigilance activities were only effectively systematized and organized in Brazil in 1999 after the creation of the Brazilian Health Regulatory Agency (ANVISA), which comprises of a technical unit in its organization(Pharmacovigilance Office), dedicated to dealing with pharmacovigilance in the country at the national level [1, 2].

Since 2018, Brazilian pharmacovigilance has undergone profound changes that have significantly impacted its workflow. From the admission of Brazil as a Regulatory Member to the International Council for Harmonization of Technical Requirements for Pharmaceuticals for Human Use (ICH) in 2016, it became mandatory to adopt ICH Guidelines. As a result, Guidelines related to pharmacovigilance matters (E2B, E2D, and M1) were among the first ones to be adopted, which led ANVISA and the pharmacovigilance team to set up some strategies and seek for solutions to fulfill this commitment by the end of 2021 [3–5]. In December 2018, Brazil started the process of replacing its electronic system for Individual Case Safety Report (ICSR) with VigiFlow, a web-based system provided by the Uppsala Monitoring Centre (UMC) to the National Pharmacovigilance Centres, which participates in the WHO Programme for International Drug Monitoring (PIDM) [6]. In addition to that, in 2020, Brazil has also updated the pharmacovigilance regulation

M. V. de Moraes (✉) · Y. S. Gonçalves
Brazilian Health Regulatory Agency (ANVISA), Brasília/DF, Brazil
e-mail: marcelo.moraes@anvisa.gov.br; yannie.goncalves@anvisa.gov.br

© Springer Nature Singapore Pte Ltd. 2025
S. R. Ahmad (ed.), *Special Issues in Pharmacovigilance in Resource-Limited Countries*, https://doi.org/10.1007/978-981-96-6154-1_7

dedicated to the Marketing Authorization Holders (MAH), in order to comply with the ICH E2D Guideline requirements.

However, there are still some challenges to be faced that remain in Brazilian pharmacovigilance. This chapter presents the NPS in Brazil, pointing out the challenges arising from its structural characteristics and other problems that are common to limited-resourced countries, as well as listing the advances achieved in recent years.

7.2 The Evolution of the National Pharmacovigilance System

As part of the Brazilian Public Health System, the NPS is a decentralized system; therefore, several public institutions end up exercising some pharmacovigilance action directly or indirectly. Brazil has more than 214 million inhabitants living in 5,570 municipalities across 26 states and the Federal District [7]. Each municipality and state has a local health authority that monitors the quality and safety of the marketed medicines. Coordinating the entire pharmacovigilance system is under the responsibility of the Pharmacovigilance Office of ANVISA, which is considered the National Medicines Monitoring Centre (CNMM) and the Brazilian representative in the PIDM since 2001, when the country joined this program (Fig. 7.1) [8, 9].

The Ministry of Health, as a component of this system, also plays an important role related to pharmacovigilance actions regarding medicines provided by Public Health Programmes, such as those for AIDS, tuberculosis, malaria, and, particularly, vaccines through the National Immunization Programme (NIP). Created in

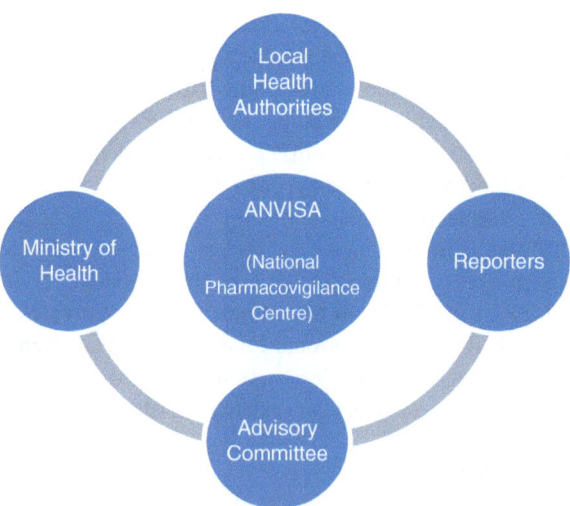

Fig. 7.1 Components of the NPS in Brazil

1975, NIP performs the public policy for national immunization and is considered one of Brazil's most successful public health interventions [10].

Currently, Brazil has several electronic systems for receiving ICSRs (small local electronic systems for ICSRs or those for specific health programs of the Ministry of Health). Still, the leading electronic system is VigiFlow, made available by UMC. Until 2018, the electronic system used for receiving ICSRs in ANVISA was NOTIVISA. However, it presented several problems, such as an unfriendly interface that discouraged citizens' notification, the absence of tools for effective signals analysis and detection, high maintenance costs, and the inability to receive improvements to the system interface. Another limitation was the impossibility of automatically sending the ICSR from NOTIVISA to VigiBase, which allowed sharing only about 10% of these due to limited human resources to perform this task manually. Besides being an alternative to solve the problems mentioned above, using VigiFlow has made it possible to standardize format and transmission pattern of the ICSRs, meeting E2B Guideline requirements, automatically sending 100% of valid ICRS to VigiBase, and incorporating ICH Guideline M1—MedDRA [6].

During the implementation of VigiFlow, the Iberian Portuguese version of MedDRA appeared to be a problem as countless medical terms in Iberian Portuguese had different meanings in Brazilian Portuguese. To solve this problem, Brazil has worked together with the MedDRA Maintenance and Support Services Organization (MSSO),[1] of ICH, in order to have a Brazilian version of the MedDRA dictionary, making it possible that the same language, Portuguese, had two versions as MedDRA options: one dedicated to the Iberian Portuguese and another specifically for Brazilian Portuguese.

The negotiations for the adoption of VigiFlow in Brazil, replacing NOTIVISA, have advanced fast, so that in just a few months, VigiFlow's e-reporting module (dedicated to citizens and health professionals) has been translated into Portuguese and made available for the first ICSR in Brazil, under the name VigiMed, on December 10, 2018 [3]. A few months later, the module designed for health institutions (hospitals and local health authorities) was also available, enabling these reporters to send and manage their ICSR. As a result, this successful initiative resulted in a 62.6% increase in the number of reports received in 2019 compared to the previous year in both electronic systems available at that time (NOTIVISA and VigiFlow) [11]. In 2020, the module dedicated to MAH was developed by UMC, and at the beginning of 2021, it started its operation. At the same time, NOTIVISA, which at that time was in operation only to receive ICSR from MAH, was discontinued.

Due to limited awareness of the importance of pharmacovigilance, underreporting is always a concern in many countries, and Brazil is no different. In addition, not all the reports are submitted by health care providers, and most of them lack clinically important information that could support causality assessment [12]. Therefore,

---

[1] Maintenance and Support Services Organization (MSSO) is responsible for maintaining, distributing and supporting MedDRA and its users.

the Pharmacovigilance Office of ANVISA has adopted strategies for publicizing and expanding the use of VigiFlow among citizens and health care professionals, who are encouraged to have access for themselves and report using VigiFlow. A Pharmacovigilance Communication Plan was also adopted. These actions were taken to maintain the increase in consistent reports each year. In addition, tutorial videos were produced and made available on ANVISA's website and social media, printed materials were distributed, and training sessions were offered to discontinue NOTIVISA and promote VigiFlow instead.

Since 2017, Brazil has had an Advisory Committee to provide technical support and advice to the NPS coordinator. Under the direction of the Pharmacovigilance Office of ANVISA, this Advisory Committee currently consists of 12 members between holders and alternates that are external to ANVISA's staff and have expert knowledge of pharmacovigilance. Among its duties, the following stand out:

• Contribute, as an advisor, to the implementation of pharmacovigilance actions
• Participate in regulation, monitoring, and evaluation of pharmacovigilance actions
• Take part in an investigation of adverse events related to medicines
• Assist in training individuals who are or intend to be part of the NPS [13, 14]

Finally, reporters are also considered NPS components, especially those whose reporting of adverse events is mandatory. In Brazil, there are legal frameworks that require MAHs, as well as health units (public, private, philanthropic, civil, and military hospitals) must report adverse events to the Pharmacovigilance Office of ANVISA according to defined criteria [15, 16]. In July 2020, the national MAH regulation on pharmacovigilance was updated and the requirements of the ICH Guidelines E2B, E2D, and M1 were incorporated [17, 18].

ANIVSA collaborates with the Sentinel Network, a group of hospitals that monitor adverse events and quality deviations related to medicines. This initiative was launched in 2001 to become an active observatory for the performance and safety profile of medical products regularly in use. Currently, it comprises more than 250 hospitals throughout the Brazilian territory [19].

7.3   Current Status of Pharmacovigilance in Brazil

With 5.3 billion unities commercialized in 2019, there is a high consumption of medicines in Brazil. In 2022, the pharmaceutical market in Brazil was seventh in income, ranking among the 20 most significant economies in the world. It resulted in a revenue of R$ 85.9 billion, equivalent to around US$ 22.2 billion at the time. Brazil is the leading market in Latin America, ahead of Mexico, Colombia, and Argentina [20–22]. These numbers reflect the size of the challenge to be faced by pharmacovigilance.

In 2020, ANVISA created a Power BI panel, available on its website. It allows visualization of the amount of the ICSR stratified by year, sex, reporter type, age range, state, name of medicine, the active ingredient, and adverse event (MedDRA—Preferred Term). The number of ICSR has been increasing during the last few years due to the adopted pharmacovigilance actions, especially the deployment of the VigiMed system, as mentioned before [23].

In Brazil, the largest number of reports are submitted by pharmacists. They represent 45% of the total submitted reports since the adoption of VigiFlow. However, the ICSR number has significantly increased in 2020 and 2021, reaching 65,120 ICSRs in 2021, probably due to the vaccinations and the indiscriminate use of medicine during the COVID-19 pandemic [23–25].

7.4   National Pharmacovigilance System and the International Organizations

To overcome the problems and difficulties faced by the pharmacovigilance system inherent in countries with limited resources, collaboration with international organizations and access to tools made available by them can be an interesting option for developing national pharmacovigilance.

The World Health Organization (WHO) permanently carries out activities, publishes references, and develops specific projects that seek to stimulate pharmacovigilance, especially in low- and middle-income countries (LMICs). Initiatives such as the publication of the WHO Pharmacovigilance Indicators: A Practical Manual for the Assessment of Pharmacovigilance Systems and 3-S Project—Smart Safety Surveillance (see Chap. 20) can add to the improvement of pharmacovigilance in these countries [12, 26].

Brazil is now participating in a new WHO initiative that, among other topics, addresses pharmacovigilance actions developed by the national regulatory authority. With the creation of the WHO Global Benchmarking Tool (GBT) for evaluating national regulatory systems, WHO and Regulatory Authorities can identify the strengths and areas for improvement. It facilitates formulating an Institutional Development Plan (IDP) to build upon strengths, address the identified gaps, prioritize IDP interventions, and monitor progress and achievements. In addition, the indicators that comprise Market Surveillance and Control can be helpful to provide ideas to improve further the pharmacovigilance systems [27].

As a member of the Pan American Health Organization (PAHO), Brazil also carries out pharmacovigilance activities with other countries within the scope of the Pan American Pharmaceutical Regulation Network (PARF Network) under the coordination of PAHO. The PARF Network was established in 1999 to support pharmaceutical regulation harmonization in the region of the Americas. Regulatory authorities of these countries and other interested entities in the area of medicines, like the pharmaceutical industry and the academic community, participate in the group [28]. Activities such as the analysis of Periodic Benefit-Risk Assessment Reports and Risk Management Plans for medicines that are marketed simultaneously in several countries of the region are performed jointly, promoting training and experience exchange between participating countries. In addition, projects encompassing active pharmacovigilance for medicines of particular interest to the network can be developed, such as that for antimalarials, providing more effective monitoring of this type of medicine whose majority of users are restricted to countries with a tropical climate [29].

All these initiatives have contributed to improving Brazilian pharmacovigilance and also emphasized the need for a closer relationship between the entities in the system, especially between ANVISA, responsible for the regulation regarding MAH, and the Ministry of Health, responsible for the acquisition and distribution of medicines, seeking the epidemiological control of diseases.

Especially in recent years, Brazilian participation has become more frequent in the proposed activities, events, and training sessions promoted by UMC and WHO. This approach provided an exchange of rich experience and greater knowledge about pharmacovigilance, as well as it has allowed Brazil to use the resources offered by the UMC, like publicity campaigns raising awareness of the importance of reporting adverse events (MedSafety Week) and VigiFlow with its related tools (VigiLyze, VigiBase, VigiGrade) [30, 31]. It can be said that the results of this partnership are visible in the number of reports per million inhabitants received by Brazil. If only ICSR sent directly to ANVISA's system were considered, there was an increase from 64 reports/million inhabitants in 2018 to 103 reports/million in 2019.

7.5 Conclusion

Brazil, like many countries, has to deal with the scarcity of budgetary resources for health. Although, in absolute terms, the amount allocated to health actions is significant, in relative terms, it did not represent more than US$ 1.09 (R $ 3.48) per capita/day in 2017 [32]. This scenario must be intensified as a result of the economic crisis that the world is experiencing due to the COVID-19 pandemic. Only in the 2nd quarter of 2020, the Brazilian GDP (Gross Domestic Product) had a 9.7% drop about the same period of the previous year [33].

However, the approach to international organizations can be a good strategy for countries with limited resources. For example, in recent years, Brazil has experienced meaningful and productive partnerships with UMC that provided significant advances for Brazilian pharmacovigilance.

Regional cooperation or even bilateral cooperation is also an excellent route for dealing with an increasingly worse scenario, which is related to the lack of resources intended for pharmacovigilance actions, since it offers a better ratio for using human resources when facing situations that are common to these countries.

Finally, cooperation between universities and the regulatory authority should be considered since there are common interests concerning knowledge gain and the safety improvement of medicines. For example, the creation of an Advisory Committee composed of academic professionals may offer full subsidies for the decision to withdraw a drug from the market as an example. In addition, the availability of these data related to adverse events, qualitatively and quantitatively, can foment knowledge to guide the actions of the Regulatory Authority better.

References

1. Castro LLC. Farmacoepidemiologia no Brasil: evolução e perspectivas. Cienc Saúde Colet. 1999;4(2):405–10. Accessed 1 Sept 2022. Available from: https://www.scielosp.org/article/csc/1999.v4n2/405-410/pt/
2. Mota DM, Vigo A, Kuchenbecker RS. Evolution and key elements of the Brazilian pharmacovigilance system: a scoping review beginning with the creation of the Brazilian Health Regulatory Agency. Cad Saude Publica. 2018;34(10). Accessed 1 Sept 2022. Available from: http://cadernos.ensp.fiocruz.br/csp/artigo/571/evolucao-e-elementos-chave-do-sistema-de-farmacovigilancia-do-brasil-uma-revisao-de-escopo-a-partir-da-criacao-da-agencia-nacional-de-vigilancia-sanitaria
3. Vogler de Moraes M. Pharmacovigilance in Brazil – a system on the move. Uppsala Reports – Covering the World of Pharmacovigilance. 2019;(81):6. Accessed 15 Sept 2020. Available from: https://view.publitas.com/uppsala-monitoring-centre/uppsala-reports-81/page/1
4. International Council for Harmonisation of Technical Requirements for Pharmaceuticals for Human Use. Effacy guidelines. E2A – E2F Pharmacovigilance. Accessed 15 Sept 2020. Available from: https://www.ich.org/page/efficacy-guidelines
5. Medical dictionary for regulatory activities. Basics. Accessed 15 Sept 2020. Available from: https://www.meddra.org/basics
6. Vogler M, Ricci Conesa H, de Araújo FK, Moreira Cruz F, Simioni Gasparotto F, Fleck K, Maciel Rebelo F, Kollross B, Silveira GY. Electronic reporting systems in pharmacovigilance: the implementation of VigiFlow in Brazil. Pharmaceut Med. 2020;34(5):327–34.
7. Instituto Brasileiro de Geografia e Estatística. Brasil. Panorama. Accessed 15 Sept 2020. Available from: https://cidades.ibge.gov.br/brasil/panorama
8. Ministério da Saúde (Brasil). Portaria n° 696, de 7 de maio de 2001. Institui o Centro Nacional de Monitorização de Medicamentos (CNMM) sediado na Unidade de Farmacovigilância da ANVISA, tendo por finalidade a notificação, registro e avaliação das reações adversas dos medicamentos registrados pelo Ministério da Saúde. Diário Oficial da União 08 may 2001; Section 1.
9. Uppsala Monitoring Centre. Members of the WHO Programme for International Drug Monitoring – full and associate member countries of the WHO Programme and the year they joined. Available from: https://www.who-umc.org/global-pharmacovigilance/who-programme-for-international-drug-monitoring/who-programme-members/. Accessed 15 Sept 2020.
10. Hochman G. Vacinação, varíola e uma cultura da imunização no Brasil. Cienc Saúde Colet. 2011;16(2):375–86.
11. Agência Nacional de Vigilância Sanitária (Brasil). VigiMed faz dois anos de existência e comemora resultados. Acessed 18 Feb 2021. Available from: https://bit.ly/2Nl8BzU
12. World Health Organization. Safety of medicines – priming resource-limited countries for pharmacovigilance – "Project 3-S": smart safety surveillance for priority medical products. WHO Drug Inf. 2017;31(4):575–80. Accessed 15 Sept 2020. Available from: http://tdr.who.int/medicines/publications/druginformation/issues/WHO_DI_31-4_Safety-Medicines.pdf
13. Agência Nacional de Vigilância Sanitária (Brasil). Portaria n° 1.856, de 7 de novembro de 2017. Diário Oficial da União 09 nov 2017. Section 2.
14. Agência Nacional de Vigilância Sanitária (Brasil). Portaria n° 222, de 8 de abril de 2022. Diário Oficial da União 13 apr 2022. Section 2.
15. Agência Nacional de Vigilância Sanitária (Brasil). Resolução – RDC N° 36, de 25 de julho de 2013. Institui ações para a segurança do paciente em serviços de saúde e dá outras providências. Diário Oficial da União, 26 jul 2013. Section 1.
16. Ministério da Saúde (Brasil). Portaria N° 1.660, de 22 de julho de 2009. Institui o Sistema de Notificação e Investigação em Vigilância Sanitária – VIGIPOS, no âmbito do Sistema Nacional de Vigilância Sanitária, como parte integrante do Sistema Único de Saúde – SUS. Diário Oficial da União, 24 jul 2009. Section 1.

17. Agência Nacional de Vigilância Sanitária (Brasil). Resolução – RDC N° 406, de 22 de julho de 2020. Dispõe sobre as Boas Práticas de Farmacovigilância para Detentores de Registro de Medicamento de uso humano, e dá outras providências. Diário Oficial da União 29 jul 2020. Section 1.
18. Agência Nacional de Vigilância Sanitária (Brasil). Instrução Normativa N° 63, de 22 de julho de 2020. Dispõe sobre o Relatório Periódico de Avaliação Benefício-Risco (RPBR) a ser submetido à Anvisa por Detentores de Registro de Medicamento de uso humano. Diário Oficial da União 29 jul 2020. Section 1.
19. Agência Nacional de Vigilância Sanitária (Brasil). Instrução Normativa N° 51, de 29 de setembro de 2014. Dispõe sobre a Rede Sentinela para o Sistema Nacional de Vigilância Sanitária. Diário Oficial da União 01 out 2020. Section 1.
20. Secretaria Executiva da Câmara de Regulação do Mercado de Medicamentos – SCMED. Anuário Estatístico do Mercado Farmacêutico – Edição Comemorativa. Brasília: 2021. Acessed 4 Agu 2022. Available from: https://www.gov.br/anvisa/pt-br/centraisdeconteudo/publicacoes/medicamentos/cmed/anuario-estatistico-2019-versao-para-impressao.pdf
21. Sindusfarma. Perfil da indústria farmacêutica e aspectos relevantes do setor. [São Paulo]: 2021. Acessed 4 Agu 2022. Available from: https://sindusfarma.org.br/uploads/files/229d-gerson-almeida/Publicacoes_PPTs/Perfil_da_IF_2021_SINDUSFARMA_po.pdf
22. Vieira FS, Santos MAB. O setor farmacêutico no Brasil sob as lentes da conta-satélite. Brasília: 2020. Acessed 4 Agu 2022. Available from: https://doi.org/10.38116/td2615.
23. Agência Nacional de Vigilância Sanitária (Brasil). Notificações de Farmacovigilância. Acessed 12 Agu 2022. Available from: https://www.gov.br/anvisa/pt-br/acessoainformacao/dadosabertos/informacoes-analiticas/notificacoes-de-farmacovigilancia
24. Melo JRR, et al. Adverse drug reactions in patients with COVID-19 in Brazil: analysis of spontaneous notifications of the Brazilian pharmacovigilance system. Cad Saude Publica. 2021;37(1). Accessed 15 Aug 2022. Available from: https://doi.org/10.1590/0102-311X00245820.
25. Melo JRR, et al. Self-medication and indiscriminate use of medicines during the COVID-19 pandemic. Cad Saude Publica. 2021;37(4). Accessed 15 Aug 2022. Available from: https://doi.org/10.1590/0102-311X00053221.
26. World Health Organization. WHO pharmacovigilance indicators: a practical manual for the assessment of pharmacovigilance systems. Geneva: World Health Organization; 2015. Accessed 15 Sept 2020. Available from: https://apps.who.int/iris/handle/10665/186642
27. World Health Organization. WHO Global Benchmarking Tool (GBT) for evaluation of national regulatory system of medical products. Accessed 13 Sept 2020. Available from: https://www.who.int/tools/global-benchmarking-tools
28. Organização Pan-Americana da Saúde. VI Conferência da Rede Pan-Americana de Regulamentação Farmacêutica. Accessed 13 Sept 2020. Available from: https://www.paho.org/bra/index.php?option=com_content&view=article&id=2165:vi-conferencia-da-rede-pan-americana-de-regulamentacao-farmaceutica&Itemid=838
29. Macías Saint-Gerons D, Rodovalho S, Barros Dias ÁL, et al. Strengthening therapeutic adherence and pharmacovigilance to antimalarial treatment in Manaus, Brazil: a multicomponent strategy using mHealth. Malar J. 2022;21:28. https://doi.org/10.1186/s12936-022-04047-3.
30. Uppsala Monitoring Centre. #MedSafetyWeek. Accessed 13 Sept 2020. Available from: https://www.who-umc.org/medsafetyweek/
31. Uppsala Monitoring Centre. Your window to a world of global safety insights. Accessed 13 Sept 2020. Available from: https://www.who-umc.org/vigibase/vigilyze/
32. Conselho Federal de Medicina (Brasil). Brasil gasta R$ 3,48 ao dia com a saúde de cada habitante. Accessed 13 Sept 2020. Available from: https://portal.cfm.org.br/index.php?option=com_content&view=article&id=27961:2018-11-12-17-57-13
33. Agência IBGE Notícias (Brasil). Contas Nacionais. PIB tem queda recorde de 9,7% no 2° trimestre, auge do isolamento social. 2020. Accessed 16 Sept 2020. Available from: https://agenciadenoticias.ibge.gov.br/agencia-noticias/2012-agencia-de-noticias/noticias/28720-pib-tem-queda-recorde-de-9-7-no-2-trimestre-auge-do-isolamento-social

Chapter 8
What Signal Detection Means in a Small Database?: Case Reports from Cabo Verde

Cálida Etezana Rodrigues da Veiga

8.1 Background

The importance of pharmacovigilance as a vital science to promote better clinical practice and public health protection is widely recognized by the regulatory authorities and public and was undeniably evident during the recent COVID-19 pandemic. The impact of pharmacovigilance activities can be seen through the improvement of access to quality, safe, and effective medicines and reflected in different health indicators [1]. However, in most resource-limited countries, pharmacovigilance is still seen as a luxury or not a priority. For example, in most of the African countries, the development of pharmacovigilance has gained attention mainly due to a) new combined therapies for antiretroviral, malaria, and tuberculosis drugs (ARV) and recently with COVID-19 vaccines, b) substandard and falsified drugs, or c) donors' requirement/technical assistance of the WHO programme [2].

Nonetheless, regardless of what drives the implementation of pharmacovigilance activities, most of the activities are essentially based on spontaneous reports, involving the systematic collection of reports of suspected adverse drug reaction (ADRs) to enable the detection of signals, their communication, and risk management. As a result, many countries have been collecting this information with the aim to ensure patient safety.

Signal detection activities are considered the cornerstone of pharmacovigilance and an indicator of the high level of maturity of a pharmacovigilance system. In general, a signal is defined as "reported information on a possible causal relationship between an adverse event and a drug, the relationship being unknown or incompletely documented previously." [1] A signal can originate from several sources including spontaneous reports, epidemiological and clinical studies, literature, and patient records. For this purpose, sophisticated approaches for signal detection have

C. E. R. da Veiga (✉)
Health Independent Regulatory Entity (ERIS), Praia, Cape Verde
e-mail: calida.veiga@gmail.com

© Springer Nature Singapore Pte Ltd. 2025
S. R. Ahmad (ed.), *Special Issues in Pharmacovigilance in Resource-Limited Countries*, https://doi.org/10.1007/978-981-96-6154-1_8

been put into place, especially in large and well-developed databases used in developed countries [1].

The problem with this common narrative of what is considered a signal detection is often misplaced in two terms "sophisticated approaches" and "large and well-developed databases," which may represent limitation for countries with small database or limited resource. This understanding can be observed in any literature search that combines the terms "signal detection" and "small database," leading to results that show that these words are infrequently associated and/or that there is a lack of broader understanding of what signal detection may mean in different context and database format/size. Until recently with the publication of the Uppsala Monitoring Center guideline for signal detection in small data sets [3], signal detection in small database was not an "official" topic to be addressed, especially when considering the use of quantitative approach, with little attempt being made to study or adapt this methodology for small database. A recent study showed that standard disproportionality analysis applied in national databases containing as few as 500 individual case reports does not yield higher rates of spurious associations than in larger national databases [4]. Increasing the knowledge about the use of quantitative methodologies in small database would assist countries to leverage signal detection tactics.

In pharmacovigilance, the use of quantitative approach such as disproportionality analysis, which is based on the difference between observed and expected numbers of reports, for any given combination of drug and adverse event, can prove very useful for automated screening of datasets for prominent statistical associations [4]. However, even with automated methodologies for signal detection, qualitative approach is still going to be used for review and interpretation of individual case safety reports (ICSRs) and is the keystone for any signal detection process [5]. The idea of facilitating the screening process does not prevent the detection process itself, which essentially consists of the qualitative review of the cases. In quantitative approach, spontaneous reports of variable quality and completeness are homogenized and provide numerical output without clinical context.

Looking at most of limited-resource countries and small databases in Africa, the ability to generate signal may be perceived by many as a long-term goal or a last wish, and this observation has been reported in studies [2, 6]. This understanding is often observed in how little discussion is promoted about the context where signal may be generated or the meaning of signal detection in absence of "sophisticated" approaches or large database. The usual endorsement is to rely on signal detected in developed countries despite the context differences such as disease prevalence and types, medicines availability, healthcare practice, and expenditure. These differences alone can lead to differences in pattern of drug use and the profile of ADRs, which makes it essential that every country establishes its own routine signal detection activities.

Signal detection can be challenging for most countries due to underreporting, or in some cases stimulated/overreporting and no denominator [5]. However, there is a common feeling these limitations are more relevant to smaller database, despite the lack of specific studies. For resource-limited context in Africa, this may also mean a relatively new database, small database, overrepresentation of certain class of medicines (e.g., antimalarial, antiretrovirals), incomplete recording of patient data, and the lack of prescription history in hospital settings, etc.

So, the aim of this chapter is to address some of the following issues through the presentation of case reports:

1- Would signal generation be a privilege only of developed countries or large database?
2- How can qualitative approach of signal detection change the dynamic of pharmacovigilance in small data sets and limited resources setting?
3- How to generate "signal" without restricting to the new or incomplete information?

8.2   Overview of Health System in Cabo Verde

Cape Verde is an archipelago located on the West African coast, composed of ten islands. The archipelago has about 491,233 inhabitants, according to the 2021 census, of which 50.1% are men. Praia is the capital with 145,378 inhabitants and is the country's largest city [7].

Regarding the organization of the healthcare system, the National Health System is designed to include all public and private entities for quality control, research, import, manufacturing, and marketing of drugs and other health-related products. At the central level, the system includes the services that assist the Minister in formulating the national health policy, supervising the healthcare service, and managing and planning resource. The decentralization of the national health system is made through the health structure whose district coincides with the county or municipality (the basis of the administrative division of the country), hospitals, and sanitary regions [8].

In terms of healthcare providers, the country has two central hospitals (tertiary care), four regional hospitals (secondary care), and thirty four health centers (primary care). It should be noted that reproductive health care is provided in all health centers. Regarding human resources, in 2022, the ratio were 7.7/ 10,000 inhabitants for physician, 16/10,000 inhabitants for nurses and 1.7/10,000 inhabitants for pharmacist [9].

The country is in the transitional phase of the epidemiological profile, where noncommunicable diseases have been overcome, in terms of prevalence and severity, for communicable disease, although acute respiratory infections diseases, diarrheal, tuberculosis, and HIV/AIDS infection continue to represent a public health concern [10].

The average life expectancy at birth, according to estimation in 2019, is 74 years for men and 80.5 years for women. In 2020, the estimated general mortality rate is around 5.3 deaths/1000 inhabitants, and the child mortality rate is around 11.6 deaths/1000 births [11].

8.3   The Pharmacovigilance System in Cabo Verde

The existence of a national pharmacovigilance centre was officially recognized in 2013 through the statutes of the then-extinct agency for the regulation and supervision of pharmaceuticals and food products (ARFA), whose competence was assumed in 2019 with the creation of the Independent Health Regulatory Entity (ERIS). ERIS is responsible, among other activities, for ensuring, in coordination with the competent bodies of the Government Department responsible for the health area, the functioning of the National Pharmacovigilance System.

The National Pharmacovigilance System (NPS) was officially created in 2017 through Decree-Law No. 17/2017 and regulated through Deliberation No. 52/2017 that approves the pharmacovigilance regulation and is responsible for the collection, management, and communication of medicine-related problems (quality defects) and adverse drug reaction (ADR), including medication errors, misuse, abuse, or use outside the approved indications. Even though the law was created in 2017, the activities for promoting the existence and functioning of the system began in 2010. In 2012, Cape Verde joined the WHO programme for international drug monitoring as a full member.

The NPS is an integrated structure composed by the National Pharmacovigilance Centre, responsible for managing and supervising the system, and other stakeholders such as National Pharmacovigilance Committee, Risk Management Centres, Healthcare facilities, Public Health Programmes, Marketing Authorization Holders, Pharmaceutical Operators (manufacturers, importers distributors, and pharmacies), and Pharmacovigilance Delegates and Healthcare Professionals. In Cabo Verde, pharmacies are required to have a designated person for pharmacovigilance activities and standard procedures for the management of ADR and medicine-related problems.

After 10 years of joining the WHO programme, the performance of the spontaneous reporting system showed a growing trend in the first five years, and in 2015 and 2017, the number of adverse reactions reports was 125 per half a million inhabitants/year, in a country with a population around 400 hundred thousand people. However, in the last 5 years, the trend in reporting has been decreasing, particularly sharpened by the COVID-19 pandemic, despite the increase seen in 2021 with the expanded vaccination against COVID-19 [12].

In terms of the profile of the reporters, around 52% of the reports received by the National Pharmacovigilance Centre were submitted by nurses, followed by physicians with 34% and pharmacists with 10%. Most of the reports come from the primary healthcare facilities (health centres) followed by hospitals [12]. The most representative pharmacotherapeutic groups of suspected or interacting drugs classified according to the Anatomical Therapeutic Chemical (ATC) include J—Anti-infectives for systemic use, D—Dermatological drugs, and S—Sensory Organs. In terms of System Organ Class (SOC), the most reported adverse reactions belong to the class of conditions of "Skin and subcutaneous tissues" followed by "General disorders and administration site conditions, "Nervous System" and "Gastrointestinal System," representing about 71% of all reported ADRs [12].

8.4   Case Examples

The following case reports illustrate how detecting aspects of known ADRs (new or otherwise) is also an important element of drug safety monitoring, despite relatively little attention given in signal detection approaches (especially data mining approaches). The need to develop pattern recognition techniques has the potential to further elucidate new aspect of known ADRs.

Signal detection and data mining in spontaneous reporting database reflect the local and regional context, despite most of the time not duly addressed. The reduced activity of marketing authorization holders (MAH) in small markets coupled with weak regulatory capacity demands regulatory authorities to consider each case reports with special attention, and at times these reports can become the "main stakeholder" in risk detection, prioritization, evaluation, and communication. The aim with these examples is to present aspects of known ADRs as an opportunity to improve medication use and ensure patient safety, which is the goal of pharmacovigilance.

8.4.1   Case 1: Cutaneous Reaction, Including Stevens-Johnson Syndrome with Nevirapine/Lamivudine/Zidovudine

The National Pharmacovigilance Centre received three spontaneous reports of cutaneous reaction, including one with Stevens-Johnson syndrome with Nevirapine/Lamivudine/Zidovudine. All patients were female aged between 37 and 51 years. All cases where assessed as serious and non-preventable ADR since the patient had no previous history of allergic reaction and the medicine was correctly prescribed and administered. The patient recovered in all these cases.

Only three cases were reported to the National Pharmacovigilance Centre, but it is likely that several more may have experienced cutaneous reaction (underreporting factor), including Stevens-Johnson syndrome. To raise awareness, the National Pharmacovigilance Centre issued a safety warning (informative circular) with the objective of advising the healthcare professional to:

(a) Intensively monitor their patients during the first 18 weeks of treatment, especially in the case of occurrence of an isolated cutaneous eruption.
(b) Alert patients to report immediately if any rash and avoid delay between the initial symptoms and medical consultation.
(c) Withdraw the treatment in any patient who has severe rash or rash accompanied by constitutional symptoms.
(d) Report any case that may arise with this class of drugs.

Observations In quantitative approaches, this information would possibly not immediately raise concern; however, in signal detection, there is no "one size fits all" approach, and realistic expectation of healthcare professional and patient is considered a strategy for signal detection, especially considering cluster reports, the type of diseases, and relevance around compliance and adequate management.

8.4.2 Case 2: Angioedema and Pulmonary Edema with Enalapril

The National Pharmacovigilance Centre received one spontaneous report of angio-edema and pulmonary edema with enalapril. The patient was a 44-year-old male. The case was assessed as serious, and the outcome was fatal.

The national centre decided to issue a safety warning with the objective of advising the healthcare professional to:

(a) Withdraw the drug and institute appropriate supervision to ensure complete resolution of symptoms prior to dismissing the patient.
(b) Intensively monitor patients with history of angioedema not related to the administration of ACE inhibitors by being at higher risk of angioedema while receiving an ACE inhibitor.
(c) Alert patients to seek immediate assistance from a healthcare professional or visit a hospital in the event of skin reactions and other allergic reactions in the form of angioedema.
(d) Report any case that may arise with this class of drugs.

Observations In cases with fatal outcome, regardless of how the drug was administered or used, the information is used to produce safety warning to prevent similar cases by raising awareness for healthcare professional and patient. The information here is not new, but some aspects of the medication use (the need to alert patient about this type of reaction, especially with angiotensin-converting enzyme inhibitors) could be improved.

8.4.3 Case 3: Gastric Irritation with Doxycycline

The National Pharmacovigilance Centre received one spontaneous report of gastric irritation with doxycycline. The patient was a 25-year-old female. The patient presented nausea and vomiting after administration of doxycycline in fasting. The case was assessed as non-serious but preventable ADR since the reaction could be avoided if the information was available on summary of product characteristics (SPC) and the package leaflet (PL). The patient recovered without medical intervention.

When considering the information in the SPC and the PL of doxycycline, it was found that none of the documents mention the need to avoid its use during fasting. When comparing the medicine with other similar products authorized in other countries, including Spain, Portugal, United Kingdom, and United States, it was found that the information in SPCs includes recommendations to avoid doxycycline administration in patients with empty stomach. For this purpose, the national centre decided to recommend the MAH to update the SPC and PL with the following recommendation "Do not administer this medicine on an empty stomach in order to avoid possible digestive disorders (nausea, vomiting)."

Observations Assessing preventability is also another signal detection strategy, as few treatments or prescription guideline exist. Furthermore, half of the drug-related harms are preventable, which means that the true signal is not only about new or incomplete information about a drug, but also about how the drug is being used.

8.4.4   Case 4: Menstrual Disturbance with COVID-19 Vaccine

National vaccination against COVID-19 began on March 19, 2021, one year after the detection of the first case of COVID-19 at national level. The vaccination schedule initially covered healthcare professionals, followed by chronically ill patients and later the general population. Until December 31, 2021, about 599,987 thousand doses of vaccines against COVID-19 were administered, of which 331,016 comprised the first dose, 260,090 to the second dose, and 8881 to the booster dose of the COVID-19 vaccines.

After the expansion of the vaccination against COVID-19, some people used social networks to report changes in the menstrual cycle after the administration of COVID-19 vaccine. The information about such reaction was rare at that time, but the recommendation was to report these cases to the National Pharmacovigilance Centre. The four cases received involved women aged between 19 and 42 years and were submitted by patients and healthcare professionals.

With the public anxiety surrounding the COVID-19 vaccination process, the cases were referred to the national safety review committee for further investigation. One year later, the European Medicine Agency (EMA) formally addressed the possibility of COVID-19 vaccines to cause menstrual bleeding abnormalities.

Observations This example can show that if active monitoring is instituted close to patient or healthcare professionals, even small pharmacovigilance database can capture unknown ADRs, especially if standardized use, medicine availability, and healthcare training were in place, as happened with COVID-19 vaccines.

These cases emphasize the need to search for information as a signal in individual context. In Africa, most of countries have accumulated large volumes of ADRs reports in hopes of generating signal while quality review of ADRs reports can improve the medication use and ensure patient safety. Furthermore, in quantitative approaches, signal detection will always end with a qualitative review of the reports.

Also, a good strategy for signal detection is to consider the expectations of different stakeholders such as patients, healthcare professional, regulators, and marketing authorization holders (MAH), etc. In resource-limited African countries, where engagement of pharmaceutical companies is scarce and government regulators on limited budget, it is informative to consider the expectations of patient and healthcare professionals as a means to increase the engagement in the pharmaco-vigilance system.

The need to reframe signal detection has never been so important if we consider the experience of COVID-19 pandemic, where several potential therapeutic options were being identified, studied, and used to address COVID-19, in which most of them had limited evidence. Therefore, despite the complexity of the situation and the time pressure to respond to demanding treatment questions, establishing a simplified approach to review safety data is a must in all types of setting.

8.5   Conclusion

Detection and reporting of ADRs are the first steps in a comprehensive and ongoing approach to drug safety monitoring. For this purpose, small data sets need to strategically consider detecting new aspects of a known ADRs, as different healthcare practice contributes to different drug utilization pattern and ADRs profile. Furthermore, what is considered a signal in resource-limited context may translate sometimes in pertinent information that may be associated to a potential public health impact of the event on public safety or the perceived impact on the overall safety profile by patient or healthcare professionals.

The functioning of a pharmacovigilance system is relatively new for most of the African countries, and this alone can have an impact on overall regulatory capacity. However, the qualitative review of case reports is the classic and reasonable method, highly recommended for small database, and an alternative for quantitative approach. Also, in limited resource context, it is essential to prioritize issues by considering some aspects such as the seriousness of the ADRs, impact on public health and public trust, healthcare or patients' realistic expectation, cluster reports, and/or preventable ADRs.

Signal detection goes beyond detecting new or incomplete information, especially when considering that half of the drug-related harm are preventable, which mean we only cover two-thirds of the problem. The drug utilization pattern is what in essence determine safety signal in national and regional context, especially in small databases. The use of quantitative approach in small dataset represents a complement to a comprehensive approach in safety monitoring, where more studies are needed to further develop data mining techniques that can be suitable for this type of database/context.

Take Away Messages
- The qualitative review of case reports is the classic and affordable method highly recommended for small database and an alternative for quantitative approach.
- Increasing the knowledge about the use of quantitative methodologies in small database would assist countries to leverage signal detection tactics.
- Strategic review pondering aspects such as seriousness, public health impact or expectation; cluster reports or the preventability of the ADRs during signal detection activities can increase the engagement in the pharmacovigilance system.
- Signal detection goes beyond detecting new or incomplete information, especially considering that half of drug-related harm are preventable.

Acknowledgments   To Entidade Reguladora Independente da Saúde (ERIS), with gratitude to Dr. Eduardo Tavares, the Chairman of board of directors, to kindly allowing the use of the necessary data. However, the opinions and conclusions of this study are not necessarily those shared by ERIS. As of May 2023, Cálida Veiga, is on leave from ERIS.

Conflict of Interests   No conflict of interest.

References

1. World Health Organization. The importance of pharmacovigilance. World Health Organization. 2002. https://apps.who.int/iris/handle/10665/42493
2. Olsson S, Pal SN, Dodoo A. Pharmacovigilance in resource-limited countries. Expert Rev Clin Pharmacol. 2015;8(4):449–60. https://doi.org/10.1586/17512433.2015.1053391. Epub 2015 Jun 3. PMID: 26041035
3. Caduff-Janosa P, Isah A, Hugman B, Norgéla G. Signal detection for national pharmacovigilance centres with small data sets. Uppsala Monitoring Centre Published by Uppsala Monitoring Centre WHO Collaborating Centre for International Drug Monitoring; 2020.
4. Caster O, Aoki Y, Gattepaille LM, Grundmark B. Disproportionality analysis for pharmacovigilance signal detection in small databases or subsets: recommendations for limiting false-positive associations. Drug Saf. 2020;43(5):479–87. https://doi.org/10.1007/s40264-020-00911-w. PMID: 32008183; PMCID: PMC7165139
5. CIOMS. Practical aspects of signal detection in pharmacovigilance. Report of CIOMS Working Group VIII. 2010. https://cioms.ch/working_groups/working-group-viii/
6. Pirmohamed M, Atuah KN, Dodoo ANO, Winstanley P. Pharmacovigilance in developing countries. Br Med J. 2007;335(7618):462. https://doi.org/10.1136/bmj.39323.586123.BE.
7. Instituto Nacional de Estatística. Relatório do Censo Populacional. 2021. https://ine.cv/censo_quadros/cabo-verde-corrigido/
8. Boletim Oficial. Decreto-lei n° 56/2021, estabelece a estrutura, organização e as normas de funcionamento do Ministério de Saúde. Serie 1, n° 91. 2021.
9. Ministério de saúde de Cabo Verde. O Índice atual de cobertura universal de saúde definido pela OMS para Cabo Verde. https://minsaude.gov.cv/noticias/**O-indice-aual-de-cob**/. Accessed at 28 Aug 2023.
10. Ministério de saúde de Cabo Verde. Plano Nacional de Desenvolvimento Sanitário 2012–2016. 2012.
11. Ministério de saúde de Cabo Verde. Relatorio Estatístico 2020. 2022.
12. ERIS. Boletim de Farmacovigilância 10 anos do Centro Nacional de Farmacovigilância: os principais resultados. Edição n.° 01/2023. 2023.

Chapter 9
Pharmacovigilance Situation in Sierra Leone in the Light of the Ebola Crisis

Wiltshire C. N. Johnson and Onome T. Abiri

9.1 Background

Sierra Leone has a tropical climate with high temperatures and humidity, with two seasons based on the agricultural cycle: dry and rainy seasons. It is located on the Western Coast of Africa, sharing borders with Guinea to the northeast, Liberia to the southeast and the Atlantic Ocean to the southwest. The country encompasses an area of 71,740 km^2 (27,699 sq. mi), with an estimated population of 7,548,702 million [1]. Sierra Leone is divided into five Geopolitical administrative regions: the Northern Province, North-West Province, Eastern Province, Southern Province and the Western Area, subdivided into sixteen districts and 186 chiefdoms.

Sierra Leone, a post-conflict country with a newly found and stable democracy since 2002, has one of the poorest health indicators globally. Life expectancy is 55 years, an infant mortality rate of 75 per 1000 live births, an under-five mortality rate of 122 per 1000 live births and a maternal mortality ratio of 443 per 100,000 births [2–4]. Revenue source is mainly the extractive industry involving diamond, gold, rutile, bauxite and iron ore. World Bank ranking is low. The health system has over 1300 healthcare facilities [5]. The physician and pharmacist ratios to patient population are 2:50,000 and 1:50,000, correspondingly [6, 7]. Free health care services exist for pregnant women, lactating mothers, children under five years and the vulnerable. Health insurance is only available in the private sector.

W. C. N. Johnson (✉)
The Faculty of Pharmaceutical Sciences College of Medicine and Allied Health Sciences, the University of Sierra Leone (Formerly with Pharmacy Board of Sierra Leone, Ministry of Health and Sanitation), Freetown, Sierra Leone
e-mail: marvic@hotmail.com

O. T. Abiri
Faculty of Basic Medical Sciences, Department of Pharmacology and Therapeutics, College of Medicine and Allied Health Sciences, University of Sierra Leone, Freetown, Sierra Leone

© Springer Nature Singapore Pte Ltd. 2025
S. R. Ahmad (ed.), *Special Issues in Pharmacovigilance in Resource-Limited Countries*, https://doi.org/10.1007/978-981-96-6154-1_9

The resilience of the health sector was tested seriously by the Ebola epidemic. In December 2013, health officials in Guinea reported cases of a strange acute illness characterised by fever, diarrhoea, vomiting and weakness and in some instances, bleeding. By 25 March 2014, the illness was confirmed to be the Ebola Virus Disease (EVD). Sierra Leone officially reported its first case on the 25 May 2014 in the Eastern part of the country bordering Guinea in a district called Kailahun. By November 2014, the disease had spread to all districts in the country. The 2014 outbreak was the largest EVD outbreak in history since the discovery of the virus in Zaire, Congo, in 1976.

The factors that contributed to the spread of the disease were:

- First outbreak to reach epidemic proportions in an urban environment.
- Recent history of armed conflicts and instabilities in Sierra Leone, Liberia and Guinea.
- Poor socioeconomic status and extreme poverty.
- Weak healthcare systems: inadequate human and infrastructural resources.
- Ebola was a new disease with limited knowledge of the disease in the outbreak region.
- Confusion of symptoms with known diseases such as malaria and typhoid.
- Delays in setting up an effective and coordinated response mechanism to the outbreak globally and nationally.
- Local and traditional socio-cultural practices and beliefs, including traditional washing of the dead, caring for the sick at home, exchanging of handshakes and hugs, healthcare-seeking behaviour of the population and blaming of witchcraft for ailments of the unknown.
- Wrong initial information on case management.
- Telling the public that there was no cure led to people refusing to come to the hospital, preferring to die at home with family around.
- False information that Ebola was man-made, or was it man-made tracing it from patient zero that was child?

The Ebola Virus Disease (EVD) was characterised by signs and symptoms that typically starts to manifest between 2 and 21 days after contact with the virus, and they include fever >38.3 ° C (101 °F), muscular pain, headaches then later, bleeding, diarrhoea and skin rash, dehydration and multiple organ failure that accounts for death [8]. Case fatality rate in the past was between 45% and 90% [9], but in Sierra Leone, a case fatality rate of 31% was reported at the Hastings Ebola Treatment Centre [10]. Ebola can spread by direct contact with the bodily fluids of symptomatic patients and may also be transmitted through sexual transmission from survivors [11].

Control of the disease required coordinated medical services and community engagement such as

- Establishing a central national coordination and response system.
- Setting up Ebola holding and treatment centres.
- Fostering partnership with local and international institutions.
- Gathering of resources.

- Recruitment of more healthcare professionals, including recalling retired health practitioners.
- Establishment of systems for notification of disease, collection of information, contact tracing, quarantine and burials.
- Prohibiting movement of the people within the affected areas and from those areas to none affected areas.

Mass public health sensitisation, acceptability of the disease and behavioural change by the general public were also key, and this involved:

- Participation of traditional and religious heads, members of the executive and parliament, local councils, professional bodies, civil society associations, trade and business entities.
- Print and electronic media and community engagement.
- Propagation of right information on the disease.
- Mass drug distribution to prevent the occurrence of malaria, whose signs and symptoms mimicked that of Ebola.

Sierra Leone experienced EVD for the very first time, and in the face of this adversary, the healthcare system was unable to cope and collapsed. The educational system and other social services, including tourism, entertainment, transportation, business, agriculture and the economy, were adversely affected as never seen in the history of the country. In low income countries like Sierra Leone where health resources were very inadequate before the Ebola and even much more compounded by the Ebola, funding a pharmacovigilance (PV) was a challenge. This is because Governments in this part of the world think it is important to focus on other competing priorities such as malaria, HIV/AIDS, tuberculosis, improving availability, access and affordability to medicines and essential health care services among others.

This scenario exemplifies the difficulties associated with conducting pharmacovigilance in an environment where medicines may be scarce or, if available, are often self-administered or improperly prescribed by both qualified and unqualified individuals due to limited diagnostic resources, healthcare personnel and infrastructure.

9.2   Pharmacovigilance Structures and Systems in Sierra Leone

9.2.1   The National Pharmacovigilance Centre

Pharmacovigilance has become an important constituent of medicines regulation. For the conceivable future in low- and middle-income countries (LMICs), this is probable to take the usual form of spontaneous monitoring, which nevertheless is not the ideal system. Many LMICs do not have rudimentary systems in place for this purpose, and even where pharmacovigilance systems do exist, active support and participation among regulators, administrators and health professionals may be lacking. Healthcare workers underreporting of ADRs is still a major problem in many countries [12–14].

According to the Sierra Leone Pharmacy and Drugs Act 2001, the Pharmacy Board of Sierra Leone (PBSL) is the National Medicines Regulatory Authority (NMRA) established by an act of parliament. It is a semi-autonomous arm of the Ministry of Health and Sanitation. The PBSL also hosts The National Pharmacovigilance Centre (NPC).

Pharmacovigilance began in Sierra Leone in the year, and in 2007, Sierra Leone was granted associate membership in the WHO Programme for International Drug Monitoring (PIDM). In September 2008, full membership was granted to Sierra Leone as the 87th member of the WHO PIDM. The NPC of the PBSL derived its mandate to ensure the safety of regulated products from the National Medicine Policy (NMP), which states that PBSL will endeavour to develop and maintain an effective and efficient drug safety monitoring system in the country. The Ministry of Health and Sanitation (MOHS), through PBSL, will establish a national drug safety committee to support the drug safety monitoring programme and control of clinical trials [15].

The vision of the NPC is to advance countrywide patient safety and well-being by decreasing the risk of medicines used by patients and consumers. The mission is to guarantee that patients and consumers get the best outcome from their treatment. This is usually accomplished through the three units of the NPC, viz., the Clinical practice unit that promotes PV in hospitals, the Public Health unit that promotes PV in public health programmes and the Clinical trial unit responsible for the regulation of clinical trials through evaluation of clinical trial applications, approval of trials, Good Clinical and Laboratory Practice (GCLP) inspection and monitoring. The general aims of the NPC are product safety monitoring, awareness raising among healthcare professionals and consumers about the need to report adverse events.

Since Sierra Leone is divided into five geographical regions, i.e., Western, Eastern, Southern, North-West and Northern regions, the NPC is supported by four regional pharmacovigilance centre's in the headquarter towns in these regions. The NPC also receives technical advice from a risk assessment and signal detection team and an expert committee on drug pharmacovigilance and clinical trials consisting of consultant physicians, a public health specialist, a consultant pathologist, consultant clinical pharmacists, a consultant quality control and quality assurance expert, an epidemiologist, a biostatistician and pharmacologists among others. This is consistent with what occurs in some sub-Saharan African countries where pharmacovigilance and medicines regulatory approvals are linked and informed by an independent technical advisory committee appointed by the national medicine regulatory authority [NMRA] [16]. The technical advisory committee may comprise experts in pharmacy, clinical medicine, epidemiology, biostatistics, paediatrics, toxicology and clinical pharmacology that are independent professionals. This arrangement instills a sense of assurance among healthcare professionals and is anticipated to significantly contribute to the safeguarding of public health.

This advisory safety committee mostly supports the NMRA in causality assessment, signal generation and evaluation [17, 18].

At the moment in Sierra Leone, the NMP recognises the need for Pharmacovigilance [15]. However, the Pharmacy and Drugs Act 2001 does not explicitly include pharmacovigilance. Legislation that requires marketing authorisation holders (MAHs) to mandatorily report all serious ADRs to the NMRA and conduct post-marketing surveillance activities is also lacking in Sierra Leone. However, a revised Pharmacy and Drugs Act, that is yet to be enacted by parliament, covers pharmacovigilance and mandates MAHs to ensure safety monitoring of their products on the market. A study conducted in 46 sub-Saharan Africa (SSA) countries revealed that 19 (41%) had a policy related to PV and 14 (30%) had a legal mandate to monitor medicine-related adverse events. With respect to legal basis that requires MAHs to report all serious ADRs to the NMRA, only 13 (28%) had provisions, while 8 (17%) required MAHs to conduct post-marketing activities. The absence of a legal provision in Sierra Leone and other SSA countries indicates inherent challenges in implementing and enforcing PV [19, 20].

The NPC has a clear mandate, defined roles, responsibilities and a formal organisational structure and some funding from the government and sometimes from donor organisations to carry out PV activities. A comprehensive national PV guideline is available that is essential to standardise the provision of PV services and processes at all levels of the health system [21]. A national medicine safety advisory committee with official terms of reference that meets regularly is also in place and is functional.

Pharmacovigilance has been incorporated in the undergraduate curriculum for pharmacy but not into training curricula of medicine, nursing and public health [22]. Medical and pharmacy students at the faculty of basic medical sciences are taught clinical toxicology, ADRs of medicines as part of pharmacology and introduction to PV. However, specific PV-related topics such as quality risk management, causality assessment, signal management and medication errors are not covered comprehensively. Absence of PV in the above pre-service curricula may be responsible for the paucity of knowledge, perception and practice of PV among healthcare professionals in Sierra Leone.

The NPC has ADR reporting forms and platforms for consumer and health care professional reporting. The passive reporting system of ADR reporting covers the full range of PV activities, which allows for the reporting of many aspects such as product quality defects, therapeutic failure, medication errors, antimicrobial resistance and other drug-related issues. However, low reporting rates and small amount of reports in the central database are currently a challenge for signal identification. Signal identification is the initial stage in PV, which is subsequently followed by the prioritisation and evaluation of these signals and the implementation of risk management strategies [23, 24].

The development of a PV information management system for receiving and processing of data from diverse sources is crucial for signal management. In Sierra Leone, the PV centre uses a central database called VigiFlow® developed and managed by the Uppsala Monitoring Centre (UMC) in Uppsala, Sweden, specially designed for NPC that are members of the WHO programme for international drug monitoring. This central database has safety reports from consumers, health professionals, hospitals, clinical trials and adverse events following immunisation (AEFIs) from the Expanded Programme on Immunization (EPI). Other PV reports include adverse drug reactions (ADRs) reported by Public Health Programmes (PHPs) such as the malaria control programme, the tuberculosis and leprosy control programme and the neglected tropical disease control programme. The NPC also received Serious Adverse Event (SAE) reports from Ebola clinical trials, providing a chance to leverage, the inherent advantage of integrating pre-marketing phases 1, 2 and 3 and post-marketing safety data. This would significantly improve the effective assessment, interpretation and use of safety-related information. A study conducted across 46 countries in SSA showed that 74% of these nations have spontaneous reporting systems. However, below 50% of them actively monitor product quality defects, medication errors and therapeutic failures. A medicine safety national database is present in 50% of these countries; nevertheless, the coordination and collation of PV data from diverse sources was deemed insufficient [20].

9.2.2   The Role of Healthcare Professionals in P.V

According to the World Health Organization (WHO) in order to provide basic access to healthcare, a country should have a minimum of 23 health professionals including doctors, nurses, pharmacists and midwives per 10,000 persons. The scarcity of health professionals is a prevalent issue in sub-Saharan Africa, with Sierra Leone being severely affected. The dearth of medical practitioners in Sierra Leone correlates with some of the most severe health outcomes globally.

The significance of health care professionals (HCPs) in the field of pharmacovigilance cannot be overstated. Nevertheless, in the context of Sierra Leone, healthcare professionals are few and frequently overwhelmed with a high patient load, leaving them with limited time to complete an ADR form and submit a report regarding a suspected ADR to the NPC [6, 7]. The nurse-to-patient ratio is twice as high as the doctor/pharmacist to patient ratio. This limits health care practitioners to detect and record ADRs. An unpublished report of an assessment that was done by the NPC of the PBSL in conjunction with the WHO country office in Sierra Leone revealed that healthcare practitioners may exhibit reluctance or unease in reporting adverse drug reactions (ADRs) associated with treatments, primarily stemming from apprehension regarding potential legal consequences for professional mistakes or liabilities. The distribution and accessibility of ADR reporting forms in healthcare facilities nationwide can pose difficulties in riverine and remote locations with limited or no access to information and communication technology (ICT). In certain instances, when certain facilities acquire the ADR forms, there tends to be significant delays in the receipt of reports at the NPC and in the overall dissemination of information.

Regarding the annaul counts of ADR reports received, WHO has developed a threshold system to ascertain if the number of ADRs reported meets the expectation for a minimally operational PV system. According to the threshold approach which considers 200 reports per million population yearly, Sierra Leone is projected to generate approximately 1400 reports annually. The number of ADR reports received in Sierra Leone recent years was 650 in 2021 and 185 in 2022 according to the pharmacovigilance departmental reports. However, about 70% of these reports were derived from large-scale medicines and vaccines campaigns with albendazole-ivermectin and COVID-19 vaccines. This implies that the ADR or adverse event following immunisation (AEFI) reports might reduce drastically in the coming years if routine PV is not boosted. Taking into consideration the fact that PV is still relatively new in Sierra Leone, it is imperative that substantial time, effort and financial resources are needed to step up sensitisation among marketing authorisation holders, health care professionals and consumers on the benefits of pharmacovigilance. A study conducted across 46 SSA countries indicated that the reporting rate of ADR is significantly low in most of these nations. The findings indicated that in 2010, only two of the countries, viz., Burkina Faso and Namibia, reported more than 100 reports per million inhabitants. Conversely, majority of countries recorded less than 20 reports per million inhabitants annually [20].

9.2.3 Hospitals and the NPC Collaborating in the Interest of Patients' Safety

Healthcare delivery systems in low-income countries like Sierra Leone are more intricate than in the high-income countries. Sierra Leone like most other low-income countries have primary, secondary and tertiary healthcare facilities. The public sector in Sierra Leone has six main tertiary hospitals that are located in the capital city Freetown, 27 secondary healthcare facilities distributed in the 16 districts with one referral facility each in the headquarter towns of the southern (Bo district), eastern (Kenema district) and northern (Bombali district) regions and over 1000 primary healthcare facilities. The private sector has diverse privately coordinated healthcare facilities, either for-profit or not for profit. The private sector has about 100 clinics and 13 hospitals [5]. Pharmacovigilance monitoring of medicinal products should be fully integrated in the health system. The extent to which physicians, pharmacists and nurses are informed about the principles and concepts of PV has a large impact on the quality of health care delivery. It has the capacity to instill faith and confidence in patients and healthcare professionals concerning the medicines they utilise, which also serves to elevate the benchmarks of clinical practice.

Most health facilities in Sierra Leone do not have an official existing PV unit. However, they have designated personnel responsible for PV-related activities available within each facility that works with the NPC. These staff are either pharmacists, nurses or medical doctors that support the NPC to promote PV in these health facilities. Drug information centres (DICs) are not available in health facilities; thus, there is no platform within the health facilities for collection and distribution of medicine information. Health facilities lack dedicated allocation of funds designated for initiatives linked to PV-related activities. Drug and therapeutic committees (DTCs) are available in some hospitals, but most of them are not engaged in PV-related activities [19]. A study conducted in Bangladesh, Cambodia, Nepal, Thailand and the Philippines found that less than 50% of the 86 health facilities assessed had a PV centre, unit or designated staff for PV-related activities within their premises. Furthermore, 15% of the facilities had DTCs, while 38% offered DIC services [25]. The process of signal detection and generation depends on the expertise and training of medical doctors, pharmacists, nurses as well as the active involvement of stakeholders who are responsible for reporting suspected adverse events. With the underutilisation of the ADR reporting forms available in the facilities, there will be low rates of reporting and delayed recognition of adverse events. As a result, there is a potential for overlooking possibilities to use the data collected to address safety concerns and identify signals.

9.2.4   The National Pharmacovigilance Centre in Collaboration with Public Health Programmes

Public health programmes (PHPs) including the malaria, HIV/AIDS, tuberculosis/leprosy, EPI and the neglected tropical diseases control programmes play a significant role in pharmacovigilance. In Sierra Leone, PHPs have traditionally prioritised the expansion accessibility to treatment as a means to accomplish their objectives of disease prevention and treatment in the population. A considerable number of PHPs engage in the distribution of substantial supplies of vaccines and medicines, occasionally employing mass drug administration methods, typically with limited regard for PV.

Among key medicines programme in Sierra Leone, namely, the national malaria, EPI, HIV/AIDS, Tuberculosis and Leprosy, Neglected Tropical Disease and the reproductive health programmes, all of them have a policy document containing essential statements on PV In an evaluation done in among 32 PHPs in Ghana, Nigeria, Senegal, Kenya, Burkina Faso, Uganda, Tanzania and Democratic Republic of Congo (DRC), only 12 (38%) possessed policy statements pertaining to PV [20]. Having PV in policy documents demonstrates government's commitment to addressing quality and safety monitoring of products used by the PHPs.

Public health programmes in Sierra Leone have designated PV focal persons for monitoring product safety within the programmes. Funding for PV-related activities is limited among the PHPs, as funding is mostly provided by donors such as United Nations Children Fund (UNICEF), World Health Organization (WHO), Global fund and Hellen Keller international more so for large-scale campaigns [19]. According to the same study conducted in SSA nations, it was found that the PV unit or a designated focal person for PV exists in a fewer than 50% of HIV/AIDS, TB and malaria programmes. On the other hand, there is a designated unit or person in most immunisation programmes [20]. Correspondingly for 32 PHPs, a specific allocation of funds was made for PV or as part of other activities in malaria and immunisation programmes, which are usually supported by organisations like the Global Fund, The Presidents Malaria Initiative, United States Centre for Disease Control and Prevention, Global Alliance for Vaccines and Immunisation [20]. The lack of devoted budget for PV. and training for health professionals is a red flag that depicts and indicates ineptitude to continually identify and address safety issues.

Over the years in Sierra Leone, these programmes rarely considered PV a priority until recently, due to the implementation of effective pharmacovigilance sensitisation and advocacy techniques by the NPC, which saw programmes starting to integrate PV in their activities. The partnership between the NPC and the National Malaria Control Programme (NMCP) resulted in a successful outcome, wherein a treatment regimen was modified based on the principles of pharmacovigilance. The NPC played an active role in the surveillance of drug safety during the mass administration of artesunate-amodiaquine, totalling more than 5,000,000 doses, in two separate cycles at the height of the Ebola outbreak. The NPC engaged in community-based activities such as searching, locating, identifying, referring and managing adverse events. The NPC conducted an analysis of the adverse responses and subsequently recommended a change in the first-line treatment for uncomplicated malaria in Sierra Leone. As a result, the use of artesunate-amodiaquine was replaced by Artemether-Lumefantrine.

The collaboration between institutions has been significantly strengthened as a result of the NPC advocacy strategies in the HIV/AIDs and EPI control programmes. This is evident by the increased submission of AEFIs reports from the EPI programme to the NPC. Furthermore, the NPC has identified and provided training to personnel in more than 40 antiretroviral therapy treatment sites. The partnership with EPI was enhanced when the vaccine safety department of WHO in Geneva conducted an evaluation of the vaccine PV system in the programme. This assessment was conducted in light of the potential introduction of a new Ebola vaccine in Sierra Leone after it is licenced. The purpose of the evaluation was to ensure that the vaccine pharmacovigilance system is robust enough to detect and manage AEFIs. The NPC aims to further augment PV in these programmes with a focus on introducing active pharmacovigilance methods like cohort event monitoring and targeted spontaneous reporting for new products.

9.2.5 Integrating PV in Traditional Complementary and Alternative Medicine (TCAM) Practice

It has been estimated that about 88% of countries use traditional medicine such as indigenous therapies and herbal medicines to prevent and treat diseases [26]. These are utilised not only in primary health care settings and rural parts of developing nations but also in developed nations where allopathic medications are primarily employed [27]. A systemic review done on traditional, complementary and alternative medicine use in SSA revealed that despite the diverse nature and limited quality of the literature, the study highlighted a substantial prevalence of TCAM usage either independently or in conjunction with allopathic medicine. This trend was observed among both the general population and individuals with specific health conditions [28, 29].

Sierra Leone is believed to possess a rich historical legacy of traditional medicine. It is observed that a significant proportion of the population relies on it for disease prevention and treatment. This preference may stem from personal choice or the limited availability of medicines in geographically isolated and inaccessible regions. The wide spread use of TCAM in Sierra Leone for medical conditions such as malaria, in pregnancy, infertility, hypertension, pneumonia, during breast-feeding and in children is a huge concern for the health authorities and especially the NPC with respect to their safety [30–36]. In Sierra Leone, like in some other parts of Africa, there is circumstantial evidence, which suggests that TCAM often contain adulterants or contaminants including conventional medicines such as corticosteroids, non-steroidal anti-inflammatory agents, antimalarial and heavy metals. This shows that there are problems relating to the use of these products. When these medicines are used concurrently with other conventional medicines, there is a possibility of significant adverse drug interactions occurring contrary to the prevailing belief among the general populace that natural therapies are inherently inert and void of adverse consequences. In addition, Peter and colleagues in a study done among EVD survivors in Sierra Leone documented that confidence and dependence on them with respect to self-medication is on the rise partly due to the fact that these products are often considered innocuous as they are considered natural and therefore thought to be safe with little or no side effects in comparison to regular allopathic medicines [37, 38].

Integrating PV in TCAM practices can sometimes be a challenge since many of the TCAM practitioners protect their methods and keep their remedies a secret. The medicinal remedies used are usually poorly elucidated and characterised, which makes causality and risk assessments very ambiguous and complex. However, as with other medicinal products proposed for human use such as medicines, vaccines and food supplements, TCAM should be incorporated within the national medicines' regulatory framework in Sierra Leone. Regulatory standards of quality, safety and efficacy that are similar to those used for medicinal products should be put in place for them. For all these reasons, integration of TCAM into the national pharmacovigilance system is very much imperative. In light of this, the Pharmacy Board of Sierra Leone has established a Department of complementary and alternative medicines to facilitate collaboration with TCAM practitioners and to promote PV. For this to succeed, it is imperative to garner the endorsement of consumers, TCAM health practitioners, providers and other knowledgeable professionals. There is a pressing need to focus on research and the provision of comprehensive training for healthcare providers and consumers in this particular domain (See Chap. 13 for another perspective on PV related to traditional medicine).

9.3   Deployment of Pharmacovigilance in Mass Medicine Administration During Public Health Emergency

Amid the Ebola crisis in Sierra Leone, the capacity of PV was severely tested in terms of assessing experimental products and the monitoring of existing medicines during mass drug distribution. The public health emergency necessitated the reevaluation of pharmacovigilance taking into consideration the absence of any prior clinical trials involving a novel therapeutic or vaccine in Sierra Leone.

Generally, public health programmes whether in normal times or in public health emergencies frequently exhibit limited interest in ADR monitoring. Alternatively they may underplay the importance of ADRs in order to protect the safety of their medicines and promote adherence. The Ebola epidemic underscored the criticality of a functional and trustworthy PV system for the sustainability of the malaria control programme in Sierra Leone. The Ebola outbreak presented a multitude of obstacles for the sustained provision of healthcare services across all levels. It imposed adverse effects on all public health programmes across the country, and there was a notable decrease in the utilisation of health facilities. Despite this, malaria, pneumonia and diarrhoea, which are the leading causes of mortality among children under the age of five in Sierra Leone, continued to be the primary causes of death during the Ebola outbreak [39, 40]. The linkages between the communities were weakened and community health workers were no longer able to play their role as expected by the community. If this trend had continued, drastic increase in malaria morbidity and mortality was to be expected. Health personnel has difficulties in detecting and managing of Ebola and malaria due to the similarity in the clinical presentation of the two infections.

Against this backdrop, the Government of Sierra Leone and the World Health Organization (WHO) recommended an antimalarial mass drug administration (MDA) campaign. The goal of the MDA with Artesunate-Amodiaquine (AS-AQ) in Sierra Leone was to actively contribute to the containment of the Ebola outbreak through:

1. Rapidly reducing the number of febrile cases in the community suspected to be Ebola. By doing so, the need for screening and isolation in the Ebola holding centres to rule out Ebola as the underlying cause of illness would be significantly reduced.

2. Mitigate the risk of Ebola transmission among individuals already afflicted with malaria.
3. Rapidly reducing malaria-related incidence and mortality rates.

The rationale for deployment of pharmacovigilance during the MDA were:

- Data regarding safety is typically gathered during clinical trials for both new and established medicines. However, it is crucial to recognise the inherent limitations of clinical trials such as limited exposure, narrow perspective, and short durations. Consequently it becomes essential to consistently monitor the safety and effectiveness of these products when they are utilised in larger populations.
- In the light of Ebola outbreak, monitoring for ADRs was imperative, since the clinical manifestations of other diseases, including malaria, as well as the ADRs resulting from the use AS-AQ, exhibited similarities with the symptoms associated with Ebola.
- Ameliorate mistrust within communities concerning the MDA with any drug especially AS-AQ or that government wanted to spread the Ebola further by giving the drug and build confidence in the health care system and government as a whole.
- Pharmacovigilance as part of Sierra Leone's national drug safety infrastructure and national Post marketing surveillance (PMS) programme was crucial to:

  – *Quantify* ADRs that have been *previously identified,*
  – *Identify signals or* ADRs that have not been previously *recognised*
  – *Evaluating the effectiveness of the medication* in *real-world contexts*
  – *Reducing both* mortality *and morbidity associated with adverse events*

The objectives of the PV monitoring during the MDA were to:

- Promote and monitor compliance with AS-AQ combination in targeted population (>80%).
- Evaluate readiness of health systems in monitoring medication safety at both district and national levels in order to identify areas where suitable responses are needed in terms of knowledge and training in PV.
- Assess the effectiveness of the drug distribution channels.
- Evaluate the seriousness, expectedness, frequency and outcome of ADRs.
- This was to help:

  – Detect adverse drug reactions not indicated in the product information leaflets or summary of product characteristics.
  – Assess association of ADR with AS-AQ combination.
  – Provide a spectrum of ADRs for AS-AQ in a larger population.
  – Provide health professionals with guidance on patient counselling and monitoring at health facility level.

- Communication of findings and recommendations to the National Malaria Control Programme, the Ministry of Health and Sanitation, policy makers, partners and the public to guide the development of future strategies in developing treatment guidelines and conducting mass drug administration (MDA) campaigns during epidemic outbreaks including that for Ebola.

The outcome of the pharmacovigilance monitoring led to the collection and assessment of thousands of ADRs. The report generated from the assessment led to the review of the malaria control treatment policy in which Artesunate-amodiaquine was replaced with artemether-lumefantrine as the first line of treatment against malaria.

9.4 Deployment of PV in Clinical Trials of Ebola Therapeutics, Vaccines and Diagnostics

In the context of public health emergencies, the Ministry of Health through PBSL made decisions about the approval of novel or established medical products. These judgements are primarily influenced by available scientific evidence, by knowledge of the product, political framework and expert professional opinion. The concept of "acceptable risk" is integral to the process of decision-making, as it pertains to the individuals or entities to which this risk is applicable.

In Sierra Leone, the national pharmacovigilance centre of the PBSL works in tandem with the clinical trial unit. The PBSL is mandated by the Pharmacy and Drugs Acts and the National Medicines Policy to define the general norms and scientific principles and to set applicable and workable standards for the approval, conduct and control of clinical trials in Sierra Leone involving medicines, medical devices, herbals, biotherapeutics and vaccines. This scope also covers the repurposing of medicines.

During the Ebola epidemic, the PBSL conducted clinical trial application (CTA) evaluation, approvals and monitoring for all experimental products (therapeutics, vaccines and diagnostics). This entails full CTA submission (protocol, chemistry manufacturing and control dossier, investigator's brochure, informed consent documents) for experimental use of therapeutics, vaccines and diagnostics in the treatment, prevention and diagnosis of new, current and emerging diseases. Reviews are normally conducted within 60 days. In public health emergency situations, PBSL expedited reviews within 10–15 working days. In exceptional circumstances, compassionate use of experimental products was also evaluated for use on a case-by-case basis. The submission of a CTA to PBSL necessitates ethics approval from the Sierra Leone Ethics and Scientific Review Committee (SLESRC) or alternatively a simultaneous submission in public health emergencies. Evaluations were conducted by an expert committee on pharmacovigilance and clinical trials appointed by the PBSL consisting of physicians, pharmacists, pathologist, pharmacologists, toxicologist, biostatistician including Public Health Specialists and the final decision is made by the Board [41].

Product approval or licensure was based on risk/benefit analysis that includes:

- Detailed review of quality (CMC) dossier.
- Pre-clinical information.
- Clinical dossier.
- GMP inspection or on-site evaluation (OSE).
- Quality control testing of product (this would be a challenge in Sierra Leone since laboratories to test vaccines are not available. However, collaboration with QC labs that have the capacity to test these products can be established.)

The Board conducted evaluations for ten repurposing applications for medical product registration and clinical trials, 21 clinical trials and compassionate use applications, together with 18 amendments for the utilisation of medical products for the purposes of treating, preventing and diagnosing EVD [41]. The NPC played a crucial role in ensuring that robust structures and systems were in place to support the evaluation of applications for clinical trials and rapid diagnostics validation and also the collection and evaluation of serious adverse events (SAEs) or suspected unexpected serious adverse reactions (SUSARs). Over 100 SAE reports were collected from these clinical trials. These reports underwent causality assessment and were subsequently submitted to VigFlow.

9.5   Pharmacovigilance During the COVID-19 Pandemic in Sierra Leone

The NPC of PSBL collaborated with the EPI to utilise the existing regulatory pathways to introduce COVID-19 vaccines in the country, viz., Comirnaty, Vaxzevria, Covishield, Sinopharm BiBBP and Janssen COVID-19 vaccines. For the introduction and approval of these new vaccines, the applicants or manufacturers were required to submit a product dossier and a comprehensive risk management plan (RMP)/pharmacovigilance plan to the PBSL for in-country review. As part of the pandemic preparedness and for emergency use approval, PBSL implemented its expedited regulatory pathway for vaccines that are WHO Prequalified, approved by WHO-listed authorities, Stringent Regulatory Authority (SRA)-approved or with WHO Emergency Use Listing predicated on the recognition and reliance framework.

Considering the paucity of information on the safety of the candidate vaccines, there was a need for effective deployment and surveillance for the detection, reporting and management of any AEFI that will occur coupled with extensive training on the expected AEFIs and reporting. The AEFI surveillance system employed in Sierra Leone was a joint endeavour involving multiple stakeholders, including the EPI, the PBSL, the National Disease Surveillance Programme, the WHO and UNICEF. Additional stakeholders encompass vaccinees, parents and caregivers (in case of child vaccine recipients), chiefs and their constituents, civil society organisations, both for-profit and non-for profit health providers, the media outlets and the general populace.

The initial and main stage in the AEFI surveillance involved the identification of cases. The primary reporter of AEFI may include individuals from various backgrounds, such as public health workers, vaccinators, health facility staff, volunteers or caregivers (such as parents) or any other person who identifies and reports the occurrence of the AEFI. Upon receiving complaints from individuals who have received vaccines or their carers or upon establishing a connection the complaints and the vaccination process, the health professional reports to the in-charge of the health facility at the primary health care level and to the AEFI focal person at the secondary and tertiary levels. All these reports from primary, secondary and tertiary levels came to PBSL for uploading into the Country's local safety database (VigiFlow) and for onward submission to the WHO global safety database (VigiBase) through Med Safety App, the WHO UMC primary reporting web-platform and Open data kit (ODK).

The AEFI committees already in existence in every district and a national committee at the central level were deployed for surveillance. In the event of serious AEFI cases, the cases were investigated by the district AEFI focal persons and the national expert Causality Assessment Committee was convened for final classification and management of the serious AEFI. The National Expert Committee on Vaccine Safety and Causality Assessment was reconstituted by the PBSL/EPI/MOH, with expertise which includes, but is not limited to specialties such as neurology, cardiology, clinical pharmacy, pharmacology, epidemiology, toxicology, public health, pathology, paediatrics and pharmacovigilance. The terms of reference of the committee in relation to vaccine pharmacovigilance were/but not limited to:

- Evaluating potential causal relationships between AEFI and a vaccine.
- Identifying signals.

Benefit-risk assessment was done for reports received by the expert committee. International experience based on data from other countries using the same vaccine, such as reports in the WHO global safety database (VigiBase), published case reports and other epidemiological studies, was considered in the analyses. Hundreds of reports were received, but the majority of them were minor AEFIs such as headache, pyrexia, dizziness, nausea, and vomiting. In addition, some people also reported asthenia, myalgia, anorexia, palpitation and severe headaches described as migraine-like headaches. These reactions occurred soon after the vaccine was administered and were related to the immunopharmacology of the vaccine. They are common to other vaccines and resolved within 5 to 7 days after the occurrence of the AEFI. Suspected Adverse Events of Special Interest (AESIs) such as ageusia, anaphylactic reactions, menstrual disorders and thrombotic thrombocytopenia syndrome were reported.

Some of the risk minimisation measures proposed and disseminated to health-care professionals and consumers included:

- Provision of rescue medications to manage suspected AEFIs in health facilities.
- Women who encountered unanticipated vaginal bleeding, particularly those who are postmenopausal or those who have concerns over protracted or severe monthly disruptions are advised to consult with their healthcare professional.
- A minimum duration of 15 minutes for observation of each vaccine following administration, due to the potentially occurrence of anaphylactic/anaphylactoid reactions that could pose a significant threat to an individual's life, is advised.
- Individuals who have previously experienced allergic reactions to vaccines such as acute allergic reaction, angioneurotic oedema, dyspnoea or similar symptoms should refrain from the second dose. Alternatively, close monitoring should be implemented for such individuals if they choose to proceed with the second dose.

9.6   Lessons Learnt

Results from the pharmacovigilance monitoring during mass medicine distribution and our activities concerning regulating clinical trials during the Ebola crisis have further highlighted the need to strengthen drug safety monitoring mechanisms across all health service delivery structures in the country. In this regard, our work provided the need and evidence for policy change to the first-line treatment of malaria in Sierra Leone. It has also become evident that there exists a necessity to enhance technical proficiency in the domains of pharmacovigilance and clinical trials.

In view of our experiences, we can confidently say that the true value and expanded role of pharmacovigilance have been clearly elucidated which includes:

- Protecting a nation in times of crisis.
- Building confidence in the health care system and government.
- Promoting PV in public health programmes and interventions.
- Identifying gaps in the drug delivery system.
- Pharmacovigilance preparedness assessment has highlighted the need for the provision of rescue medications for future mass drug administration.
- Providing an evidence base for policy change in drug selection and use in the interest of better patient outcomes.
- Pharmacovigilance can be used as a tool to monitor the quality of pharmaceutical services in the country.

9.7   Conclusion

The Pharmacy Board of Sierra Leone, which hosts the NPC, has the basic pharma-covigilance structures and processes in place. However, the system is still in its primordial stage and requires adequate funding to optimise it, coupled with the need for a definite legislation to ensure industry assumes responsibility and liability for their products on the market and to ensure that appropriate actions are taken when required.

Health facilities and PHPs have PV systems and structures that exhibit fragility. Moreover, the ability to create signals, assess them, and utilise the resulting infor-mation for risk management and communication is restrained. Integration of both spontaneous reporting and active approaches is relevant to improve patient safety.

The impression that PV is a luxury and can only be realised in high-income countries should be changed taking into consideration that PV is important for the prudent and economically efficient utilisation of medicines in all countries. As a result, it plays a crucial role in safeguarding public health.

9.8   Recommendations

Specific legislation should be put in place to adequately address medicine safety monitoring. Active pharmacovigilance methods like cohort event monitoring, use of registries and targeted spontaneous reporting should be incorporated into the national PV system through close collaboration with public health programmes, research institutions and health care training institutions due to the fact that new vaccines and medicines especially for Ebola will not be deployed in the developed world, but rather in resource-limited settings like Sierra Leone for the first time on a huge scale.

There should be a stronger collaboration with health professional associations and institutions offering health-related subjects to ensure relevant PV topics are incorporated in pre- and in-service training curricula. Comprehensive risk-mitigation plan targeting high-risk medicines should be developed and implemented by PHPs and health facilities in collaboration with the national pharmacovigilance centre. Drug and Therapeutics Committees and Drug Information Centres should be estab-lished where they are not in existence and where they exist, capacity to carry out PV activities should be strengthened, and the safety information collected should be used to ensure patient safety at the level of health facilities in collaboration with national PV centre.

In order to accomplish this objective, it is imperative to eliminate the conven-tional schism between the domains of medicine safety and public health. The Ministry of Health must rely on the NPC for the ongoing evaluation of the safety of medical products undergoing clinical trials and approved medicines. This is particularly important for promoting rational medicines use, especially those utilised within the public sector.

9.9 The Future of PV in Sierra Leone

In 2023, the Pharmacy Board of Sierra Leone introduced requirements mandating marketing authorisation holders (MAHs) to appoint Qualified Persons for Pharmacovigilance (QPPV). These individuals will be responsible for establishing operational pharmacovigilance systems, thereby assuming accountability and legal liability for their marketed products. The primary objective of this requirement is to ensure that appropriate measures are promptly undertaken when deemed necessary. Instituting such requirements would favour strengthening of the national PV system and guarantee the country to adopt the fundamental aspects of PV that align with international best practices. The Paul Ehrlich Institute (PEI) in Germany through collaboration with the Food and Drug Authority in Ghana has provided technical support to ensure that this is brought to fruition. The PEI has been working with the NPC and is providing technical and financial support to ensure that it attains a WHO maturity level 3 before the end of 2025.

The inclusion of pharmacovigilance training in the undergraduate curriculum for pharmacists at College of Medicine and Allied Health Sciences, University of Sierra Leone that hosts the only pharmacy school (faculty) in the country has been implemented. The NPC will work with the faculties of clinical sciences, nursing, Laboratory medicine and public health for incorporation of PV in their curricula.

The NPC has requested technical support from the Uppsala Monitoring Centre in Sweden and PEI in Germany for the deployment of the VigiMobile. This is a new offline application that aims to enhance accessibility and user-friendliness for health care professionals and consumers in a bid to increase the ADR and AEFI reporting rate in Sierra Leone.

References

1. Statistics Sierra Leone. Sierra Leone mid-term housing and population census. Provisional result [online]. 2021. Available at: https://www.statistics.sl/. Accessed 1 Nov 2022.
2. Statistics Sierra Leone (Stats SL) and ICF. Sierra Leone demographic and health survey 2019. Freetown, Sierra Leone, and Rockville, Maryland, USA: Stats SL and ICF; 2020.
3. World Bank Group. Maternal Mortality Ratio (Modeled estimate per 100,000 live births) – Sierra Leone. 2023. Available at https://data.worldbank.org/indicator/SH.STA. MMRT?locations=SL. Accessed 30th May 2023.
4. World Bank Group. Live expectancy at birth (total years) – Sierra Leone. 2022. Available at https://data.worldbank.org/indicator/SP.DYN.LE00.IN?locations=SL. Accessed 20 Oct 2022.
5. World Health Organisation. 2018. World Health Organisation Sierra Annual Report. Available at https://www.afro.who.int/sites/default/files/2019-09/WHO%20Sierra%20Leone%20 2018%20Annual%20Report.pdf. Accessed 12 Aug 2022.

6. Government of Sierra Leone. The Sierra Leone gazette (extraordinary): pharmacy Board of Sierra Leone. Government of Sierra Leone: Freetown; 2021. Available at https://pharmacy-board.gov.sl/admin/gallery/3b0646cca6ebb51a29a37af7cca15ae8.pdf. Accessed 12 Oct 2022

7. Sierra Leone Medical Dental Association. Sierra Leone medical and dental association annual congress and scientific meeting. Freetown: Sierra Leone Medical and Dental Association; 2021.

8. Kortepeter MG, Bausch DG, Bray M. Basic clinical and laboratory features of filoviral hemorrhagic fever. J Infect Dis. 2011;204(suppl 3):S810–6.

9. Kuhn JH, Dodd LE, Wahl-Jesnsen V, et al. Evaluation of perceived threat differences posed by filovirus variants. Biosecur Bioterror. 2011;9(4):361–71.

10. Ansumana R, Jacobsen KH, Idris M, et al. Ebola in Freetown area, Sierra Leone—a case study of 581 patients. N Engl J Med. 2015;372(6):587–8.

11. Deen GF, et al. Ebola RNA persistence in semen of Ebola virus disease survivors—preliminary report. Mass Medical Soc; 2015.

12. Avong YK, Jatau B, Gurumnaan R, Danat N, Okuma J, Usman I, Mordi D, Ukpabi B, Kayode GA, Dutt S, El-Tayeb O. Addressing the under-reporting of adverse drug reactions in public health programs controlling HIV/AIDS, tuberculosis and malaria: a prospective cohort study. PLoS One. 2018;13(8):e0200810.

13. Hailu AD, Mohammed SA. Adverse drug reaction reporting in Ethiopia: systematic review. Biomed Res Int. 2020;2020:1–12.

14. Paudyal V, Al-Hamid A, Bowen M, Hadi MA, Hasan SS, Jalal Z, Stewart D. Interventions to improve spontaneous adverse drug reaction reporting by healthcare professionals and patients: systematic review and meta-analysis. Expert Opin Drug Saf. 2020;19(9):1173–91.

15. Ministry of Health and Sanitation [MOHS]. National Medicine Policy. Freetown: Directorate of Drugs and Medical Supplies, Ministry of Health and Sanitation; 2012.

16. Hughes ML, Whittlesea CM, Luscombe DK. Review of national spontaneous reporting schemes. Adverse Drug React Toxicol Rev. 2002;21(4):231–41.

17. Barry A, Olsson S, Minzi O, Bienvenu E, Makonnen E, Kamuhabwa A, Oluka M, Guantai A, Bergman U, van Puijenbroek E, Gurumurthy P. Comparative assessment of the national pharmacovigilance systems in East Africa: Ethiopia, Kenya, Rwanda and Tanzania. Drug Saf. 2020;43:339–50.

18. Collet JP, MacDonald N, Cashman N, et al. Monitoring signals for vaccine safety: the assessment of individual adverse event reports by an expert advisory committee. Bull World Health Organ. 2000;78(2):178–85.

19. Abiri OT, Johnson WC. Pharmacovigilance systems in resource-limited settings: an evaluative case study of Sierra Leone. J Pharma Policy Pract. 2019;12(1):1–8.

20. Strengthening Pharmaceutical Services (2011). Safety of Medicines in Sub-Saharan Africa: Assessment of Pharmacovigilance Systems and their Performance. Arlington, VA: US Agency for International Development by the Strengthening Pharmaceutical Systems (SPS) Program.

21. Pharmacy Board of Sierra Leone. A Guide for Safety Monitoring of Medicines in Sierra Leone. 2019. Available at: https://pharmacyboard.gov.sl/admin/gallery/41a7813d75c1bbd77cf0d9e9a3421d57.pdf. Accessed 1st Feb 2023.

22. College of Medicine and Allied Health Sciences [COMAHS]. Curriculum for the bachelor of pharmacy with honours programme. Freetown: Faculty of Pharmaceutical Sciences, College of Medicine and Allied Health Sciences, University of Sierra Leone; 2015.

23. Chan CL, Ang PS, Li SC. A survey on pharmacovigilance activities in Asean and selected non-Asean countries, and the use of quantitative signal detection algorithms. Drug Saf. 2017;40:517–30.

24. Malikova MA. Practical applications of regulatory requirements for signal detection and communications in pharmacovigilance. Ther Adv Drug Saf. 2020;11:2042098620909614.

25. System for Improved Access to Pharmaceuticals and Services [SIAPS]. Comparative analysis of pharmacovigilance systems in five Asian countries. Arlington, VA: Systems for Improved Access to Pharmaceuticals and Services. Management Sciences for Health; 2013. Available

at https://siapsprogram.org/wp-content/uploads/2014/02/Asia-PV-report.pdf. Accessed 4th May 2023

26. World Health Organisation. Catalysing ancient wisdom and modern science for the health of people and the planet; why is it needed? 2023. Available at https://www.who.int/initiatives/who-global-centre-for-traditional-medicine. Accessed 22 June 2023.

27. World Health Organisation (WHO). WHO guidelines on safety monitoring of herbal medicines in pharmacovigilance systems. Geneva: World Health Organisation; 2004.

28. James PB, Wardle J, Steel A, Adams J. Traditional, complementary and alternative medicine use in sub-Saharan Africa: a systematic review. BMJ Glob Health. 2018a;3(5):e000895.

29. Liwa AC, Smart LR, Frumkin A, Epstein HAB, Fitzgerald DW, Peck RN. Traditional herbal medicine use among hypertensive patients in sub-Saharan Africa: a systematic review. Curr Hypertens Rep. 2014;16(6):437.

30. Bakshi SS, McMahon S, George A, Yumkella F, Bangura P, Kabana A, Diaz T. The role of traditional treatment on health care seeking by caregivers for sick children in Sierra Leone: results of a baseline survey. Acta Trop. 2013;127(1):46–52.

31. Diaz T, George AS, Rao SR, Bangura PS, Baimba JB, McMahon SA, Kabano A. Healthcare seeking for diarrhoea, malaria and pneumonia among children in four poor rural districts in Sierra Leone in the context of free health care: results of a cross-sectional survey. BMC Public Health. 2013;13(1):157.

32. James PB, Kaikai AI, Bah AJ, Steel A, Wardle J. Herbal medicine use during breastfeeding: a cross-sectional study among mothers visiting public health facilities in the Western area of Sierra Leone. BMC Complement Altern Med. 2019a;19(1):66.

33. James PB, Bah AJ, Tommy MS, Wardle J, Steel A. Herbal medicines use during pregnancy in Sierra Leone: an exploratory cross-sectional study. Women Birth. 2018b;31(5):e302–9.

34. James PB, Taidy-Leigh L, Bah AJ, Kanu JS, Kangbai JB, Sevalie S. Prevalence and correlates of herbal medicine use among women seeking Care for Infertility in Freetown, Sierra Leone. Evid Based Complement Alternat Med. 2018c;2018:9493807.

35. James PB, Kamara H, Bah AJ, Steel A, Wardle J. Herbal medicine use among hypertensive patients attending public and private health facilities in Freetown Sierra Leone. Complement Ther Clin Pract. 2018d;31:7–15.

36. Ranasinghe S, Ansumana R, Lamin JM, Bockarie AS, Bangura U, Buanie JA, Stenger DA, Jacobsen KH. Herbs and herbal combinations used to treat suspected malaria in Bo, Sierra Leone. J Ethnopharmacol. 2015;166:200–4.

37. James PB, Wardle J, Steel A, Adams J. Utilisation of and attitude towards traditional and complementary medicine among Ebola survivors in Sierra Leone. Medicina. 2019b;55(7):387.

38. James PB, Wardle J, Steel A, Adams J. Pattern of health care utilisation and traditional and complementary medicine use among Ebola survivors in Sierra Leone. PLoS One. 2019c;14(9):e0223068.

39. Brolin Ribacke KJ, Saulnier DD, Eriksson A, Von Schreeb J. Effects of the West Africa Ebola virus disease on health-care utilization–a systematic review. Front Public Health. 2016;4:222.

40. Mulenga-Cilundika P, Ekofo J, Kabanga C, Criel B, Van Damme W, Chenge F. Indirect effects of Ebola virus disease epidemics on health Systems in The Democratic Republic of the Congo, Guinea, Sierra Leone and Liberia: a scoping review supplemented with expert interviews. Int J Environ Res Public Health. 2022;19(20):13113.

41. Abiri OT, Bah AJ, Lahai M, Lisk DR, Komeh JP, Johnson J, Johnson WC, Mansaray SS, Kanu JS, Russell JB, Thomas F. Regulating clinical trials in a resource-limited setting during the Ebola public health emergency in Sierra Leone. Trials. 2022;23(1):466.

Chapter 10
New Tuberculosis Drugs and the Role of Pharmacovigilance: Issues in Resource-Limited Countries

Edine W. Tiemersma, Susan van den Hof, and Michael Kimerling

Abbreviations

aDSM	Active drug safety management and monitoring
AE	Adverse event
AIDS	Acquired immuno-deficiency syndrome
ALT	Alanine aminotransferase
ATP	Adenosine tri-phosphate
AST	Aspartate aminotransferase
CEM	Cohort event monitoring
CIOMS	Council for International Organizations of Medical Sciences
BPaL	Regimen containing bedaquiline, pretomanid, and linezolid
DOT(S)	Directly observed treatment (short course)
DR	Drug-resistant

E. W. Tiemersma (✉)
KNCV Tuberculosis Foundation, Technical Division of TB elimination and Health Systems Innovations, The Hague, The Netherlands
e-mail: edine.tiemersma@kncvtbc.org

S. van den Hof
KNCV Tuberculosis Foundation, Technical Division of TB elimination and Health Systems Innovations, The Hague, The Netherlands

National Institute for Public Health and the Environment, Bilthoven, The Netherlands
e-mail: susan.van.den.hof@rivm.nl

M. Kimerling
KNCV Tuberculosis Foundation, Technical Division of TB elimination and Health Systems Innovations, The Hague, The Netherlands

Independent Consultant, The Hague, The Netherlands
e-mail: mekimcorp2@gmail.com

© Springer Nature Singapore Pte Ltd. 2025
S. R. Ahmad (ed.), *Special Issues in Pharmacovigilance in Resource-Limited Countries*, https://doi.org/10.1007/978-981-96-6154-1_10

DST	Drug susceptibility testing
EMA	European Medicines Agency
FDA	Food and Drug Administration (USA)
GRADE	Grading of Recommendations Assessment, Development, and Evaluation
HIV	Human immuno-deficiency virus
ICH	International Conference on Harmonisation of Technical Requirements for Registration of Pharmaceuticals for Human Use
MDR	Multidrug-resistant
NTP	National Tuberculosis Programme
PAS	Para-aminosalicylic acid
PMDT	Programmatic management of drug-resistant tuberculosis
PV	Pharmacovigilance
RR	Rifampicin-resistant
SAE	Serious adverse event
STR	Shorter treatment regimen
TB	Tuberculosis
ULN	Upper limit of normal
UMC	Uppsala Monitoring Centre
USAID	United States Agency for International Development
WHO	World Health Organization
XDR	Extensively drug-resistant

10.1 Introduction

Rifampicin-resistant (RR), particularly multidrug-resistant (MDR), tuberculosis (TB) (see Table 10.1 for definitions) is difficult to treat and requires a combination of different drugs given for a period of at least 6 months, and sometimes much longer, depending on the resistance pattern of the MDR-TB strain that causes the disease [1, 2]. Additional resistance to two potent classes of drugs (fluoroquinolones and second-line injectables (kanamycin, amikacin, and capreomycin)), for decades left limited options for cure, as these drugs formed the core MDR-TB treatment regimens [3, 4].

Since 2013, three new anti-TB medicines were approved by the Food and Drug Administration (FDA) of the USA and the European Medicines Agency (EMA), and several other legal bodies, providing new opportunities for treatment of DR-TB: bedaquiline (first received accelerated approval in November 2012 by the FDA), delamanid (first conditionally approved by the EMA in April 2014), and pretomanid as part of a fixed regimen was approved in 2019 by the FDA for the treatment of

Table 10.1 Definitions of drug-resistant tuberculosis[a]

Term	Abbreviation	Description
Drug-resistant TB	DR-TB	TB disease caused by an organism that is resistant to any TB medicine.
Multidrug-resistant TB	MDR-TB	(TB disease caused by) an organism that is resistant against at least the two most effective anti-TB drugs in the first-line TB regimen: rifampicin and isoniazid.
Isoniazid-resistant TB	Hr-TB	(TB disease caused by) an organism is susceptible to rifampicin, but resistant to isoniazid.
Rifampicin-resistant TB	RR-TB	(TB disease caused by) an organism is resistant to rifampicin. It may be susceptible or resistant to isoniazid, and/or to other first- or second-line TB medicines.
Extensively resistant TB[b]	XDR-TB	RR-TB organism that is additionally resistant to one or more fluoroquinolone (moxi- or levofloxacin) and at least one other "group A" drug.

[a]Source: WHO, 2020 [1]
[b]Disease caused by an RR-TB strain that is resistant to moxifloxacin and/or levofloxacin, but not to another "group A" drug, is referred to as pre-XDR-TB

adults with pulmonary XDR-TB or MDR-TB that is treatment-intolerant or non-responsive. In June 2013, the World Health Organization (WHO) issued an interim policy guidance on the use of bedaquiline as part of MDR-TB treatment [5]. A similar interim guidance document on delamanid was published in October 2014 [6]. In 2022, WHO published new guidance on the treatment of drug-resistant (DR) TB, in which bedaquiline plays a central role in any regimen [2].

The approvals received from regulatory drug authorities were conditional, because at the time, no full drug safety profiles were established as efficacy and safety data were only available from Phase IIb studies with inclusion of limited numbers of carefully selected patients. Particularly concerning bedaquiline, there were safety concerns, based on increased mortality and QT prolongation during the phase II trials [7]. Therefore, in its guidance document, the WHO included the requirement that treatment implementation of bedaquiline and delamanid must be accompanied by active pharmacovigilance (PV) [5, 6] to safeguard the early detection and prompt reporting of adverse events (AEs) during use of these new drugs under programmatic conditions.

In this chapter, we first discuss TB, drug-resistant TB disease and its treatment options, and the safety of that treatment. We then discuss PV for TB treatment (focusing on MDR-TB), highlighting issues in the resource-limited country context where the burden of TB is highest. We conclude with examples of the PV systems for patients with drug-resistant (DR) TB in two of the countries where we are providing technical assistance.

10.2 Tuberculosis

10.2.1 A Brief History of the Treatment of Tuberculosis

Skeletal artifacts indicate that TB has affected human beings at least as early as 3000–5000 B.C. Until Robert Koch discovered the infectious agent *Mycobacterium tuberculosis* in 1882, the cause of TB remained unknown [8]. His discovery opened opportunities for further investigations, including treatment of TB disease. However, it took more than 60 years before the first effective anti-TB drug was discovered and used in the successful treatment of TB. In November 1944, the first patients received streptomycin and subsequently were declared cured. Other anti-TB drugs soon followed: thioacetazone and para-aminosalicylic acid (PAS) in 1948, isonicotinic hydrazide (isoniazid) in 1951, pyrazinamide and cycloserine in 1952, ethionamide in 1956, rifampin in 1957, and ethambutol in 1962 [9]. After 1962, no new anti-TB drugs were developed until very recently. This was partially due to the fact that the core four-drug "DOTS" (directly observed treatment, short course) regimen proved to be effective and partially to the fact that TB funding was dramatically reduced in the 1970s when TB had disappeared as a major public health threat in the affluent world, and because its confinement in developing countries was judged too distant, complicated, and costly [10].

It should be noted that all these drugs had been developed and marketed before there was much attention to drug safety—the first systematic international initiatives to address drug safety concerns started in the mid-1960s after thousands of children whose mothers had taken thalidomide during pregnancy were born with deformations [11]. Moreover, since TB is a life-threatening disease with a high case-fatality rate if left untreated [12], the benefits of treatment were felt to outweigh the risks of potential AEs due to the toxicity of the drugs employed [4].

However, the TB world had its own experience showing the need of structural PV for TB drugs in the example of thioacetazone [13]. Since its discovery, thioacetazone had been widely applied in TB treatment regimens, although there was a well-established relationship with cutaneous hypersensitivity [14]. Despite this, thioacetazone remained a popular anti-TB drug because it was cheap and easy to administer. With the surge of the HIV-epidemic, an increase in severe and serious adverse drug reactions related to thioacetazone was seen, including Stevens-Johnson syndrome or toxic epidermal necrolysis [15]. By that time, HIV was already an epidemic in Africa. This led to the WHO recommendation in 1991 to replace thioacetazone with ethambutol for TB patients coinfected with HIV [16]. Currently, thioacetazone is no longer recommended for use in the treatment of TB [17].

The emergence and recognition of MDR-TB resulted in the need for developing longer and more toxic regimens, further underlining the urgent need for PV systems. The subsequent approval of new drugs for the treatment of M/XDR-TB that had not yet gained sufficient evidence of efficacy and safety past phase II studies has made active PV an imperative.

10.2.2 Multidrug-Resistant Tuberculosis: Emergence and Development of Treatment

Already in 1942, Rene Dubos postulated the hypothesis that selection toward resistant variants of bacteria would occur with the use of antibiotic drugs [18]. Indeed, soon after the introduction of streptomycin, streptomycin resistance was appreciated to cause TB relapse among previously cured patients. Thereafter, resistance was shown to all existing anti-TB drugs, including rifampicin and isoniazid, the two most potent drugs [19, 20]. Combined resistance to these core drugs was defined as multidrug resistance (MDR). Outbreaks of drug-resistant TB were reported from several (affluent) countries since the 1970s. A well-documented MDR-TB outbreak in New York City, in the 1990s, was successfully contained by applying the principles of routine drug susceptibility testing (DST), appropriate (individualized) treatment, and good case holding (using DOT, social support, and an emphasis on management of AEs to ensure treatment completion). Also, infection control was upgraded to prevent nosocomial transmission [21]. However, in many resource-constrained settings, first- and second-line DST are not readily available, and thus, until recently, most MDR-TB patients either were treated with ineffective first-line regimens or empiric, low-cost, standardized second-line regimens. Many of the drugs in such regimens were known for their risk of causing serious and severe AEs (Table 10.2). In fact, more than half of the patients treated with MDR-TB regimens were thought to experience one or more AEs during treatment [22], some of which have serious and lifelong consequences (e.g., severe hearing loss due to the use of injectable drugs [23, 24], depression/suicide due to cycloserin [25], and myelosuppression due to linezolid [26]. Although some of these events may seem non-life threatening or severe, such as nausea, such complications may still lead to treatment discontinuation and patient dropout [27, 28], and in that way, further contribute to amplification and transmission of resistant TB [29, 30].

Despite the introduction of new, less toxic regimens, DR-TB patients are still treated with multiple drugs, some of which are associated with a high rate of severe AEs, such as cycloserin and linezolid [31, 32]. Some of these drugs were repurposed for the treatment of DR-TB, and for these, the safety profiles for treatment in multidrug regimens for a lengthy period are not yet fully understood, like clofazimine [33] and linezolid [32].

10.2.3 Three New Drugs for Treatment of (MDR)TB, the First in Over 40 Years

In the past 15 years, three new drugs were introduced which have led to a series of newly recommended regimens for patients who previously had little treatment options, including patients with allergies or adverse reactions to certain classes of drugs.

Table 10.2 List of first- and second-line anti-TB drugs and their most common side effects [22, 33, 36, 62–64, 87][a]

Adverse event (AE)	Potential causative anti-TB drugs	Proportion of patients on MDR-TB treatment suffering from the AE: mean [22] or range
Nausea/vomiting	Ethionamide, PAS (isoniazid, pyrazinamide, fluoroquinolones, bedaquiline)	70 [67]–97% [65]
Diarrhea	Ethionamide, PAS (isoniazid, pyrazinamide, fluoroquinolones) (most often not caused by drugs)	9% [66]–39% [67]
Arthralgia	Pyrazinamide, fluoroquinolones	8%[b]
Dizziness/vertigo	Aminoglycosides, capreomycin, fluoroquinolones	14% [85]–24% [65]
Hearing loss	Aminoglycosides, capreomycin	15%
Tinnitus	Aminoglycosides, capreomycin	5% [85]–12% [65]
Headache	Fluoroquinolones, cycloserine	10% [65]–12% [85]
Sleep disturbances	Aminoglycosides, fluoroquinolones	12% [85][c]
Electrolyte disturbance (hypokalemia)	Capreomycin, aminoglycosides	3% [c]
Abdominal pain	High-dose isoniazid, ethambutol, clofazimine, PAS, ethionamide/proteonamide, fluoroquinolones, pyrazinamide	11% [85]–24% [65]
Anorexia	Ethionamide, PAS (isoniazid, pyrazinamide, fluoroquinolones, bedaquiline)	9% [85]–58% [65]
Gastritis	High-dose isoniazid, ethambutol, clofazimine, PAS, ethionamide/proteonamide, fluoroquinolones, pyrazinamide	9% [85][d]
Peripheral neuropathy	Linezolid, cycloserine, high-dose isoniazid, ethionamide	8%
Depression	Cycloserine, high-dose isoniazid (most often not caused by drugs)	6 [85]–13% [66]
Allergic reaction	Any anti-TB drug in MDR-TB regimen	5% [85][d]
Rash	Any anti-TB drug in MDR-TB regimen	4% [66]–14% [67]
Visual disturbances	Ethambutol, linezolid	2%
Seizures	Cycloserine, high-dose isoniazid	3 [66]–9% [67]
Hypothyroidism	Ethionamide/proteonamide, PAS	4%
Psychosis	Cycloserine, high-dose isoniazid	2% [66]–9% [67]
Hepatitis (hepatotoxicity)	Pyrazinamide, PAS, (other second-line drugs)	7%

(continued)

Table 10.2 (continued)

Adverse event (AE)	Potential causative anti-TB drugs	Proportion of patients on MDR-TB treatment suffering from the AE: mean [22] or range
Renal failure (nephrotoxicity)	Aminoglycosides, capreomycin	4%
QT prolongation[e]	Moxifloxacin, clofazimin, bedaquiline, delamanid	11% [36][f]
Hematologic disorders	Linezolid	2%[g]
Skin discoloration	Clofazimine	97% [33][h]

[a] Where available, data from the systematic review by Wu et al. [22] are presented; otherwise, specific references are mentioned. All references include cohorts after the year 1999 of greater than 500 patients except reference [36]

[b] The larger cohorts generally reported higher proportions of 13% [62]–50% [64]

[c] Keshavjee et al. [64] reported a proportion as high as 38%

[d] Only reported by one study [87]

[e] Note that QT prolongation is a risk factor of torsade de pointes

[f] Data of 45 patients on bedaquiline-containing regimens; QTcF >500 ms, considered dangerous and a reason for stopping QT-prolonging drugs

[g] Bloss et al. [62] reported this proportion at 11%

[h] The larger cohorts did not report this side effect; the proportion was reported from a randomized controlled trial comparing a clofazimine-containing MDR-TB regimen to a regimen not containing clofazimine

Bedaquiline is a diarylquinoline that inhibits mycobacterial ATP synthetase, thereby depleting cellular energy stores. Since this mechanism differs from those of other approved anti-TB drugs, it can remain active against *M. tuberculosis* strains that are resistant to (most) other anti-TB drugs, thereby providing treatment options for those patients for whom otherwise no effective treatment regimen can be constructed. The conditional approval of the drug by the FDA was based on the efficacy data of the phase IIb trial available at week 72 of treatment, not on the final treatment outcomes available 120 weeks after starting the treatment [4] that showed a higher overall mortality in the treatment arm that received bedaquiline (10 of 79 patients) compared to the placebo arm (2 of 81 patients) [7]. There was no clear relationship between these deaths and bedaquiline, and most deaths occurred more than a year after the last dose of bedaquiline had been administered. The FDA approved bedaquiline only for patients with smear-positive MDR-TB for whom there were no effective treatment options, because in this group, the benefits of effective treatment outweigh the risk of excess mortality [4]. However, subsequent observational studies including cohorts of patients on compassionate use and programmatic implementation of bedaquiline have not shown excess mortality among patients receiving bedaquiline as compared to other patients with MDR-TB, and generally showed that this drug can be safely applied in MDR/RR-TB regimens despite its long half-life [34–39]. Using the GRADE approach [40],[1] the WHO expert group judged the quality of the evidence of the efficacy of the drug to be low, and the quality of the evidence of the safety of the drug to be low to very low [5]. Accumulating evidence on the efficacy and safety of bedaquiline has led the WHO to recommend that the drug is part of any DR-TB regimen, including the 6-month BPaL(M) regimen, the 9-month all-oral regimen, and the longer individualized MDR-TB regimens (alongside linezolid and levofloxacin or moxifloxacin, which together with bedaquiline are called "group A medicines"), unless it cannot be used due to resistance or intolerance [1].

Bedaquiline is associated with QT prolongation. A QT value of >500 ms and QT values higher than 60 ms from the patient's pre-treatment value are regarded as potentially life threatening (and thus, a serious AE (SAE) as this may lead to ventricular arrhythmia and is a risk factor for torsade de pointes causing sudden death); it is recommended to stop bedaquiline if such prolongation occurs.

Based on evidence from two ongoing trials and individual data from 24,231 individual pediatric MDR/RR-TB patient records, the WHO now recommends prescription of bedaquiline to patients of all ages [41].

Delamanid is an antimycobacterial drug of the nitro-dihydro-imidazooxazole class of compounds which inhibit mycolic acid synthesis, and thus interferes with the *M. tuberculosis* bacteria's cell wall construction process. The drug was conditionally approved by various drug and medical authorities, and WHO conditionally recommends it with very low confidence in the estimates of effect, to be added to a WHO-recommended regimen in adult patients with pulmonary MDR-TB. The overall evidence available on the safety of the drug was graded as "low" by the WHO Expert Group using the GRADE approach [6]. The evidence base for the recommendation was from two trials and one observational study, which were in fact all based on the same randomized, double-blind, placebo-controlled multicenter trial; 399 (81%) of the patients participating in one or both trials were followed for 24 months [42]. The data showed that delamanid was effective and safe [6]. After 2 months of treatment with delamanid, significantly more patients reached culture conversion (i.e., no growth of *M. tuberculosis* on culture) than patients treated with an optimized background regimen plus placebo [43]; after 6 months of treatment, 74% of the patients treated with any dose of delamanid had successful treatment outcomes, compared to 55% of patients who had not received delamanid, or for 2 months or less [42].[2] Although generally, cohort studies and clinical trials have found high treatment success rates for delamanid-containing regimens [44], a multi-country phase III trial including 511 patients did not succeed in showing noninferiority of delamanid compared to a WHO-recommended background regimen

---

[1] See also http://gradeworkinggroup.org/

[2] The WHO Expert group redid these analysis, and showed a 35% increase in culture confirmed cure among patients who received at least 6 months of delamanid compared to patients who had not received any dose of delamanid [6] WHO. The use of delamanid in the treatment of multidrug-resistant tuberculosis. Interim policy guidance. Geneva: World Health Organization; 2014. Contract No.: WHO/HTM/TB/2014.23.

[45]. Due to this potential lack of efficacy, the WHO is currently recommending to use the drug only to complement individualized MDR-TB regimens, or if higher priority drugs cannot be used [1]. The safety profile of delamanid is favorable, also for young children [46, 47].

The only AE reported more often from patients in the delamanid arms than patients in the placebo arms was (mild) QT prolongation [6, 42], with a 11–13 ms increase from baseline in the group receiving 100 mg of delamanid twice daily; 3% of these patients had a prolongation of >60 ms. Patients treated with daily doses of 200 mg delamanid had a slightly higher incidence of AEs than patients on 100 mg delamanid daily or placebo [43]. No clinically relevant drug-drug interactions were observed when delamanid was co-administered with anti-HIV medication [48]. Ongoing trials on the safety and efficacy of delamanid in children (6–17 years of age) showed that the drug can be safely provided to children of this age group; recently published results from a phase I/II trial showed similar safety profile [47]. Delamanid is considered safe for treating children of all ages [41].

Pretomanid is currently only approved for use in a fixed three-drug, 6-month, all-oral regimen, containing another new drug (bedaquiline) and a repurposed drug (linezolid): the BPaL regimen, which may be combined with clofazimine (BPaLC) or moxifloxacin (BPaLM) [1, 2]. Pretomanid is a nitroimidazooxine. It requires metabolic activation by the *Mycobacterium tuberculosis* bacteria for antibacterial activity through a complex mechanism, which is not yet fully understood. The drug has shown to interfere with cell wall composition and to trigger respiratory poisoning. In an open-label, single-arm study including 109 patients diagnosed with either XDR-TB, or treatment intolerances, or non-responsive MDR-TB treated for 6 months with BPaL, 90% (95% confidence interval, 83–95%) of the patients experienced a favorable treatment outcome, which is much higher than usually reported for such patients [49]. AEs most commonly reported included peripheral neuropathy (occurring in as much as 81% of the patients) and myelosuppression (48%), but these remained manageable by lowering linezolid dosage according to the study group. Other commonly reported AEs included skin disorders (acne, rash), gastrointestinal disorders (nausea, vomiting, dyspepsia, diarrhea), increased liver and pancreatic enzymes (transaminases, gamma-glutamyltransferase, hyperamylasemia), visual impairment, and hypoglycemia [49]. A phase III follow-up trial among patients with (pre-)XDR-TB using different doses of linezolid showed that with a lower dose of linezolid (600 mg instead of 1200 mg used earlier) for 26 weeks, similar efficacy (91%) could be achieved with much lower rates of peripheral neuropathy (24%) and myelosuppression (2%) [50]. These results were confirmed by another, open-label phase II/III trial providing 600 mg linezolid daily for 16 weeks and then 300 mg for 8 weeks for a regimen that also contained moxifloxaxin (BPaLM) among RR-TB patients. The treatment outcomes among those treated with BPaL-containing regimens were so much better than those obtained with the then-standard-of-care regimens, leading to the trial being ended early [51]. These results have led to the new WHO recommendation that all patients with MDR/RR-TB may be treated with BPaLM [1].

The WHO guideline development group, combining data from several studies (the endTB observational cohort study [52], and MSF-supported site in India [53] and the DELIBERATE trial [46] concluded that there are no additional safety concerns when bedaqiline and delamanid are administered together [1]. This is in line with data presented in two systematic reviews [54, 55].The treatment of difficult-to-treat variants of tuberculosis also requires the off-label use of drugs, such as clofazimine and linezolid [56]; the interactions of these drugs and the other drugs in the multidrug regimen are not yet fully understood [32].

In summary, the results to date show that (a) AEs and SAEs occur very frequently among MDR-TB patients, even in those with "uncomplicated" MDR-TB, and (b) evidence is accumulating that bedaquiline and delamanid are well tolerated. However, there are some concerns related to particularly linezolid. Also, there is limited evidence of the safety of several other repurposed drugs when provided for lengthy periods in multidrug regimens. This calls for active PV. To date, in many countries with a high burden of TB, systematic assessment and routine recording and reporting of AEs are not routinely done, although AEs are usually managed on case-by-case basis.

10.2.4   PV Is Part of Good Clinical Practice and Is Recommended in PMDT Guidelines

The first comprehensive guidelines for the programmatic management of drug-resistant TB (PMDT) were published in 2006 [57]. These guidelines contained recommendations for the treatment of drug-resistant TB, with a focus on MDR-TB, including MDR-TB/HIV co-management. Updates followed in 2008 [58] (including programmatic management of XDR-TB), 2011 [31] (using the GRADE approach), 2016 [2] (including new regimens and drugs), 2019 [1] (including a new classification of TB medicines), 2020 [59] (including the BPaL regimens), and 2022 [1]. While monitoring and management of AEs occurring during treatment were recommended in the 2006 and 2008 guidelines [57, 58], there was no requirement or recommendation of recording and reporting them. The priority was on systematic and regular screening of symptoms of common AEs through patient interviews and periodic laboratory assessments. The 2011 update did not provide updates on monitoring, management, and recording and reporting of AEs [31]. The 2016 update recommend that the WHO framework for active TB drug-safety monitoring and management (aDSM) [60] should be applied to "ensure appropriate action to monitor and respond promptly to AEs" [2]. These guidelines describe the situation whereby systematic monitoring of AEs was not routinely done under programmatic conditions until recently with the increasing availability of new and repurposed drugs and regimens, and that experience in implementing systematic monitoring was still being gained. Thus, the implementation of PV by TB programmes has been fueled by the introduction of bedaquiline and delamanid, for which the drug safety profiles are currently incomplete. The recommendation included in the interim policy guidance documents for bedaquiline and delamanid were to implement "active PV" [5, 6]. However, at the time of publication of the first document (on bedaquiline), it was not defined what was meant by "active PV," though cohort event monitoring (CEM) was recommended as the best method [5]. CEM was also included as the preferred method in the WHO PV Handbook for TB programmes [61]. However, CEM requires the systematic recording and reporting of all AEs occurring in the included patient cohort, irrespective of their seriousness, severity, or clinical significance, which is challenging for a cohort in which 70–80% of the patients will experience one or multiple AEs [62–64], foremost in settings which experience serious constraints regarding human resource constraints, patient support, and PV systems [65]. This raised immediate concerns that the introduction of bedaquiline and delamanid may be delayed because of the requirement of active PV. Therefore, the WHO developed the aDSM framework [58]. The guidance document confirms and illustrates the core PMDT recommendation of active and systematic monitoring of common AEs as part of proper patient management, provides guidance on the recording and reporting of AEs, and recommends coordination of aDSM activities with existing PV structures in-country. Details of the WHO aDSM guidance are presented below (Sect. 10.3.2 and further).

10.3 Pharmacovigilance for MDR-TB Treatment

One could question why separate recommendations for recording and reporting of AEs are needed: Is the monitoring and management of AEs, as recommended since 2006, not sufficient? There are several advantages to recording and reporting AEs. First, consistent recording of clinical actions taken, including the identification and management of AEs, should be conducted as part of good clinical practice [66]. This is included in the International Standards of TB Care [67]. Reactions and allergies to specific drugs should be carefully recorded to ensure that patients will not receive drugs that they cannot tolerate. Second, a systematic overview of the incidence of (common) AEs, and the drugs used to treat these, is needed to enable careful planning of the procurement of ancillary drugs [68]. Third, post-marketing surveillance of AEs is needed to detect and describe rare AEs [69] that cannot be detected in the small-scale clinical trials on which most (conditional) approvals from drug regulatory authorities are based. Fourth, clinical trials are usually conducted on adults without significant comorbidities. There is limited knowledge about how the drug behaves in children, pregnant and lactating women, the elderly and patients with comorbidities (although some persons infected with HIV and children were included in ongoing and finalized bedaquiline and delamanid trials [41, 42, 47, 70]), whereas such populations may require specific dosing and may have altered drug responses [71]. For example, preliminary data showed lower levels of delamanid in children than was expected based on pharmacokinetic models [47]. Though the phase II trials for bedaquiline and delamanid were conducted in multiple countries [7, 42, 43, 72], they did not cover the full geographical diversity of MDR-TB patients. It is well known that drug-disease interactions and drug-drug interactions, together with factors such as nutritional status, genetics, and age, may alter pharmacokinetic characteristics and pharmacodynamic relationships [71]. Fifth, the lack of drug safety data means that there is limited knowledge of the extent to which the occurrence of AEs leads to unfavorable treatment outcomes (such as untimely death, treatment failure) and loss to follow-up in programmatic settings, especially in resource-constrained countries with a high burden of TB [73] and limited options for and expertise in clinical management.

There is a wide variation in the frequency and type of AEs among MDR- and XDR-TB patients reported [22] (see also Table 10.2). Such variation is the result of differences in treatment regimens and differential management of AEs, but it probably also illustrates cultural differences, omissions, and mistakes in reporting and recording by patients and health care workers. It should be noted most AEs reported by patients will be mild and nonspecific. Very low concordance was found between types of AE reported and recorded by clinicians and patient's reports in a cross-sectional study of 121 South African MDR-TB patients [74].

10.3.1 *Pharmacovigilance in Resource-Constrained Settings*

While MDR-TB is found in every country investigated, much of the burden is in resource-constrained settings or highly populated regions [75]. Such settings frequently suffer from poor public health infrastructures and shortages in human resources due to a combination of high work load, low payments, limited education, and few possibilities for personal development, leading to low motivation and high staff turn-over [76]. In these settings, it is hard to ensure collection of good safety data. Moreover, in many high MDR-TB countries, there are major limitations in terms of human and financial resources for PV [65]. While many countries do have a system of spontaneous reporting of AEs using so-called suspect adverse reaction forms or individual case safety reports (also often referred to as yellow forms or yellow cards) [77], in practice, spontaneous reporting rarely occurs [78], notably also for TB [79, 80, 81]. This suggests that health care workers do not routinely connect with the national PV centres and do not understand the value of their work. Of 46 sub-Saharan African countries included in a situational analysis, 74% had spontaneous reporting systems in place, but only two countries collected more than 100 reports per million population in 2010 (all diseases included), while most countries generated less than 20 reports per million population per year. Also, the majority of the countries did not act upon the reports received to improve patient safety [65]. A PV database existed in only half of the countries (while this is one of the five minimum requirements formulated for PV by the WHO [82]) and data analysis was judged inadequate [65]. Also, there was little collaboration between national PV centres and disease-specific public health programmes (notably also with TB programmes). A similar analysis in five Asian countries (Bangladesh, Cambodia, Nepal, the Philippines, and Thailand) showed that the PV systems were stronger in the more affluent countries (notably Thailand, and to a lesser extent the Philippines), but significant underreporting of AEs occurred in all public health programmes for malaria, HIV/AIDS, and TB, while reporting was not coordinated with the national PV system [83]. Only four of the 46 African countries [65], and one of the five Asian countries [83], studied had a PV system functional to detect, evaluate, and prevent medicine safety issues. Specifically TB programmes had not conducted active surveillance of AEs. Although these reports have been published about a decade ago, a recently published review shows that little has changed in the last decade [84].

There is a wealth of literature about the occurrence of AEs from different study cohorts [64, 85, 86], and data about the prevalence of AEs in MDR-TB patients treated under programmatic conditions is gradually accumulating [62, 87–94]. These studies did not assess the relationship between the AEs reported and the drugs administered, and did not include nor discuss links to the national PV centre.

10.3.2 Active Drug Safety Management and Monitoring (aDSM)

Because of the limited capacity of PV systems to actively monitor drug safety, and because of the lack of collaboration between TB programmes and national PV centres, it was judged impossible to conduct full CEM. Thus, the WHO proposed another approach called aDSM [60] for all XDR-TB patients treated with any second-line drugs and all MDR-TB patients treated with new TB drugs and regimens. Since 2019, WHO recommends to apply aDSM to all patients on any type of MDR-TB regimen [1]. aDSM is defined as the "active and systematic clinical and laboratory assessment of patients on treatment with new anti-TB drugs, new MDR-TB regimens or XDR-TB regimens, in order to detect, manage and report suspected or confirmed drug toxicities" [60]. The WHO guidance document describes three essential activities: 1) proper patient monitoring by periodic systematic clinical and laboratory assessments to detect AEs, 2) timely and proper management of the detected AEs (as described in the Companion handbook to the WHO PMDT guidelines [68], and 3) systematic and standardized data recording and reporting for all SAEs. As WHO indicates, the first two elements of aDSM were already included in the standard PMDT documents, published and updated since 2006 [1, 2, 57, 58]. The third element was added. Specifically regarding recording and reporting, the document defines three-tiered monitoring "packages": the core package, in which only the SAEs are recorded and reported, the intermediate package, requiring additional recording and reporting of AEs of special interest (see Text Box 10.1), and the advanced package, including recording and reporting of all AEs deemed clinically significant [60].

Text Box 10.1 Suggested List of Adverse Events that Should Be Recorded and Reported in TB Programmes Applying the Intermediate aDSM Package

Peripheral neuropathy (paresthesia)

Psychiatric disorders and central nervous system toxicity (e.g., depression, psychosis, suicidal intention, seizures)

Optic nerve disorder (optic neuritis) or retinopathy

Ototoxicity (hearing impairment, hearing loss)

Myelosuppression (manifested as anemia, thrombocytopenia, neutropenia, or leukopenia)

Prolonged QT interval

Lactic acidosis

Hepatitis (defined as increases in alanine aminotransferase (ALT) or aspartate aminotransferase (AST) $\geq 5\times$ the upper limit of normal (ULN), or increases in ALT or AST $\geq 3\times$ ULN with clinical manifestations, or increases in ALT or AST $\geq 3\times$ ULN with concomitant increase in bilirubin $\geq 1.5\times$ ULN)

Hypothyroidism

Hypokalemia

Pancreatitis

Phospholipidosis

Acute kidney injury (acute renal failure)

Source [60]

The aDSM approach should be integrated into PMDT cohort monitoring and is the primary responsibility of the national TB programmes (NTPs). aDSM should be established engaging the national PV centre and using the expertise of local and/or international experts in drug safety issues. A link needs to be established to ensure that (as per national regulations) the PV centre receives reports for at least the SAEs and supports causality assessment and signal detection. Eight key steps are described in the aDSM framework document: (1) creation of a national aDSM coordinating mechanism, (2) development of a national aDSM implementation plan, (3) definition of roles and responsibilities for management and supervision of the system, (4) creation of standardized data collection tools (the document provides some suggested examples of these in annexes), (5) training on data collection of all staff involved, (6) definition of monitoring schedules and reporting routes, (7) development of an electronic database for storage of the collected data, and (8) development of capacity for signal detection and causality assessment.

10.3.3 Implementation of aDSM

Translating policy into practice, the KNCV Tuberculosis Foundation (KNCV), in the framework of the Challenge TB programme, has prepared a generic implementation guide for the introduction of shorter regimens and new drugs for the treatment of MDR- and XDR-TB [95], offering practical guidance on all aspects that need to be addressed when introducing new drugs and regimens, including aDSM. KNCV follows a comprehensive approach meant to ensure that patients are given a quick and correct diagnosis and treatment: right diagnosis/right treatment, using the patient triage concept. For a quick and accurate diagnosis of TB disease, including the differentiation of patterns of anti-TB drug resistance, rapid molecular tests are recommended [96].

With regard to aDSM, while building on the WHO policy [60], the KNCV generic implementation guide provides practical guidance on how to implement aDSM (described below). While acknowledged by WHO that monitoring, recording, and management of AEs is part of good clinical practice [68], the aDSM guidance recommends to include all MDR-TB patients on new drugs and regimens, as well as all XDR-TB patients in aDSM [60]. At KNCV, we recommend including all patients on drug-resistant TB treatment in aDSM as aDSM is primarily meant to improve MDR- and XDR-TB patient safety, implementation of aDSM should be incorporated into the routine PMDT. This is now also recommended by the WHO [1]. If possible, the intermediate package is the preferred package by KNCV, as the core package is judged to be the bare minimum and the advanced package is usually not feasible in the countries where shortage of staff and other resources are common. We emphasize that also previously unknown or unexpected AEs outside the package should be reported. National PV authorities, if available in the country, should play a central role in aDSM [95, 97].

At the *health centre level* (or designated most decentralized level of care), incorporation of aDSM into standard PMDT means that health care workers should carefully monitor all patients for AEs in a systematic and timely manner. Early detection with timely and proper management of AEs may prevent more severe or serious adverse outcomes, and help build a relationship of trust with the patient and prevent treatment dropout. During every DOT visit, the health worker should ask the patient about clinical symptoms of common AEs including skin rashes, gastrointestinal disturbances, psychiatric disturbance (headache, anxiety, depression, irritability, behavior change), jaundice, vestibular toxicity (nausea, vertigo, ataxia), potential symptoms of specific AEs, such as long QT (palpitations, dizziness, seizures, sudden fainting), peripheral neuropathy (numbness or muscle weakness in hands or feet, imbalance, reduced coordination), and electrolyte wasting (muscle cramping, palpitations). Additional laboratory tests should be conducted according to schedule (see [2], for an example) to detect occult adverse effects. As several drugs commonly included in MDR- and XDR-TB treatment (such as moxifloxacin, gatifloxaxin, clofazimine, bedaquiline, and delaminid) may induce QT prolongation, the monitoring of electrocardiograms is advised.

Apart from daily DOT encounters, all patients are seen by an MDR-TB clinician at enrollment (before the start of MDR-TB treatment) and starting from 2 weeks after MDR-TB treatment initiation, then on a monthly basis until treatment completion. At each of these visits, a clinical assessment is done, including an evaluation of treatment efficacy and an assessment of AEs. We advise that at these follow-up visits, treatment safety data will be collected by the doctor and/or nurse (see reference [60] for example forms). Ideally, any relevant clinical event and any required additional diagnostic testing and/or therapy is recorded. It depends on the aDSM package that the country is implementing[3] which adverse events need to be reported to the authorities managing the aDSM data. While still much of the data collection is paper-based, in some countries, digital applications via computer and/or mobile phone have been adopted in which clinicians and/or nurses can enter AEs which can then be directly sent to the PV centre, or are even sent automatically [84]. Paper reports may be entered into electronic data solutions at the health centre at regular intervals (e.g., at the end of every day or week) or at a central location. In the latter case, alternative processes need to be defined, for example, periodic visits by data management staff or periodic forwarding of forms to a national data management unit for data-entry. Ideally, adverse event data is collected in the national PV database.

AEs should be managed taking the safety of the patient and the treatment possibilities into account. For minor AEs, reassurance of the patient to make sure treatment is adhered to will be needed. For AEs that need additional evaluation and/or medical treatment, a treatment decision structure (consultation backup for DOT provider), additional tests, and ancillary medicines[4] should be available and accessible, free of charge. Drugs may have to be provided at lower dose or withdrawn. Drugs that are withdrawn from the regimen due to an AE may need to be replaced, especially in the intensive phase of treatment, when the bacillary load is high. Clinical panels should act in accordance with the WHO recommendations for replacement of drugs, taking into account the patient's condition and bacteriological status [1, 2]. This requires careful case review.

Data on safety can be collected from routinely used electronic recording and reporting systems, from routine registers (laboratory registers, TB registers), patients' medical records, or yellow forms as necessary. WHO has proposed lists of minimal data elements in its aDSM guidelines [60]. To capture all PV data, patient registers and records, as well as the routine electronic recording and reporting system, may need adaptation. Routine data collection best includes registration of all

---

[3] Within the Challenge TB program, we advise that at minimum an "intermediate package" (i.e. including SAEs and AEs of special interest, depending on the drugs that the patients receive) is implemented.

[4] See WHO recommendations outlined in the Companion Handbook to the WHO PMDT guidelines [68].

SAEs and AEs of special interest—in line with the intermediate aDSM package.[5] Within the scope of active PV, it is vital that not only AEs suspected to be related to the MDR-TB treatment be recorded and reported, but also *all* AEs that are either SAEs or AEs of special interest, as well as all AEs that occur unexpectedly or were not previously recorded, even if not thought to be related with the treatment. This will prevent previously unknown adverse drug reactions from being missed. The reported (S)AEs need to be clearly described, so that a careful assessment can be done by the national PV centre (see below). To enable international comparisons, we recommend coding the AEs using a standardized international coding system (MedDRA developed by the International Conference on Harmonisation of Technical Requirements for Registration of Pharmaceuticals for Human Use (ICH) (http://www.meddra.org). Also the WHO Programme for International Drug Monitoring   (https://www.who-umc.org/global-pharmacovigilance/global-pharmacovigilance/) currently recommends to use MedDRA. Since coding can be time-consuming and difficult for individual clinicians, this is best done at the national level by staff of the PV centre. Also, the type of SAE (congenital anomaly or birth defect; persistent or significant disability; death; required hospitalization; prolonged hospitalization; life threatening) should be described. Other data to be recorded and reported are a short description of the AE, the onset date of the AE, and clinical action(s) taken (such as (temporary) withdrawal of the drug suspected of having caused the AE, or lowering its dosage, provision of ancillary drugs, or other actions).

At the *national level*, the collected safety data should be compiled to enable programmatic analysis on the indicators. It should be noted that high-quality and regular monitoring and evaluation of data collection is crucial to obtain and maintain high data quality. We advise to involve the national PV centre from the moment that PV data collection is being set up. As collection and analysis of safety data is the core business of the national PV centre, we also recommend that the national PV centre be in charge of this. Alternatively, the safety data should be shared with the national PV centre in real time or at regular intervals (e.g., monthly or quarterly). Note that sharing of SAEs within a short time frame after occurrence (usually 24, 48, or 72 hours) is mandatory in most countries because of legal requirements for reporting these to the national PV centre. Also, collaboration with the PV centre is needed to ensure participation in regular expert committee meetings, in which the reported (S)AEs are reviewed and assessed for potential relationship with any drug used for the treatment of MDR-TB. The result of this causality assessment (the likelihood that the (S)AE is attributable to one or more anti-TB or concomitant

---

[5] Countries may decide to implement the advanced aDSM package with recording and reporting of all AEs of clinical significance. In that case the same information will be recorded for those AEs, including type of AE of clinical significance. Countries are encouraged to also systematically collect data on other adverse events (e.g. adverse events leading to drug or dosage change or discontinuation, adverse events requiring ancillary drugs).

drugs) should be added to the (S)AE report. As stated above, the national PV centre may be responsible for coding of the AEs using the MedDRA. The national PV centre is also responsible for data analysis including the detection of safety signals.

We consider the frequency of SAEs by MDR-TB regimen group, and the frequency of AEs of special interest, by MDR-TB treatment group, as the primary safety indicators [98]. Additional indicators of interest are the frequency of probable adverse drug reactions, by type of drug, the median time to SAE, and the median time to AE of special interest, both by MDR-TB regimen group and the median time to adverse drug reaction by type of drug. Involvement of experts from other disciplines, including the national PV centre and pharmacologists, is required to enable analysis including adverse drug reactions caused by any (or multiple) drugs used for the treatment of MDR-TB. Most countries have a national medicine safety advisory board consisting of highly qualified experts of a range of disciplines that meets at regular intervals to discuss potential safety issues. To keep the reporters (i.e., the health facility staff) motivated, regular feedback reports should be sent to the health facilities reporting.

Data sent to the national PV centre are usually shared with the UMC at *supranational level*. A global aDSM database was developed by the Special Programme for Research and Training in Tropical Diseases in collaboration with WHO [99]. In 2019, data from this database from 658 patients in 26 countries, including several high burden countries, were presented [100]. However, there were no updates after 2019. Thus, the system cannot be used for early warning purposes, as there are (significant) delays in reporting (depending on the country), there is variation in data quality and completeness. Also judgment of the causal relationship between treatment and effect and coding of the AEs vary by country [99], as the latter are not necessarily done by trained PV staff [60].

10.4   aDSM in Practice: Examples from Indonesia and Kyrgyzstan

10.4.1   Indonesia

Endang Lukitosari, Cicilia Gita Parwati, Yusie Permata, Tiar Salman,
Rahma Handari and Edine W. Tiemersma

In *Indonesia* prior to the introduction of bedaquiline, the national PV centre conducted spontaneous reporting only. The number of reports received from health care workers had steadily increased from 137 in 2010 to 345 in 2014 for a population of over 250 million people. In parallel, reporting from pharmaceutical companies was made mandatory in 2010 and rapidly increased from 7 in 2010 to 1871 in 2014. Few reports, however, were received from the TB programme: six in 2013, and 54 in 2014. Most of these concerned dermatological reactions such as rash ($n = 17$) or vomiting and nausea ($n = 21$).

With technical assistance from the WHO and KNCV, the NTP of Indonesia introduced bedaquiline-containing regimens in Indonesia in August 2015. The WHO aDSM guidance document [60] was not yet available, and therefore, CEM was chosen as the standard for PV. To conduct CEM, it was a requirement that all patients be treated in the pilot centre for the full duration of their treatment. As feared when bedaquiline became available for treatment of MDR-TB under programmatic conditions [60], this requirement has been a major obstacle in the rollout of bedaquiline.

Between 1 August 2015 and 1 October 2017, 120 patients who started on bedaquiline-containing regimens were included in CEM, initially in three MDR-TB treatment centres (in May 2016, one, and in October 2016, two additional centres were added). It was anticipated that collection of safety data would require large efforts that the MDR-TB clinicians would not take due to their already high workload. Moreover, in the university hospitals, clinicians-in-training rather than MDR-TB specialists did the routine clinical checkups. Therefore, a PV officer with a medical doctor's or pharmacist's degree was hired for each centre to systematically collect and record safety data. A schematic presentation of the data flow is provided in Fig. 10.1 (left panel). All patients in whom bedaquiline was initiated as part of the MDR or XDR-TB treatment were included in CEM. Initially, all AEs were recorded and reported; by May 2017, the number of AEs had amounted to 746 from 62 patients included in the project at that time (median 8 AEs per patient, IQR: 4–16). There was variation between the types of AEs and the number of AEs reported per patient between centres; this variation was most pronounced for the non-serious AEs. The variation was largely due to differences in treatment regimens and differences in the relationship that PV officers had with the MDR-TB patients.

A major challenge of the programme in Indonesia is the limitation in human resource capacity of the national PV centre. Currently, the centre has eight permanent staff members being responsible for all PV-related activities in Indonesia, including spontaneous reporting, of whom only three have a permanent position. This workload has contributed to delays in the conduct of causality assessments. It is also the main reason for downscaling CEM to only include recording and reporting of SAEs and AEs of special interest in the second half of 2017.

By August 2018, 389 AEs of special interest had been reported, among which were 80 SAEs, but only part of the SAEs had been assessed by the PV centre with the clinical review team for their potential causal relationships with bedaquiline. SAEs have been assessed for 28 of 120 patients; one of the SAE was judged to be related to bedaquiline (probable causal relationship).

In August 2018, of the 120 patients, 32 had completed their bedaquiline-containing treatment, and 22 of these had proof of cure. Thirteen (11%) patients died and one patient was shifted to another regimen because of SAEs judged to be probably related to bedaquiline (QT prolongation, arrhythmia, and torsade de pointes). All deaths were assessed for causal relationship with the treatment; none was found to be due to bedaquiline. Informal feedback to the treating clinician was given directly during the causality assessment meetings, but no written individual feedback reports are being shared. No signals have been observed thus far.

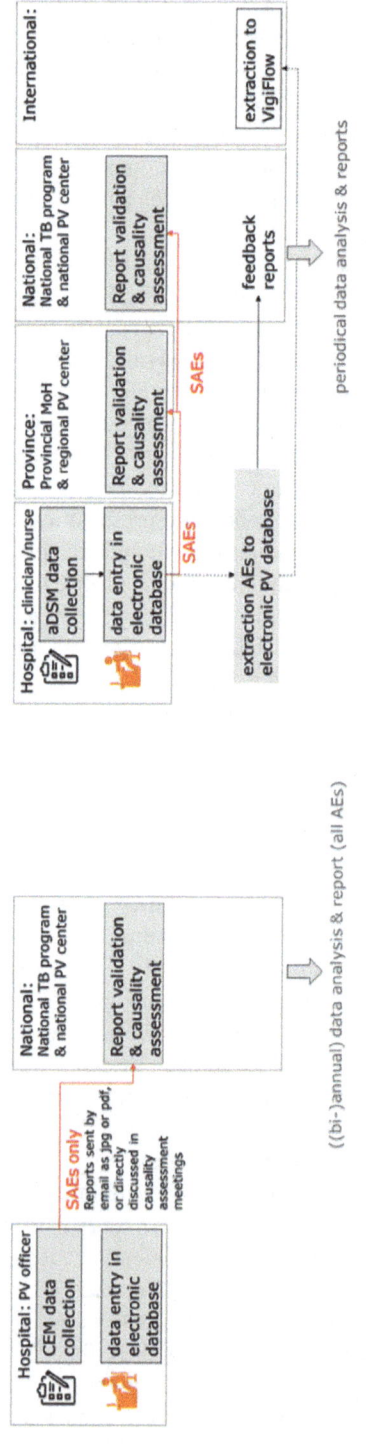

Fig. 10.1 Data flow for pharmacovigilance in Indonesia. Left panel: data flow in the cohort event monitoring project for 100 patients treated in pilot sites introducing new drugs and regimens (2015–2017). Note that data on all AEs were sent to the national pharmacovigilance centre, but only reports of SAEs were validated and assessed for causal relationships by the centre due to understaffing. Right panel: proposed data flow for scaling up to include all sites treating patients with new drugs and regimens (2017). Abbreviations used: aDSM—active drug safety monitoring and management; AE—adverse event; CEM—cohort event monitoring; MoH—Ministry of Health; PV—pharmacovigilance; SAE—serious adverse event; TB—tuberculosis

Because of these challenges, further scaling up of new drugs and regimens is envisioned to include the regional PV authorities. Also, the focus will likely be on SAEs rather than full CEM, thus following the core aDSM package (Fig. 10.1, right panel).

10.4.2 Kyrgyzstan

A. Duishekeeva, M. Sulaimanova, A. Sooronbaeva, G. Dravniece, M. Idrissova, S. van den Hof, A. Kadyrov, Z. Karasartova and B. Myrzaliev

In *Kyrgyzstan*, another country where KNCV has been engaged for PMDT, the national PV centre also only had experience with spontaneous reporting. In 2016, 146 reports of adverse drug reactions were received for a population of six million people. A third of the received reports were related to drugs used for the treatment of TB. The treating physicians recognized the known adverse drug reactions that their patients experienced, and managed these adequately from a clinical point of view. However, awareness about the usefulness of reporting new, unknown adverse drug reactions and clinically well-known but rather rare reactions of well-established drugs not yet described in the summaries of product characteristics was low. Within the scope of the USAID-funded Challenge TB project, KNCV supported programmatic introduction of the shorter treatment regimen (STR) and individualized regimens containing bedaquiline and/or delamanid. One of the key components supported is aDSM. To introduce aDSM, KNCV organized several joint trainings for clinical staff and staff from the PV unit to improve their understanding of PV and processes related to this, including on the detection, management and reporting of AEs and on causality assessment. In addition, KNCV helped arranging the access to monitoring tests required for safe introduction of new drugs and regimens. The reporting form for AEs was adjusted to align with international standards and to make reporting less time-consuming. On the initiative of KNCV, a technical working group on PV was established, with all stakeholders represented. This group facilitated aDSM introduction in the country and collaboration between the NTP and PV centre in conducting aDSM.

Since the start of the project, the number of TB treatment-related AE reports has been steadily rising: from 45 in the first half year of 2017, to 69 in the second half year, and up to 201 in the first half year of 2018. A first joint meeting on causality assessment was held in May 2017, thereby utilizing complementary expertise from clinical and drug safety experts. Since May 2017, causality meetings are organized every quarter. Over the last 18 months, the number of patients newly enrolled on the new drugs and regimens has also increased, but not as steeply as the number of AEs reported: in the first half year of 2017, 69 patients had been initiated on the STR and 127 on individualized regimens with inclusion of bedaquiline, whereas this was 92 and 127 in the first half year of 2018.

10.5　Conclusion

The introduction of new drugs and regimens for the treatment of MDR-TB has come with the requirement of conducting active PV. New guidance for active drug safety monitoring and management has led to the introduction of active PV in the form of aDSM in many low- and middle-income countries. As the capacity regarding PV is low in most of these countries, this requires development of the capacity of TB programmes and PV centres. As this process is still in an early phase, the effects of active PV for TB patients are yet to come.

Acknowledgments The Global Health Bureau, Office of Infectious Disease, US Agency for International Development, financially supported this project through Challenge TB under the terms of Agreement No. AID-OAA-A-14-00029. This project is made possible by the generous support of the American people through the United States Agency for International Development (USAID). The contents are the responsibility of Challenge TB and do not necessarily reflect the views of USAID or the United States Government.

Conflicts of Interest The authors declare that they have no conflicts of interest

References

1. WHO. WHO consolidated guidelines on drug-resistant tuberculosis treatment. Report No: WHO/CDS/TB/2019.7. Geneva: World Health Organization; 2019. Available at: https://apps.who.int/iris/bitstream/handle/10665/311389/9789241550529-eng.pdf?ua=1. Date last accessed: 27 July 2020.
2. WHO treatment guidelines for drug-resistant tuberculosis. 2016 update. Report No.: WHO/HTM/TB/2016.04. Geneva: World Health Organization; 2016. Available at: http://apps.who.int/iris/bitstream/handle/10665/250125/9789241549639-eng.pdf;jsessionid=F86064624275EB8C3DD33D52A0C49F70?sequence=1. Date last accessed: 18 September 2018.
3. WHO. Multidrug and extensively drug-resistant TB (M/XDR-TB): 2010 global report on surveillance and response. Report No.: WHO/HTM/TB/2010.3. Geneva: World Health Organization; 2010. Available at: http://apps.who.int/iris/bitstream/handle/10665/44286/9789241599191_eng.pdf?sequence=1. Date last accessed: 18 Sept 2018.
4. Cox E, Laessig K. FDA approval of bedaquiline--the benefit-risk balance for drug-resistant tuberculosis. N Engl J Med 2014;371(8):689–691.
5. WHO. The use of bedaquiline in the treatment of multidrug-resistant tuberculosis. Interim policy guidance. Report No.: WHO/HTM/TB/2013.6. Geneva: World Health Organization; 2013. Available at: http://apps.who.int/iris/bitstream/handle/10665/84879/9789241505482_eng.pdf?sequence=1. Date last accessed: 18 Sept 2018.
6. WHO. The use of delamanid in the treatment of multidrug-resistant tuberculosis. Interim policy guidance. Report No.: WHO/HTM/TB/2014.23. Geneva: World Health Organization; 2014. http://apps.who.int/iris/bitstream/handle/10665/137334/WHO_HTM_TB_2014.23_eng.pdf?sequence=1. Date last accessed: 18 Sept 2018
7. Diacon AH, Pym A, Grobusch MP, de los Rios JM, Gotuzzo E, Vasilyeva I, et al. Multidrug-resistant tuberculosis and culture conversion with bedaquiline. N Engl J Med. 2014;371(8):723–32.
8. Koch R. The aetiology of tuberculosis. New York: National Tuberculosis Association; 1932.

9. Keshavjee S, Farmer PE. Tuberculosis, drug resistance, and the history of modern medicine. N Engl J Med. 2012;367(10):931–6.
10. Walsh JA, Warren KS. Selective primary health care: an interim strategy for disease control in developing countries. N Engl J Med. 1979;301(18):967–74.
11. WHO. The importance of pharmacovigilance. Safety monitoring of medicinal products. Geneva: World Health Organization; 2002. Available at: https://apps.who.int/iris/bitstream/handle/10665/42493/a75646.pdf?sequence=1&isAllowed=y. Date last accessed: 18 Sept 2018.
12. Tiemersma EW, van der Werf MJ, Borgdorff MW, Williams BG, Nagelkerke NJ. Natural history of tuberculosis: duration and fatality of untreated pulmonary tuberculosis in HIV negative patients: a systematic review. PLoS One. 2011;6(4):e17601.
13. Falzon D, Hill G, Pal SN, Suwankesawong W, Jaramillo E. Pharmacovigilance and tuberculosis: applying the lessons of thioacetazone. Bull World Health Organ. 2014;92(12):918–9.
14. Miller AB, Nunn AJ, Robinson DK, Fox W, Somasundaram PR, Tall R. A second international cooperative investigation into tioacetazone side effects. Bull World Health Organ. 1972;47(2):211–27.
15. Nunn P, Kibuga D, Gathua S, Brindle R, Imalingat A, Wasunna K, et al. Cutaneous hypersensitivity reactions due to thiacetazone in HIV-1 seropositive patients treated for tuberculosis. Lancet. 1991;337(8742):627–30.
16. WHO. Guidelines for tuberculosis treatment in adults and children in national tuberculosis programmes. Report No.: WHO/TB/91.161. Geneva: World Health Organization; 1991. Available at: http://apps.who.int/iris/bitstream/handle/10665/59121/WHO_TB_91.161. pdf?sequence=1&isAllowed=y. Date last accessed: 18 Sept 2018.
17. WHO. Treatment of tuberculosis: guidelines, 4th ed. Report No.: WHO/HTM/TB/2009.420. Geneva: World Health Organization; 2010. Available at: http://apps.who.int/iris/bitstream/handle/10665/44165/9789241547833_eng.pdf?sequence=1. Date last accessed: 18 Sept 2018.
18. Moberg CL. Rene Dubos: a harbinger of microbial resistance to antibiotics. Microb Drug Resist. 1996;2(3):287–97.
19. Manten A, Van Wijngaarden LJ. Development of drug resistance to rifampicin. Chemotherapy. 1969;14(2):93–100.
20. Fox W, Ellard GA, Mitchison DA. Studies on the treatment of tuberculosis undertaken by the British Medical Research Council tuberculosis units, 1946-1986, with relevant subsequent publications. Int J Tuberc Lung Dis. 1999;3(10 Suppl 2):S231–79.
21. Frieden TR, Fujiwara PI, Washko RM, Hamburg MA. Tuberculosis in New York City–turning the tide. N Engl J Med. 1995;333(4):229–33.
22. Wu S, Zhang Y, Sun F, Chen M, Zhou L, Wang N, et al. Adverse events associated with the treatment of multidrug-resistant tuberculosis: a systematic review and meta-analysis. Am J Ther. 2016;23(2):e521–30.
23. Seddon JA, Godfrey-Faussett P, Jacobs K, Ebrahim A, Hesseling AC, Schaaf HS. Hearing loss in patients on treatment for drug-resistant tuberculosis. Eur Respir J. 2012;40(5):1277–86.
24. Seddon JA, Thee S, Jacobs K, Ebrahim A, Hesseling AC, Schaaf HS. Hearing loss in children treated for multidrug-resistant tuberculosis. J Infect. 2013;66(4):320–9.
25. Behera C, Krishna K, Singh HR. Antitubercular drug-induced violent suicide of a hospitalised patient. BMJ Case Rep. 2014;2014:bcr2013201469.
26. Agyeman AA, Ofori-Asenso R. Efficacy and safety profile of linezolid in the treatment of multidrug-resistant (MDR) and extensively drug-resistant (XDR) tuberculosis: a systematic review and meta-analysis. Ann Clin Microbiol Antimicrob. 2016;15(1):41.
27. Tupasi TE, Garfin AM, Kurbatova EV, Mangan JM, Orillaza-Chi R, Naval LC, et al. Factors associated with loss to follow-up during treatment for multidrug-resistant tuberculosis, The Philippines, 2012–2014. Emerg Infect Dis. 2016;22(3):491–502.
28. Shringarpure KS, Isaakidis P, Sagili KD, Baxi RK, Das M, Daftary A. "When treatment is more challenging than the disease": a qualitative study of MDR-TB patient retention. PLoS One. 2016;11(3):e0150849.

29. Temple B, Ayakaka I, Ogwang S, Nabanjja H, Kayes S, Nakubulwa S, et al. Rate and amplification of drug resistance among previously-treated patients with tuberculosis in Kampala. Uganda Clin Infect Dis. 2008;47(9):1126–34.

30. Shin SS, Keshavjee S, Gelmanova IY, Atwood S, Franke MF, Mishustin SP, et al. Development of extensively drug-resistant tuberculosis during multidrug-resistant tuberculosis treatment. Am J Respir Crit Care Med. 2010;182(3):426–32.

31. WHO. Guidelines for the programmatic management of drug-resistant tuberculosis – 2011 update. Report No.: WHO/HTM/TB/2011.6. Geneva: World Health Organization; 2011. Available at: http://apps.who.int/iris/bitstream/handle/10665/44597/9789241501583_eng.pdf?sequence=1. Date last accessed: 18 Sept 2018.

32. Mafukidze A, Harausz E, Furin J. An update on repurposed medications for the treatment of drug-resistant tuberculosis. Expert Rev Clin Pharmacol. 2016:1–10.

33. Tang S, Yao L, Hao X, Liu Y, Zeng L, Liu G, et al. Clofazimine for the treatment of multidrug-resistant tuberculosis: prospective, multicenter, randomized controlled study in China. Clin Infect Dis. 2015;60(9):1361–7.

34. Borisov SE, Dheda K, Enwerem M, Romero Leyet R, D'Ambrosio L, Centis R, et al. Effectiveness and safety of bedaquiline-containing regimens in the treatment of MDR- and XDR-TB: a multicentre study. Eur Respir J. 2017;49(5):1700387.

35. Pym AS, Diacon AH, Tang SJ, Conradie F, Danilovits M, Chuchottaworn C, et al. Bedaquiline in the treatment of multidrug- and extensively drug-resistant tuberculosis. Eur Respir J. 2016;47(2):564–74.

36. Guglielmetti L, Jaspard M, Le Du D, Lachatre M, Marigot-Outtandy D, Bernard C, et al. Long-term outcome and safety of prolonged bedaquiline treatment for multidrug-resistant tuberculosis. Eur Respir J. 2017;49(3):1601799.

37. Guglielmetti L, Le Du D, Jachym M, Henry B, Martin D, Caumes E, et al. Compassionate use of bedaquiline for the treatment of multidrug-resistant and extensively drug-resistant tuberculosis: interim analysis of a French cohort. Clin Infect Dis. 2015;60(2):188–94.

38. Ndjeka N, Conradie F, Schnippel K, Hughes J, Bantubani N, Ferreira H, et al. Treatment of drug-resistant tuberculosis with bedaquiline in a high HIV prevalence setting: an interim cohort analysis. Int J Tuberc Lung Dis. 2015;19(8):979–85.

39. Ferlazzo G, Mohr E, Laxmeshwar C, Hewison C, Hughes J, Jonckheere S, et al. Early safety and efficacy of the combination of bedaquiline and delamanid for the treatment of patients with drug-resistant tuberculosis in Armenia, India, and South Africa: a retrospective cohort study. Lancet Infect Dis. 2018;18(5):536–44.

40. Guyatt GH, Oxman AD, Vist GE, Kunz R, Falck-Ytter Y, Alonso-Coello P, et al. GRADE: an emerging consensus on rating quality of evidence and strength of recommendations. BMJ. 2008;336(7650):924–6.

41. WHO consolidated guidelines on tuberculosis. Module 5: management of tuberculosis in children and adolescents. Geneva: World Health Organization; 2022. Licence: CC BY-NC-SA 3.0 IGO. Available via https://www.who.int/publications/i/item/9789240046764. Date last accessed: 6 Jan 2023.

42. Skripconoka V, Danilovits M, Pehme L, Tomson T, Skenders G, Kummik T, et al. Delamanid improves outcomes and reduces mortality in multidrug-resistant tuberculosis. Eur Respir J. 2013;41(6):1393–400.

43. Gler MT, Skripconoka V, Sanchez-Garavito E, Xiao H, Cabrera-Rivero JL, Vargas-Vasquez DE, et al. Delamanid for multidrug-resistant pulmonary tuberculosis. N Engl J Med. 2012;366(23):2151–60.

44. Nasiri MJ, Zangjabadian M, Arabpour E, Amini S, Khalili F, Centis R, et al. Delamanid-containing regimens and multidrug-resistant tuberculosis: a systematic review and meta-analysis. Int J Infect Dis. 2022;124(Suppl 1):S90–103.

45. Von Groote-Bidlingmaier F, Patientia R, Sanchez E, Balanag V Jr, Ticona E, Segura P, et al. Efficacy and safety of delamanid in combination with an optimised background regimen for treatment of multidrug-resistant tuberculosis: a multicentre, randomised, double-blind, placebo-controlled, parallel group phase 3 trial. Lancet Resp Med. 2019;7(3):249–59.

46. Dooley KE, Rosenkranz SL, Conradie F, Moran L, Hafner R, Von Groote-Bidlingmaier F, et al. QT effects of bedaquiline, delamanid or both in patients with rifampicin-resistant-TB: a randomized controlled trial. Lancet Inf Dis. 2021;21(7):975–83.
47. Garcia-Prats AJ, Frias M, Van der Laan L, De Leon A, Gler MT, Schaaf HS, et al. Delamanid added to an optimized background regimen in children with multidrug-resistant tuberculosis: Results of a phase I/II clinical trial. Antimicrob Agents Chemother. 2022;66(5):e0214421.
48. Mallikaarjun S, Wells C, Petersen C, Paccaly A, Shoaf SE, Patil S, et al. Delamanid coadministered with antiretroviral drugs or antituberculosis drugs shows no clinically relevant drug-drug interactions in healthy subjects. Antimicrob Agents Chemother. 2016;60(10):5976–85.
49. Conradie F, Diacon AH, Ngubane N, Howell P, Everitt D, Crook AM, et al. Treatment of highly drug-resistant pulmonary tuberculosis. N Engl J Med. 2020;382(10):893–902.
50. Conradie F, Bagdasaryan TR, Borisov S, Howell P, Mikiashvili L, Ngubane N, et al. Bedaquiline-pretomanid-linezolid regimens for drug-resistant tuberculosis. N Engl J Med. 2022;387(9):810–23.
51. Nyang'wa BT, Berry C, Kazounis E, Motta I, Parpieva N, Tigay Z, et al. A 24-week, all-oral regimen for rifampicin-resistant tuberculosis. N Engl J Med. 2022;387(25):2331–43.
52. Das M, Dalal A, Laxmeshwar C, Ravi S, Mamnoon F, Meneguim AC, et al. One step forward: successful end-of-treatment outcomes of patients with drug-resistant tuberculosis who received concomitant bedaquiline and delamanid in Mumbai. India Clin Infect Dis. 2021;73(9):e3496–504.
53. Padmapriyadarsini C, Vohra V, Bhatnagar A, Solanki R, Sridhar R, Anande L, et al. Bedaquiline, delamanid, linezolid and clofazimine for treatment of pre-extensively drug-resistant tuberculosis. Clin Infect Dis. 2022:ciac528.
54. Pontali E, Sotgiu G, Tiberi S, Tadolini M, Visca D, D'Ambrosio L, et al. Combined treatment of drug-resistant tuberculosis with bedaquiline and delamanid: a systematic review. Eur Respir J. 2018;52(1):1800934.
55. Holmgaard FB, Guglielmetti L, Lillebaek T, Andersen AB, Wejse C, Dahl VN. Efficacy and tolerability of concomitant use of bedaquiline and delamanid for multidrug- and extensively drug-resistant tuberculosis: a systematic review and meta-analysis. Clin Infect Dis. 2022;76:ciac876.
56. Gualano G, Capone S, Matteelli A, Palmieri F. New Antituberculosis Drugs: From Clinical Trial to Programmatic Use. Infect Dis Rep. 2016;8(2):6569.
57. WHO. Guidelines for the programmatic management of drug-resistant tuberculosis. Report No.: WHO/HTM/TB/2006.361. Geneva: World Health Organization; 2006. Available at: http://apps.who.int/iris/bitstream/handle/10665/246249/978?sequence=2. Date last accessed: 18 Sept 2018.
58. WHO. Active TB drug-safety monitoring and management (aDSM). Framework for implementation. Report No.: WHO/HTM/TB/2015.28. Geneva: World Health Organization; 2015. Available at: http://apps.who.int/iris/bitstream/handle/10665/204465/WHO_HTM_TB_2015.28_eng.pdf?sequence=1. Date last accessed: 18 September 2018.
59. WHO consolidated guidelines on tuberculosis. Module 4: treatment – drug-resistant tuberculosis treatment. Geneva: World Health Organization; 2020. Licence: CC BY-NC-SA 3.0 IGO. Available via https://www.who.int/publications/i/item/9789240007048. Date last accessed: 6 Jan 2023.
60. WHO. Active TB drug-safety monitoring and management (aDSM). Framework for implementation. Report No.: WHO/HTM/TB/2015.28. Geneva: World Health Organization; 2015. Available at: http://apps.who.int/iris/bitstream/handle/10665/204465/WHO_HTM_TB_2015.28_eng.pdf?sequence=1. Date last accessed: 18 Sept 2018.
61. WHO. A practical handbook on the pharmacovigilance of medicines use in the treatment of tuberculosis. Enhancing the safety of the TB patient. Geneva: World Health Organization; 2012. Available at: https://www.who.int/medicines/publications/Pharmaco_TB_web_v3.pdf?ua=1&ua=1. Date last accessed: 18 Sept 2018.

62. Bloss E, Kuksa L, Holtz TH, Riekstina V, Skripconoka V, Kammerer S, et al. Adverse events related to multidrug-resistant tuberculosis treatment, Latvia, 2000–2004. Int J Tuberc Lung Dis. 2010;14(3):275–81.
63. Akshata JS, Chakrabarthy A, Swapna R, Buggi S, Somashekar M. Adverse drug reactions in management of multi drug resistant tuberculosis, in tertiary chest institute. J Tuberc Res. 2015;3:27–33.
64. Keshavjee S, Gelmanova IY, Farmer PE, Mishustin SP, Strelis AK, Andreev YG, et al. Treatment of extensively drug-resistant tuberculosis in Tomsk, Russia: a retrospective cohort study. Lancet. 2008;372(9647):1403–9.
65. Strengthening Pharmaceutical Systems (SPS) Program. Safety of medicines in Sub-Saharan Africa: assessment of pharmacovigilance systems and their performance. Submitted to the US Agency for International Development by the SPS Program. Arlington, Virginia: Management Sciences for Health; 2011. Available at: https://www.msh.org/sites/msh.org/files/Safety-of-Medicines-in-SSA.pdf. Date last accessed: 18 Sept 2018.
66. Maher D, Raviglione MC. Why is a recording and reporting system needed, and what system is recommended? In: Frieden TR, editor. Toman's tuberculosis. 2nd ed. Geneva: World Health Organization; 2004. p. 270–3. Available at: http://apps.who.int/iris/bitstream/handle/10665/42701/9241546034.pdf?sequence=1. Date last accessed: 18 Sept 2018.
67. TBCARE I. International Standards for Tuberculosis Care. 3rd ed. The Hague: TBCARE I; 2014. Available at: http://www.who.int/tb/publications/ISTC_3rdEd.pdf?ua=1. Date last accessed: 18 Sept 2018.
68. WHO. Companion handbook to the WHO guidelines for the programmatic management of drug-resistant tuberculosis. Report No.: WHO/HTM/TB/2014.11. Geneva: World Health Organization; 2014. Available at: http://apps.who.int/iris/bitstream/handle/10665/130918/9789241548809_eng.pdf?sequence=1. Date last accessed: 18 Sept 2018.
69. Pal SN, Duncombe C, Falzon D, Olsson S. WHO strategy for collecting safety data in public health programmes: complementing spontaneous reporting systems. Drug Saf. 2013;36(2):75–81.
70. Hughes J, Solans B, Draper HR, Schaaf HS, Winckler JL, Van der Laan L, et al. Pharmacokinetics and safety of bedaquiline in human immunodeficiency virus (HIV)-positive and negative older children and adolescents with rifampicin-resistant tuberculosis. Clin Infect Dis. 2022;75(10):1772–80.
71. McIlleron H, Abdel-Rahman S, Dave JA, Blockman M, Owen A. Special populations and pharmacogenetic issues in tuberculosis drug development and clinical research. J Infect Dis. 2015;211(Suppl 3):S115–25.
72. Diacon AH, Pym A, Grobusch M, Patientia R, Rustomjee R, Page-Shipp L, et al. The diarylquinoline TMC207 for multidrug-resistant tuberculosis. N Engl J Med. 2009;360(23):2397.
73. WHO. Global tuberculosis report 2016. Report No.: WHO/HTM/TB/2016.13.Geneva: World Health Organization; 2016. Available at: http://apps.who.int/medicinedocs/documents/s23098en/s23098en.pdf. Date last accessed: 18 Sept 2018.
74. Kelly AM, Smith B, Luo Z, Given B, Wehrwein T, Master I, et al. Discordance between patient and clinician reports of adverse reactions to MDR-TB treatment. Int J Tuberc Lung Dis. 2016;20(4):442–7.
75. WHO. Global tuberculosis report 2022. Licence: CC BY-NC-SA 3.0 IGO Geneva: World Health Organization; 2022. Available via: https://www.who.int/teams/global-tuberculosis-programme/tb-reports/global-tuberculosis-report-2022. Date last accessed: 6 Jan 2023.
76. Pozo-Martin F, Nove A, Lopes SC, Campbell J, Buchan J, Dussault G, et al. Health workforce metrics pre- and post-2015: a stimulus to public policy and planning. Hum Resour Health. 2017;15(1):14.
77. Singh A, Bhatt P. Comparative evaluation of adverse drug reaction reporting forms for introduction of a spontaneous generic ADR form. J Pharmacol Pharmacother. 2012;3(3):228–32.
78. Hazell L, Shakir SA. Under-reporting of adverse drug reactions: a systematic review. Drug Saf. 2006;29(5):385–96.

79. Jakasania A, Shringarpure K, Kapadia D, Sharma R, Mehta K, Prajapati A, Kathirvel S. "Side effects – part of the package": a mixed methods approach to study adverse events among patients being programmatically treated for DR-TB in Gujarat, India. BMC Inf Dis. 2020;20(1):918.
80. Krishnappa L, Gadicherla S, Chidambaram P, Anuradha HV, Somanna SN, Naik PR, et al. 'Have we missed reporting adverse drug reactions under Revised National TB Control Programme?' – a mixed method study in Bengaluru, India. Indian J Tuberc. 2020;67(1):20–8.
81. Krasniqi S, Neziri B, Jakupi A, Shurdhaj I, Daci A, Jupolli-Krasniqi N, Pira M. Tuberculosis drug safety and pharmacovigilance in health system of Kosova: a cross-sectional analysis. Pharmacoepidemiol Drug Saf. 2020;29(9):1037–45.
82. WHO. Minimum requirements for a functional pharmacovigilance system. Geneva: World Health Organization; 2010. Available at: http://www.who.int/medicines/areas/quality_safety/safety_efficacy/PV_Minimum_Requirements_2010_2.pdf. Date last accessed: 18 Sept 2018.
83. Systems for Improved Access to Pharmaceuticals and Services (SIAPS) Program. Comparative analysis of pharmacovigilance systems in five Asian countries. Submitted to the US Agency for International Development by the SIAPS. Arlington, Virginia: Management Sciences for Health; 2013. Available at: http://siapsprogram.org/wp-content/uploads/2014/02/Asia-PV-report.pdf. Date last accessed: 18 September 2018.
84. Kiguba R, Olsson S, Waitt C. Pharmacovigilance in low- and middle-income countries: a review with particular focus on Africa. Br J Clin Pharmacol. 2022:1–19.
85. Furin JJ, Mitnick CD, Shin SS, Bayona J, Becerra MC, Singler JM, et al. Occurrence of serious adverse effects in patients receiving community-based therapy for multidrug-resistant tuberculosis. Int J Tuberc Lung Dis. 2001;5(7):648–55.
86. Carroll MW, Lee M, Cai Y, Hallahan CW, Shaw PA, Min JH, et al. Frequency of adverse reactions to first- and second-line anti-tuberculosis chemotherapy in a Korean cohort. Int J Tuberc Lung Dis. 2012;16(7):961–6.
87. Nathanson E, Gupta R, Huamani P, Leimane V, Pasechnikov AD, Tupasi TE, et al. Adverse events in the treatment of multidrug-resistant tuberculosis: results from the DOTS-Plus initiative. Int J Tuberc Lung Dis. 2004;8(11):1382–4.
88. Avong YK, Isaakidis P, Hinderaker SG, Van den Bergh R, Ali E, Obembe BO, et al. Doing no harm? Adverse events in a nation-wide cohort of patients with multidrug-resistant tuberculosis in Nigeria. PLoS One. 2015;10(3):e0120161.
89. Ahmad N, Javaid A, Syed Sulaiman SA, Afridi AK, Zainab, Khan AH. Occurrence, management, and risk factors for adverse drug reactions in multidrug resistant tuberculosis patients. Am J Ther. 2018;25(5):e533–40.
90. Sagwa EL, Ruswa N, Mavhunga F, Rennie T, Leufkens HG, Mantel-Teeuwisse AK. Comparing amikacin and kanamycin-induced hearing loss in multidrug-resistant tuberculosis treatment under programmatic conditions in a Namibian retrospective cohort. BMC Pharmacol Toxicol. 2015;16:36.
91. Schnippel K, Berhanu RH, Black A, Firnhaber C, Maitisa N, Evans D, et al. Severe adverse events during second-line tuberculosis treatment in the context of high HIV co-infection in South Africa: a retrospective cohort study. BMC Infect Dis. 2016;16(1):593.
92. Ngoc NB, Dinh VH, Thuy NT, Quang DV, Huyen CTT, Hoa NM, et al. Active surveillance for adverse events in patients on longer treatment regimens for multidrug-resistant tuberculosis in Viet Nam. PLoS One. 2021;16(9):e0255357.
93. Atif M, Ahmed W, Iqbal MN, Ahmad N, Ahmad W, Malik I, Al-Worafi YM. Frequency and factors associated with adverse events among multi-drug resistant tuberculosis patients in Pakistan: a retrospective study. Front Med. 2022;8:790718.
94. Trubnikov A, Hovhannesyan A, Akopyan K, Ciobanu A, Sadirova D, Kalandarova L, et al. Effectiveness and safety of a shorter treatment regimen in a setting with a high burden of multidrug-resistant tuberculosis. Int J Environ Res Public Health. 2021;18(8):4121.

95. KNCV Tuberulosis Foundation for ChallengeTB. Generic programmatic and clinical guide for introduction of new drugs and shorter regimens for treatment of multi/extensively drug resistant tuberculosis. The Hague: KNCV Tuberculosis Foundation; 2017. Available at: https://www.challengetb.org/publications/tools/pmdt/Generic_programmatic_and_clinical_guide_for_the_introduction_of_new_drugs_and_shorter_regimens.pdf. Date last accessed: 18 Sept 2018.

96. WHO consolidated guidelines on tuberculosis. Module 3: diagnosis: rapid diagnostics for tuberculosis detection, 2021 update. Geneva: World Health Organization; 2021. Licence: CC BY-NC-SA 3.0 IGO. Available via https://www.who.int/publications/i/item/9789240029415. Date last accessed: 6 Jan 2023.

97. Tiemersma E, Van den Hof S, Dravniece G, Wares D, Molla Y, Permata Y, et al. Integration of drug safety monitoring in tuberculosis treatment programs: country experiences. Eur Resp Rev. 2019;28(153):180115.

98. WHO. Inter-regional workshop on pharmacovigilance for new drugs and novel regimens for the treatment of drug-resistant tuberculosis. Meeting report, 12–14 November 2014, Hanoi, Vietnam. Report No: WHO/HTM/TB/201507 Geneva: World Health Organization; 2015 Available at: http://wwwwhoint/tb/challenges/meeting_report_pv_workshop_hanoi_2014pdf. Date last accessed: 18 Sept 2018.

99. Halleux CM, Falzon D, Merle C, Jaramillo E, Mirzayev F, Olliaro P, et al. The World Health Organization global aDSM database: generating evidence on the safety of new treatment regimens for drug-resistant tuberculosis. Eur Resp J. 2018;51(3):1701643.

100. Borisov S, Danila E, Maryandyshev A, Dalcolmo M, Miliauskas S, Kuksa L, et al. Surveillance of adverse events in the treatment of drug-resistant tuberculosis: first global report. Eur Resp J. 2019;54:1901522.

Chapter 11
The Public Health Issue of Falsified and Substandard Medicines in Resource-Limited Settings

Céline Caillet and Paul N. Newton

11.1 Introduction

Although the problem of substandard and falsified medical products has probably been with us since the beginning of the trade in medicines, there has been a seemingly recent increase in their frequency on the global pharmaceutical market. The problem is not limited to lower-resources countries, but it appears to be of greater scale there than in wealthier countries. In wealthy countries, it is likely that those with fewer financial resources suffer disproportionately from this problem.

Poor-quality medical products are categorized by the World Health Organization (WHO) since 2017 as falsified and substandard (SF) [1]. Falsified (aka fake) medicines are the result of criminal activity. They purport to be genuine, authorized medicines, but they 'deliberately/fraudulently misrepresent their identity, composition or source.' Copies of packaging of a genuine product is a common feature. Falsified medicines may contain the correct active pharmaceutical ingredients (but usually the wrong amount), incorrect active pharmaceutical ingredients (API) or, more commonly, they may contain no API at all. There has been lots of controversies around the term 'counterfeit' that, when used technically, refers to trademark infringement, rather than public health violation. It is increasingly replaced by the term 'falsified medicines', which takes into account the public health issue of SF

C. Caillet (✉) · P. N. Newton
Medicine Quality Research Group, Centre for Tropical Medicine and Global Health, Nuffield Department of Medicine, University of Oxford, Oxford, UK

Infectious Diseases Data Observatory, University of Oxford, Oxford, UK

Lao-Oxford-Mahosot Hospital-Wellcome Trust Research Unit, Microbiology Laboratory, Mahosot Hospital, Vientiane, Lao People's Democratic Republic

Centre for Tropical Medicine and Global Health, Nuffield Department of Medicine, University of Oxford, Oxford, UK
e-mail: Celine.caillet@ndm.ox.ac.uk

© Springer Nature Singapore Pte Ltd. 2025
S. R. Ahmad (ed.), *Special Issues in Pharmacovigilance in Resource-Limited Countries*, https://doi.org/10.1007/978-981-96-6154-1_11

medicines, rather than intellectual property aspects [2]. The term makes it clear that the consequences on people are far more serious than buying fake shoes or watches. Substandard medicines, on the other hand, result from errors and/or negligence during the manufacturing of the products. They are defined as 'authorized medical products that fail to meet either their quality standards or their specifications, or both' [1]. The WHO definition also includes degraded medicines within the substandard category and are medicines that left the factory good quality but deteriorate in the supply chain due to improper storage, such as without refrigeration in hot climates. It can be difficult to distinguish degraded medicines from those which left the factory as substandard. Inspection of the packaging is required to determine whether a medicine is falsified, but this is not always performed. In many reports, it is thus unclear whether the tested medicines are falsified, or are substandard resulting from errors in manufacturing or in supply chains. However, as corrective and regulatory actions vary according to the type of 'defect', understanding the differences is essential. Confusing SF medical products with generic medicines is dangerous for public health, as these latter play a substantial role in making medicines accessible. Their affordability has been essential in many health programmes globally.

Analysis of risks for substandard and falsified medicines suggests that cost cutting of production to ensure profit is a key driver of the former and medicine shortages and medicine expense key drivers of the latter [3]. However, it is not only expensive medicines that are falsified. Relatively inexpensive anti-infectives such as the antimalarials chloroquine and artemisinin derivatives, or the widely used antibiotic amoxicillin are also falsified. The high demand and economy of scale of these medicines presumably gives criminals significant profit. Many medicines regulatory agencies have limited capacities, in terms of technical resources and funding. There is often infrequent legislation and enforcement, corruption, inadequate penalties, and low awareness of SF medicines among the population and healthcare professionals. All these factors contribute to the current dire situation. During the COVID-19 pandemic, impaired access to medicines; shutdown of land, sea, and air transports; and limited access to disrupted health services within countries contributed to a surge of SF issues [4].

Few low- and middle- income countries (LMICs) have medicines regulatory authorities with adequate capacities. This makes it difficult for national authorities to investigate and to act when SF medical products are found. Researchers have only recently started to investigate this issue, and unfortunately most of those who have looked have found falsified and substandard medicines. Given the poor health consequences for patients and the community, the issue of SF medical products has been described as a 'pandemic'. There has been increased interest in pharmacovigilance in LMICs over the last decade, and such enhanced systems will be important for preventing, detecting, and responding to SF medicines [1].

11.2   The Problem of Poor-Quality Medicines

11.2.1   Short History

The quality of medicines has been a problem since the start of the trade in medicines in antiquity. The detection of drug adulteration performed by organoleptic tests was described by classical writers such as Pedanius Dioscorides. This first-century Greek physician, botanist, and pharmacologist described using characteristics of taste, colour, odour, and feel [5] in his book *De Materia Medica* to evaluate medicines. He described various types of adulteration, especially for plants not grown locally. Herbal products have a long history of being adulterated. In the seventeenth century, Peruvian Cinchona barks—from which quinine, the first effective treatment of malaria, is extracted—were widely marketed in Europe but were adulterated on a large scale with other barks [6, 7]. Congeners were also used to adulterate *Valeriana officinalis* root used for treating cholera [7]. Two centuries later, poor-quality quinine remedies were repeatedly reported, with adulteration by substances such as salicilin [8]—a compound closely related to acetylsalicylic acid, starch, the useless and less expensive Gentianae or spermaceti [9]. Given this widespread adulteration of early industrialized 'modern' medicine, the first regulation of the importation of medicines and guides on the detection of falsified medicines appeared in Europe and the USA in the mid-nineteenth century, building on earlier systems in the Middle East [7]. Later, in the early twentieth century, anti-tuberculous remedies were accused of being 'mixtures of inert drugs' or 'made of cocaine, opium, hasheesh and cheap whisky' [10]. Elixirs of sulfanilamide containing diethylene glycol in the 1930s, resulted in the death of many people in the USA [11], and led to the strengthening of the US Food and DDrugs Administration (FDA).

Despite this history, the World Health Assembly adopted a resolution to address the issue of counterfeit and substandard pharmaceuticals only in 1988 [12].

11.2.2   Epidemiology: A Paucity of Trustworthy Evidence

The extent of the problem of SF medicines is uncertain with scarce and poor-quality data [13]. However, the burgeoning literature over the last few decades suggests that there is a significant increasing issue. The number of articles published on SF medicines in Pubmed using relevant keywords almost tripled between 2010 (263 articles) and 2021 (755 articles). More and more pharmacological classes and geographic regions have been described as affected, as illustrated by findings on erectile dysfunction medicines in Europe [14], anticancer medicines in the USA [15, 16] and Vietnam [17], cardiovascular [18] and antiepileptic [19] medicines in sub-Saharan Africa, and emergency contraceptives in Nigeria and Peru [20, 21].

In 2006, the International Medical Products Anti-counterfeiting Task (IMPACT) force gave a global estimate of 10% of the global supply being falsified and suggested that '*many developing countries of Africa, parts of Asia, and parts of Latin America have areas where more than 30% of the medicines on sale can be counterfeit. Other developing markets, however, have less than 10%; overall, a reasonable estimate is between 10 and 30%*' [22]. However, the evidence base supporting these estimates was poor.

A decade later, a review of the scientific literature by the WHO, of papers published between 2007 and 2017, estimated that ~10.5% and 10.6% of medical products circulating in low- and middle-income countries, respectively, were either substandard or falsified. This estimate was based on the analysis of 48,218 samples collected in 88 WHO Member States. Another review including 96 studies published in five scientific databases until November 2017, including testing of more than 50 samples of essential medicines, showed an overall proportion of samples failing of 13.6% [23]. More than a decade after the first estimate by IMPACT, these estimates should still be cautiously interpreted because of methodological flaws of the included studies.

Estimations of the prevalence of SF medicines suffer from other important limitations such as the large unpublished inaccessible 'grey' literature held by medicines regulatory authorities (MRAs) and the pharmaceutical industry, the lack of standardization of reporting, the variable techniques used to assess the quality, and the diverse definitions used.

Considering the large extent of the global pharmaceutical industry and ill health, as 'little' as 1% of SF medicines is unacceptable, potentially implying millions of casualties. In addition to increasing reports or field surveys on the quality of medicines in the scientific literature, there has also been a large increase in lay literature reports. There were, as an illustration, 58 cases of seizures/incidents/thefts/recalls of SF medicines reported in more than 30 countries in Google (French and English searches) and some websites such as the IRACM just between July and December 2015 (Table 11.1). In these 6 months, medicine regulatory authorities seized from several boxes to tons of putative SF medicines.

The Medicine Quality Monitoring Globe, which was made publicly available in March 2020, includes data describing a wide range of incidents related to the quality of medical products globally, retrieved from online newspapers (GoogleNews searches) in multiple languages, with viewable on-screen results in French, English, Spanish, Vietnamese, and Mandarin (Fig. 11.1). Since 2022, an additional feature added to the Globe allows users a direct access to webpages of recalls/alerts on SF medical products from MRA.

Just before the pandemic, between just October 1 and December 31, 2019, the Globe captured events that occurred in 329 locations around the world. During the COVID-19 pandemic, up to March 2022, the Globe captured 1028 relevant articles on quality problems with COVID-19 medical products in the English language lay press alone. Examples of issues identified were substandard COVID-19 test kits giving false results in Ireland; falsified vaccines containing only saline solution in India, China, and Singapore; unregistered medicines (that often had not proven

Table 11.1 Examples of the issues: reports of incidents related to the quality of medicines available in the lay literature between July and December 2015

Country	Seizure/theft/recall/diversion	Type of medicines	Source
Algeria	Seizure of 766 boxes of medicines	Not specified	L'Expression- Le Quotidien (1)
Angola	Seizure of 11,000 kg of medicines	Antimalarials, antibiotics, sexual stimulants and anabolic steroids	AllAfrica (2)
Argentina	Recall of one medicine	Antiseptic for topical application	Anmat - Ministerio de Salud Presidencia de la Nation (3)
Bangladesh	Seizure of five trucks of adulterated medicines valued at Tk5 crore	Not specified	Dhaka Tribune (4)
Belgium	Increase by 60% of seizures compared to 2014	Erectile dysfunction medicines, antibiotics, weight loss supplements	RTL Info (5)
Brazil	Theft of $3 m-worth of pharmaceutical from a warehouse	Not specified	Securing Industry (6)
Cameroon	Seizure of 5 tons of medicines (value of 20 millions of francs CFA = about 34,000 USD)	Not specified	StarAfrica (7)
	Seizure, unknown number of medicines	Not specified	StarAfrica (8)
Canada	Seizure of 2 millions of tablets	Anxiolytic medicine (alprazolam)	Ici Radio Canada (9)
China	Seizure of 20,000 boxes of medicines and several tons of raw products (value of 100 million yuan = about 16.1 million US dollars)	Weight loss and analgesics	Xinhuanet.com (10)
	Seizure of 7000 kg of medicines (value of 150 million yuan = about 23.5 million US dollars)	Veterinary medicines	Shangai Daily (11)
	Seizure of 900,000 of medicines (value of more than 1 million yuan = about 160,000 USD)	Erectile dysfunction medicines	ECNS (12)
	Seizure of 1.5 million of erectile dysfunction medicines and thousands of antibiotics	Erectile dysfunction medicines and antibiotics	SCMP (13)

(continued)

Table 11.1 (continued)

Country	Seizure/theft/recall/diversion	Type of medicines	Source
Colombia	Seizure of 600 products	Cardiovascular medicines, antibiotics…	IRACM (14)
	Seizure of 2000 vials, 500 capsules, 500 ointment tubes, 4000 tablets and 2000 capsules, 400 drug labels and leaflets (worth 1 billion Colombian pesos = about 315,300 USD)	Not specified	Entorno Inteligente (15)
	Dismantling of a gang selling poor-quality medicines (worth 3 billion pesos = about 1 million USD)	Not specified	IRACM (16)
	Seizure of 2 tons of medicines	Various medicines including antiretrovirals	IRACM (17)
Democratic Republic of Congo	Expired medicines circulating on the market	Antimalarial, antibiotics and medicines for cough	IRACM (18)
	Alert, two falsified medicines	Antibiotics	E-med discussion forum November 3, 2015
Costa Rica	Alert by Ministry of Health	Medicine for general anaesthesia	Ministerio De Salud Republica de Costa Rica (19)
Dominican Republic	Dismantling of an international network, 40,000 kg of medicines seized	Analgesics (including opioids) and cardiovascular medicines	IRACM (20)
	Dismantling of a criminal organization	Not specified	IRACM (21)
	Recall of 22 batches of falsified medicines	Analgesics, antibiotics, anti-inflammatory, sexual stimulants and condoms	Ministerio De Salud Publica (22)
Dubai	Alert, one medicine	Drug supplement (marketed for the treatment of erectile dysfunction, diabetes and hypertension)	Gulf Today (23)
Ecuador	Seizure, one medicine, unknown number of medicines	Treatment for joint pain	IRACM (24)
France	Seizure of 1000 products	Sexual enhancement products	Le Dauphin (25)
Ghana	Alert, two batches of a medicine	Medicine for the treatment of worm infestation	FDA Ghana (26)
	Dismantling of a network selling falsified medicines	Antimalarials and other anti-infectives, one syrup for cough	Guinee News (27)

(continued)

Table 11.1 (continued)

Country	Seizure/theft/recall/diversion	Type of medicines	Source
India	Seizure of six medicines (value of Rs. 5 lakh = 500,000 USD)	Antibiotics, sleeping pills for pregnant women, medicines for psychiatric patients, anti-rabies vaccine	Times of India (28)
	Recall of four medicines	Antibiotics, anti-inflammatory medicines, analgesics, anti-histamine medicine	Nyoooz (29)
	Recall of 21 spurious medicines	Antibiotics, medicines for diabetes, cardiovascular medicines	Times of India (30)
	Seizure of medicines (value of Rs. 50 lakh = 5 millions USD), unknown number	Erectile dysfunction medicines, anti-depressants	Times of India (31)
	Recall of seven medicines	Not specified	Times of India (32)
	Fake medicines factory 'busted'	Not specified	News Web India (33)
	Seizure of 39,980 tablets of Rabeprazole, and 19,400 tablets of Aceclofenac and Paracetamol	Medicines for stomach pain relief, anti-inflammatory medicine, and analgesics	Times of India (34)
Italy	Seizure of 600,000 products	Condoms made with noxious chemicals	Vice (35)
Liberia	Seizure of a *'huge consignment'* of medicines	Various medicines including eye drops, cough candies	Liberian Observer (36)
Nigeria	Seizure, unknown number (worth 40 million Naira = about 200,000 US$)	Antimalarials, analgesics, medicines for stomach pain relief, antifungals drug	Leadership (37)
Pakistan	A racket involving the sale of poor-quality medicines was 'busted'	Anti-asthmatics, cardiovascular medicines, analgesics, antidiabetics	The News (38)
Peru	50 illegal pharmacies selling falsified medicines uncovered	Not specified	Rpp (39)
The Philippines	Seizure of several boxes of medicines	Various medicines including vitamins	SunStar (40)
	Recalls, warnings unknown number	Antibiotics	BusinessWorld Weekender (41)
Portugal	29 falsified medicines sold online	Not specified	IRACM (42)
El Salvador	Several seizures, unknown number of medicines	Mainly vitamins	IRACM (43)
	Seizure of 900 products	Not specified	IRACM (44)

(continued)

Table 11.1 (continued)

Country	Seizure/theft/recall/diversion	Type of medicines	Source
Senegal	Seizure of a large batch of medicines	Not specified	IRACM (45)
	Seizure of 991 kg of medicines	Antibiotics, analgesics, vitamins	DakarActu (46)
	Seizure of 200 kg of medicines	Antibiotics, antihypertensives, and aphrodisiac medicines	Zoom Infos (47)
South Africa	Giboia operation: Three clandestine factories manufacturing falsified medicines were closed	Not specified	IRACM (48)
Spain	Seizure of 1.8 million doses	Sexual enhancement products and anabolic steroids	Securing Industry (49)
Tanzania	Seizure of medicines, unknown number (value of 135,994,950 shillng kenyan = about 1.3 million US$)	Not specified, illegal drugs and cosmetics	IPP Media (50)
Togo	Seizure of 22 tons of medicines	Antibiotics, analgesics, and antimalarial drugs	Securing Industry (51)
Turkey	Alert, one product	Antiepileptic	Bundesinstitut für Arzneimittel und Medizinprodukte (BfArM) (52)
Uganda	Seizure of 1000 boxes of medicines	Antibiotics	E-med discussion forum, July 20, 2015
The United Arab Emirates	Warning	Sexual enhancement products	Maktoob News (53)
The USA	Not specified, many recalls by FDA	Dietary supplements (weight loss sexual enhancement products)	US FDA (54)
	Death of two persons because of falsified Xanax	Anxiolytic medicine (alprazolam)	Securing Industry (55)
Zimbabwe	Giboia operation: Seizure of 424,257 tablets	Various products including antiretrovirals	Chronicle (56)

1. Saisie de six détecteurs de métaux et des quantités de carburant et de médicaments. http://www.lexpressiondz.com/actualite/228395-saisie-de-six-detecteurs-de-metaux-et-desquantites-de-carburant-et-de-medicaments.html; 2. Angola: Over 11.000 Kilograms of Counterfeit Medicines Seized. http://allafrica.com/stories/201509142142.html. 3. Anmat recuerda sobre unidades apócrifas de pervinox. http://www.anmat.gov.ar/comunicados/Pervinox-comunicado-disposicion.pdf; 4. Merchants of death. http://www.dhakatribune.com/crime/2015/sep/10/merchants-death; 5. Forte hausse des saisies de médicaments illégaux ou contrefaits. http://www.msn.com/fr-be/video/celeb-rites/forte-hausse-des-saisies-de-médicaments-illégaux-ou-contrefaits/vi-BBlifbO; 6. Thieves raid pharmaceutical warehouse in Brazil. http://www.securingindustry.com/pharmaceuticals/-thieves-raid-pharmaceutical-warehouse-in-brazil/s40/a2409/#.VgpSzBu3BBQ; 7. Saisie au Cameroun d'un important stock de médicaments périmés - Afrique - Actualités - StarAfrica.com. http://fr.starafrica.com/actualites/saisie-au-cameroun-dun-important-stock-demedicaments-perimes.html;

(continued)

Table 11.1 (continued)

8. Des faux médicaments et des plastiques non biodégradables saisis au Cameroun. http://fr.starafrica.com/actualites/des-faux-medicaments-et-des-plastiques-non-biodegradables-saisis-au-cameroun.html; 9 Saisie de 2 millions de comprimés de médicaments contrefaits. http://ici.radio-canada.ca/nouvelles/societe/2015/10/08/003-medicaments-contrefaits-davidson-reseau-saisie-police-canada.shtml; 10. Chine: au moins 20 personnes arrêtées dans une campagne visant des médicaments contrefaits—french.xinhuanet.com. http://french.xinhuanet.com/2015-07/20/c_134427622.htm; 11. Twelve caught in east China for faking animal drugs I Shanghai Daily. http://www.shanghaidaily.com/article/article_xinhua.aspx?id=298736; 12. Counterfeit Viagra pills raise their ugly head in China. http://www.ecns.cn/2015/10-22/185310.shtml; 13. Police in southern China raid labs churning out fake Viagra and antibiotics. http://www.scmp.com/news/china/society/article/1862425/police-southern-china-raid-labs-churning-out-fake-viagra-and; 14. Seizure of 600 counterfeit medicines in Santander pharmacies in Colombia. http://www.iracm.com/en/2015/09/seizure-of-600-counterfeit-medicines-in-santander-pharmacies-in-colombia/; 15. COLOMBIA: Cae red de traficantes de medicamentos falsificados. http://entornointeligente.com/articulo/6763996/COLOMBIA-Cae-red-de-traficantes-de-medicamentos-falsificados-21082015; 16. Six members of an expired drugs smuggling gang arrested in Colombia. http://www.iracm.com/en/2015/08/six-members-of-an-expired-drugs-smuggling-gang-arrested-in-colombia/; 17. Two tons of counterfeit medicines including treatments against HIV-AIDS seized in Colombia. http://www.iracm.com/en/2015/11/two-tons-of-counterfeit-medicines-including-treatments-against-hiv-aids-seized-in-colombia/; 18. Expired quinine, amoxicillin and noscapine found on the market of Bunia in the Democratic Republic of Congo (DRC). http://www.iracm.com/en/2015/09/expired-quinine-amoxicillin-and-noscapine-found-on-the-market-of-bunia-in-the-democratic-republic-of-congo-drc/; 19. Ministerio de salud dirección de regulación de productos de interés sanitario. https://www.ministeriodesalud.go.cr/index.php/alertas/alerta-por-productos-en-el-mercado/2756-11-de-septiembre-de-2015-alerta-sobre-la-falsificacion-del-producto-propofol/file; 20. Dismantling of an international network dedicated to counterfeit medicines in Santo Domingo. http://www.iracm.com/en/2015/07/dismantling-of-an-international-network-dedicated-to-counterfeit-medicines-in-santo-domingo/; 21. Operation to dismantle a criminal organization involved in trafficking of counterfeit drugs in the Dominican Republic. http://www.iracm.com/en/2015/10/operation-to-dismantle-a-criminal-organization-involved-in-trafficking-of-counterfeit-drugs-in-the-dominican-republic/; 22. Dirección General de Medicamentos Alimentos y Productos Sanitarios-Alerta N°003/15. http://www.sespas.gov.do/nivo-slider/demo/docs/AlertaMedicamentos.pdf; 23. Drug supplement testing yields low efficacy levels: MoH. http://gulftoday.ae/portal/ba97cf47-1bd5-4ae6-ac94-9c5290eff74a.aspx; 24. Ecuador stops import of a drug suspected of being counterfeit. http://www.iracm.com/en/2015/10/ecuador-stops-import-of-a-drug-suspected-of-being-counterfeit/; 25. Avignon I Des contrefaçons et des munitions saisies. http://www.ledauphine.com/vaucluse/2015/09/21/des-contrefacons-et-des-munitions-saisies; 26. Press release - Fake/Counterfeit Vermox. http://www.fdaghana.gov.gh/images/stories/pdfs/Pressrelease/2015/COUNTERFEIT VERMOX.pdf; 27. Les services spéciaux démasquent un réseau de contrefaçon à Conakry. http://guineenews.org/les-services-speciaux-demasquent-un-reseau-de-contrefacon-a-conakry/; 28. Test nails it: Drugs seized in raid found fake. http://timesofindia.indiatimes.com/city/chandigarh/Test-nails-it-Drugs-seized-in-raid-found-fake/articleshow/47904616.cms; 29. In 90 days, 35 firms given notices over sub-standard medicines. http://www.nyoooz.com/jaipur/157679/in-90-days-35-firms-given-notices-over-substandard-medicines; 30. DCA recalls 21 spurious drugs. http://timesofindia.indiatimes.com/city/hyderabad/DCA-recalls-21-spurious-drugs/articleshow/48383148.cms; 31. Fake pharmacist held with drugs worth 50L. http://timesofindia.indiatimes.com/city/delhi/Fake-pharmacist-held-with-drugs-worth-50L/articleshow/49051709.cms; 32. 7 drug samples found to be fake. http://timesofindia.indiatimes.com/city/meerut/7-drug-samples-found-to-be-fake/articleshow/49278170.cms; 33. Fake drugs factory busted in MP. http://news.webindia123.com/news/Articles/India/20151005/2694699.html; 34. Dodgy drugs: Rs. 3 lakh seizure takes

(continued)

Table 11.1 (continued)

month's count to Rs. 45 lakh. http://timesofindia.indiatimes.com/city/chandigarh/Dodgy-drugs-Rs-3-lakh-seizure-takes-months-count-to-Rs-45-lakh/articleshow/49514258.cms; 35. Italy Seizes 600 K Counterfeit Condoms Made with Noxious Chemicals | VICE News. https://news.vice.com/article/italy-seizes-600k-counterfeit-condoms-made-with-noxious-chemicals; 36. Huge 'Counterfeit Drugs' Seized at Ganta Border. http://www.liberianobserver.com/news/huge-'counterfeit-drugs'-seized-ganta-border; 37. NAFDAC's War Against Fake Drugs, Foods In South-South. http://leadership.ng/news/469805/nafdacs-war-against-fake-drugs-foods-in-south-south; 38. FIA busts counterfeit medicines racket. http://www.thenews.com.pk/Todays-News-4-335517-FIA-busts-counterfeit-medicines-racket; 39. Detectan 50 boticas ilegales. http://rpp.pe/peru/arequipa/detectan-50-boticas-ilegales-noticia-908412; 40. Fake meds seized in Cebu. http://www.sunstar.com.ph/cebu/local-news/2015/07/09/fake-meds-seized-418061; 41. Citizens must take part in fight against fake medicines. http://www.weekender.bworldonline.com/2015/12/04/citizens-must-take-part-in-fight-against-fake-medicines/; 42. 29 cases of counterfeit drugs found on online sales sites in Portugal. http://www.iracm.com/en/2015/10/29-cases-of-counterfeit-drugs-found-on-online-sales-sites-in-portugal/; 43. Seizures of vitamins falsified and unfit for consumption on markets in El Salvador. http://www.iracm.com/en/2015/09/seizures-of-vitamins-falsified-and-unfit-for-consumption-on-markets-in-el-salvador/; 44. El Salvador: seizure of counterfeit drugs at the airport. http://www.iracm.com/en/2015/07/el-salvador-seizure-of-counterfeit-drugs-at-the-airport/; 45. Operation 'clean sweep' to illegal and counterfeit drugs in Senegal. http://www.iracm.com/en/2015/11/operation-clean-sweep-to-illegal-and-counterfeit-drugs-in-senegal/; 46. 991 kg de médicaments frauduleux et 275 kg de chanvre indien saisis par la Douane. http://www.dakaractu.com/991-kg-de-medicaments-frauduleux-et-275-kg-de-chanvre-indien-saisis-par-la-Douane_a99646.html; 47. Vente illicite de medicaments à yeumbeul: 200 kg de produits contrefaits et frauduleux saisis. http://www.zoominfos.net/vente-illicite-de-medicaments-a-yeumbeul-200kg-de-produits-contrefaits-et-frauduleux-saisis/; 48. 3 factories dismantled and 150 tons of illicit drugs seized during the Interpol international operation Gibioa II in southern Africa. http://www.iracm.com/en/2015/09/3-factories-dismantled-and-150-tons-of-illicit-drugs-seized-during-the-interpol-international-operation-gibioa-ii-in-southern-africa/; 49. Pharma crime: news in brief. A round-up of international cargo theft and counterfeiting incidents from Liberia, Brazil, Italy and Togo. http://www.securingindustry.com/pharmaceuticals/pharma-crime-news-in-brief/s40/a2540/#.VtUIxk2kpBR; 50. TFDA exposes sellers of govt drugs. http://www.ippmedia.com/frontend/index.php?l=84313; 51. TOGO: SEIZED 20 TONS OF COUNTERFEIT MEDICINES. http://linkis.com/www.youtube.com/Tkhfk (accessed 28 Sep 2015); 52. Weitere Arzneimittelrisiken – Petnidan® Saft, 50 mg/ml Lösung zum Einnehmen: Möglicherweise Fälschungen des Arzneimittels in der legalen Vertriebskette in Deutschland. http://www.bfarm.de/SharedDocs/Risikoinformationen/Pharmakovigilanz/DE/RI/2015/RI-petnidan.html; 53. MoH warns of fake herbal medicines and products – Yahoo Maktoob News. https://en-maktoob.news.yahoo.com/moh-warns-fake-herbal-medicines-products-054031141.html; 54. Recalls, Market Withdrawals, & Safety Alerts. http://www.fda.gov/Safety/Recalls/; 55. Fake Xanax claims two more lives in California. http://www.securingindustry.com/pharmaceuticals/fake-xanax-claims-two-more-lives-in-california/s40/a2581/#.VtUKX02kpBR; 56. 'Operation Giaboia'…395 drug traffickers nabbed, 424,000 pills recovered. http://www.chronicle.co.zw/operation-giaboia-395-drug-traffickers-nabbed-424000-pills-recovered/

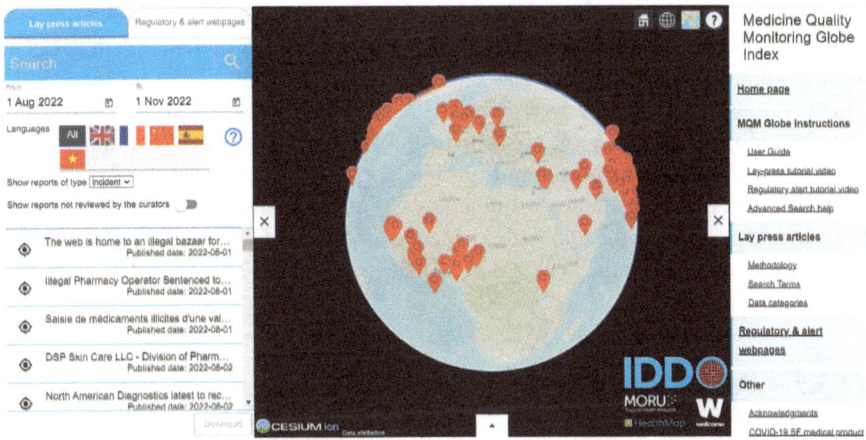

Fig. 11.1 The Medicine Quality Monitoring Globe: screenshot taken on November 24th, 2022, shows events captured by the system from August 1, 2022, to November 1, 2022, in English, French, Mandarin, Vietnamese, and Spanish

efficacy against COVID-19) in Pakistan; and substandard hand sanitizers and anti-septics in the USA, some containing toxic ingredients such as methanol. Those were described throughout the pandemic in publicly available reports [24].

Severe problems were exacerbated because of the lack of information sharing between key stakeholders [25]. Since the launch of the WHO Medical Product Alert system in 2013, 126 Member States had been trained to use the system, and 1500 suspected products incidents were reported globally as of July 2017 (World Health Organization, 2017b). Most of these reports were about anti-infective medicines.

In countries with strong regulatory systems, for example in Europe or North America, reports of SF medicines are relatively rare [27]. Most reports involve high value products such as 'lifestyle medicines' (erectile dysfunction, weight loss medications) that often circulate via the internet [28, 29]. However, there have been reports of severe public health problems, such as falsified Durex condoms in the Italian pharmaceutical market [30], falsified version of the anticancer medicine Avastin in the US supply chain [31], falsified hepatitis C antivirals in Germany and Japan [32, 33], poor-quality heparin administered to many patients in the USA [34], and 64 deaths due to contaminated intrathecal steroids in the USA [35]. Products containing valsartan, and other products containing other sartans, pioglitazone, ranitidine, and more recently metformin products [36], were found to contain low levels of potentially carcinogenic impurities and led to the recalls of hundreds of batches all around the world between 2018 and 2020 [37, 38]. The impurities appeared during the production of the raw active ingredients but were not identified by finished products manufacturers for many years.

Repeated yearly, the international week of action to tackle the online sale of falsified medicines coordinated by INTERPOL, called Operation Pangea that started in 2008, resulted in the seizure of millions of illegal medicines. In 2021 alone, 113,020 websites were taken down [39].

Fragmented research networks, limited number of researchers per network and cross-country collaborations, especially in countries where problems seem to occur more commonly, slow down progress on the understanding of the problem [40]. There is an urgent need for good-quality data, including sufficient sample size of the samples being tested, objective consensus study designs to obtain the samples (mystery shopping) and formal random sampling approaches, to more reliably estimate the proportion of SF medicines within countries and to allow objective evaluation of time trends. However, the available evidence—both scientific and lay literature—increasingly recognizes the problem as a 'pandemic' [41, 42].

11.2.3   Data on Anti-Infectives

In contrast to developed countries where a large proportion of falsified medicines are costly, relatively inexpensive poor-quality medicines more frequently make newspaper headlines in LMICs. Because of the tremendous challenge of infectious diseases, and of antimicrobial resistance (AMR), researchers have primarily focused on the problem of the quality of anti-infective medicines, although only few studies describing their prevalence have adopted a robust methodology to allow the generalization of the findings [43].

Almuzaini et al. reported a median prevalence of SF anti-infectives of 28.5% in 25 LMICs in a systematic review in 2013 [44]. In 2022, Zabala et al. observed a failure frequency for the 13,555 antibiotic samples tested for quality in 106 reports, published between 1992 and 2020, of 17.4% [45]. Early-generation antibiotics, such as amoxicillin, ampicillin, tetracycline, and sulfamethoxazole-trimethoprim, are often targeted [46–51]. SF antiviral agents such as oseltamivir and antiretrovirals have also been reported [52–55].

Throughout history, antimalarials have been particularly attractive for falsifiers. However, this may be an artefact of public health interest, as there are relatively limited data for other medicines and as chemical analyses for antimalarials have become relatively accessible. Almost all of the different types of marketed antimalarials have been reported as falsified and/or substandard. The WorldWide Antimalarial Research Network, which tabulates and maps accessible reports of the quality of antimalarials, summarized the data on the quality of antimalarials collected in 130 surveys globally from 1946 to 2013 [56]. Worryingly, they found 'no publicly available reports for 60.6% (63) of the 104 malaria-endemic countries'. In total, almost one-third of the antimalarials tested over 67 years failed chemical and/or packaging analysis. Oral artesunate was the most commonly reported as falsified. These results, and those of other reviews on medicine quality, should be interpreted with caution because of the often poor methodology of the surveys. For example, many of the surveys included in these reviews use 'convenience' sampling rather than random sampling to select health facilities where to collect the medicines investigated for quality, potentially leading to under- or over-estimations of the prevalence of SF medicines [57].

In surveys in Laos, Cambodia, and Tanzania, there was no evidence of the presence of falsified artemisinin-based combination therapies (ACTs) on the market in several studies [58–60]. ACTs have been recommended by WHO to treat *P. falciparum* malaria since 2006 [61]. Unfortunately, the findings in Laos, Cambodia, and Tanzania cannot be extrapolated to other low- and middle-income countries as falsified ACTs with none of the expected antimalarial ingredient(s) have been reported, especially in African countries where malaria is endemic. Falsified dihydroartemisinin-piperaquine that were found to contain sildenafil (the API of the erectile dysfunction medicine Viagra) due to be shipped to Africa from China in 2007 [62] were intercepted. In 2012, 1.4 million packs of falsified medicines—mostly labelled as the antimalarial artemether-lumefantrine—that contained no API and were hidden in loudspeakers were intercepted on arrival in Angola from China. Falsified artemether-lumefantrine was found in Ghana in 2009 [62], in Nigeria in 2011 [63], in Cameroon and Senegal in 2013 [64, 65], in Ivory Coast and Gabon in 2015 [66], and in Chad, Côte d'Ivoire, and Mali in 2021. In 2015, in Myanmar, falsified intravenous/intramuscular artesunate—a vital medicine for the treatment of severe falciparum malaria—was found to contain no artesunate [67]. That there are so many reports of falsified key antimalarials in high malaria burden countries is of great concern.

It is noteworthy that, although no falsified ACTs were found in the Laos, Cambodia, and Tanzania surveys (above), unacceptable proportions of the samples tested were substandard, either due to factory errors of degradation in supply chains. Indeed, in Laos and Tanzania, one-fourth and 30% of the antimalarials tested, respectively, were outside the 90–110% pharmacopeial range of the stated API; in Cambodia, almost one-third were outside the 85–115% range.

Although the API content is the most commonly tested component of medicines quality, incorrect excipient(s), excipient formulations, or poor manufacturing procedures may result in low bioavailability of medicines with correct %API, which consequently decreases the efficacy of the medicine. In Afghanistan, all antimalarials tested contained the correct amount of API, but 26% failed dissolution testing [68]. In Ethiopia, 18% and 42% of tinidazole and albendazole tablets, respectively, failed dissolution tests [69]. However, in a systematic review of the literature, researchers found that only one-fourth of the surveys on antimalarial quality over 67 years included dissolution testing [56], highlighting the limited data on dissolution defects, '*presumably because of the large investments in equipment, funds and laboratory time required*'. More investment in dissolution testing is needed.

11.2.4 Awareness of the Population and Healthcare Professionals

Raising community awareness of SF medicines is essential, as they can notice if medications change in either appearance or taste, and they are in the first line to note adverse drug reactions. There is little information on the public perception and understanding of the issues in different settings and societies, and on which interventions may be the most effective to increase their awareness without discouraging patients from taking genuine medicines. The limited available evidence suggests a rather low awareness of the problem of SF medicines, and low knowledge on how to identify and how and to who to report them. Only half of citizens interviewed in Vientiane Capital in Laos in 2013 had heard of poor-quality medicines, mainly through media or through relatives/friends [70]. Sanofi conducted a study in 2015 in six Asian countries, China, Indonesia, Malaysia, the Philippines, Thailand, and Vietnam [71], finding that only 67% of those surveyed considered 'counterfeit' medicines to be harmful. In addition, the purchase of medicines online was quite common in Asia, although 58% of those who had purchased medicines online were aware of the risks. Reporting to the authorities is essential, but in Poland, 92% of lay persons interviewed did not know that there is a necessity to report suspicious medicines [72].

To be better prepared for harm from suspicious products, healthcare providers should have access to information on the problem, which should allow faster and more efficient reactions. Medicine quality should be suspected in the face of unexpected treatment failure or puzzling clinical syndromes [73]. In Poland, where numerous seizures of SF medicines were reported in 2010 [74], one-third of physicians and nurses did not know the procedures for reporting suspicious medicines [72]. In western India, only 1 in 5 of the dental and medical practitioners, and medical wholesale distributors, interviewed knew about falsified medicines [75].

Awareness campaigns through media, involving diverse partners, have been the main initiatives so far to raise public awareness [76–78]. However, as far as we are aware, their effect on public awareness and perception of the issue has only been evaluated in one study. This showed that after a 9-month campaign on the dangers of 'counterfeit' medicines from illicit drug markets in Benin, mainly using TV and radio announcements, those interviewed who received the awareness messages about the dangers of the street medicine markets were six times more likely to avoid the illicit drug market than those who did not [79]. Some institutions such as Fight The Fakes [80] and The Partnership for Safe Medicines [81] have played significant roles in the communication of the issue, but mostly in wealthier anglophone countries and concerning falsified and not substandard medicines. The MedsWeCanTrust campaign launched in 2018 involved 300 partners in 45 countries around the world [82]. Describing the physical characteristics of fakes was probably effective in Cambodia, where a poster and radio education campaign educated patients to distinguish falsified tablets and the sale of falsified antimalarials was driven underground [83]. However, this may result in giving criminals valuable information to boost the sophistication of their 'products'. Understanding how to create public awareness in diverse communities without assisting criminals requires more engagement research. Raising awareness of people on the risks of buying medicines on the illicit market is needed.

11.3   The Consequences of SF Medicines for Patients and the Community

SF medicines represent a major risk to human health, not just for those who use them, but also for their communities [84]. A statistical model estimated that ~122,350 malaria deaths among children under 5 years in 39 countries in sub-Saharan Africa in 2013 were from SF antimalarials, representing almost 4% of all under-five deaths in these countries [85]. Investigations into the impact of the use of SF antibacterials on childhood pneumonia, and antimalarials on uncomplicated *Plasmodium falciparum* malaria in sub-Saharan Africa were commissioned by the WHO and results were published in 2017 [86]. In a context of 10% prevalence of SF antibiotics, from 72,430 (assuming reduced antibiotic activity) to 169,271 deaths (assuming no antibiotic activity) were attributed to the use of SF antibiotics. Using data on the prevalence of SF antimalarials in sub-Saharan Africa, based on results from a systematic review of the literature, it was estimated that excess SF antimalarial deaths in sub-Saharan Africa comprise approximately 2.1 to 4.9% of total malaria deaths.

11.3.1   Lack of Efficacy

The API in a medicine is usually the most costly component of the medicine formulation. Therefore, falsifiers may not add, or add a limited amount of the API in the product in order to increase their profit margins. Subtherapeutic dosage, such as may occur in SF medicines containing lower amount of API or in degraded products, risks therapeutic failure.

Indeed, isolated reports of therapeutic failures have been published. For example, either a substandard or degraded vial of intramuscular artemether containing only 74% artemether may have been involved in the poor clinical outcome of an adult with uncomplicated *P. falciparum* in Laos [87]. Ceftriaxone injection vials containing only half of the stated strength were likely to have contributed to the death of an adolescent patient treated for meningitis in Kampala [88]. Falsified oral artesunate may have led to the death of a young man suffering severe malaria on the Thai/Myanmar border [89].

Isolated cases of failure to a treatment may go under the radar in most cases, unlike series of cases when several patients treated in a defined area and in a limited period of time do not respond to the same batches of a medicine. There are numerous examples in the literature, such as the meningitis epidemic in Niger in 1995 when over 50,000 people were injected with falsified vaccines—with no traces of active vaccine component, received as a donation from Nigeria which were thought to be safe [90]. That incident resulted in an estimated 2500 deaths. Falsified phenobarbital was reported in Guinea Bissau and Nigeria in 2013 and 2014 [91]. Of 117 patients treated for epilepsy, 74 (63%) had more frequent seizures and 2 patients died in Guinea. Higher seizure frequencies were reported in 105 of 120 (88%) patients in Nigeria. Dissolution failure of poor-quality sulfadoxine-pyrimethamine (SP) has been linked to an epidemic of *Plasmodium falciparum* malaria on the Afghanistan/Pakistan border [92].

However, most of the poor treatment outcomes related to SF medicines are likely unrecognized, especially in limited-resources settings where diagnostic facilities are rarely available. When facing a therapeutic failure, healthcare workers usually first think of misdiagnosis rather than of a quality defect of the medicine, especially for anti-infectives. In addition, effectiveness of a medicine depends on the adherence of patients with the prescription.

11.3.2   Resistance of Pathogens

Poor-quality medicines are increasingly mentioned as a potentially important factor in the emergence and spread of drug resistance to anti-infectives [93–96] and worries are increasing, as the anti-infective development pipeline is diminishing. However, there is no robust evidence base for this and there is uncertainty about how important a driver it is, in comparison to the other AMR drivers in different communities. The relationships between anti-infectives and drug-resistant pathogens are complex, given that drug resistance is a multifactorial issue. Anti-infectives containing subtherapeutic amounts of the active ingredient, whether falsified, substandard, or degraded, may increase the risk of selection and spread of drug-resistant pathogens [97–100]. The subject is reviewed in the literature [94, 96, 101, 102], but more evidence-based modelling is needed to understand the issue better [103]

11.3.3   Adverse Drug Reactions: The Ears of the Hippopotamus

In some instances, falsifiers may replace expensive active ingredients with less expensive ones, or by any active or inactive substance available at the time of the 'manufacture'. Sometimes the substitution of the active ingredient by another appears to be made intelligently in order to fool the user. For example, paracetamol that may lower fever was found in falsified antimalarials [62, 104]. However, wrong ingredients may cause severe adverse effects. For example, in the late 1990s, aspirin, an important contributor to acidosis and a cause of Reye's syndrome in children [105], had been deliberately mislabelled as chloroquine in Africa [106]. Indomethacin, a non-steroidal anti-inflammatory drug, was found, at the recommended dosage for treating rheumatic patients, in a herbal medicine advertised as

100% 'natural' [107]. Generic atorvastatin was recalled from the US market in 2012, by one of the largest generic companies in India, because of the presence of small glass particles. Fortunately, this 'inactive' ingredient was judged as low-risk by the US medicine regulatory authority (FDA) that received no reports of patient harm [108].

A wide range of other wrong and potentially harmful active ingredient(s) have been described. Falsified artesunate containing sulfadoxine, noramido-pyrine, pyrimethamine, erythromycin, chloramphenicol, or even dimethyl fumarate [109], exposed patients to blood conditions such as agranulocytosis with noramidopyrine or leukopenia with pyrimethamine, especially when they are used at high doses and over long treatment courses. But even small quantities of some unexpected active ingredients, such as dimethyl fumarate or sulfadoxine, expose patients to severe outcomes such as anaphylaxis or toxic epidermal necrolysis.

This wide range of unexpected components that can find their way into SF medicines, and the clinically surprising and confusing symptoms or conditions they may induce, render the 'diagnosis' very difficult for a healthcare professional that is blinded to the real active ingredients contained in the products; knowing their composition relies on expensive chemical analyses that are not available at the distal end of the supply chain.

Outbreaks of adverse drug reactions and treatment failures are the 'ears of the hippopotamus' of the consequences of SF medicines on patients' health. Contamination of paediatric syrups (labelled paracetamol and cough syrups mainly) by the toxic anti-freeze diethylene glycol led to the death of 107 people in the USA (many of whom were children) in 1937 [11], with outbreaks since then in South Africa [110], Nigeria [111, 112], Bangladesh [113], Haiti [114], and India [114, 115]. Unfortunately, history has recently repeated itself, with dozens of children dying in the Gambia and Indonesia because of unacceptable levels of diethylene glycol (DEG) and ethylene glycol (EG) in different paracetamol and cough syrups [116, 117]. In 2015, in the Democratic Republic of Congo over 900 patients, mainly children, suffered painful and distressful reactions of the face, neck, and tongue or 'acute dystonic reactions' because of falsified diazepam that actually contained between 10 mg and 20 mg of the antipsychotic haloperidol per tablet [118]. In Pakistan, in 2011–2012, a manufacturer inadvertently added large amounts of the antimalarial pyrimethamine (known for causing severe haemato-logical adverse reactions at high doses) to isosorbide-5-mononitrate tablets, leading to ~200 deaths from bone-marrow suppression [119]. Other notorious examples include hundreds of reports of acute hypersensitivity-like reactions associated with the use vials of heparin contaminated by oversulfated chondroitin sulfate imported from China by the US firm Baxter Pharmaceuticals, which led to many deaths in the USA in 2008 [34], and the hospitalization of 150 non-diabetic men with severe hypoglycaemia in Singapore in 2008 after they used erectile dysfunction medicines containing up to 100 mg of the sulfonylurea glyburide, resulting in the death of four [120].

11.3.4   Beyond Health Consequences

Beyond the mortality and morbidity resulting from SF medicines described above, they can undesirably influence the way patients think about the quality of their healthcare system and treatment options. Health practitioners may also lose trust in the medications that they rely upon.

Economic consequences are also of great concern. The Center for Medicines in the Public Interest estimated the worldwide falsified medicines trade to be worth $75 billion in 2010 [121]. Models estimated a total annual economic impact of substandard and falsified antimalarials due to additional treatment-seeking and further care between $12.1 million and $44.7 million [86]. However, these results should be considered as 'tentative and illustrative' only, given the assumptions that had to be made because of limited data and more research on methods to assess the health, economic and social impacts of SF medical products is needed [122, 123]. In addition, several factors could not be taken into account in the estimates (e.g. the economic impact of adverse drug reactions) because of the lack of data. A review of the literature published in 2018 found only eight studies analysing economic harms of SF medical products, all either old or lacking methodological details or both. They concluded that the economic losses due to poor-quality medicines ranged between USD 10 to 200 billion [23]. Spending money on SF medicines is a waste of the limited financial resources reserved for health. It is particularly problematic for countries and vulnerable communities already suffering from limited resources, especially but not only in LMICs. Money is lost for patients and their families because they must bear the costs of increased suffering, healthcare costs, and sometimes death. The availability of falsified medicines on the market also induces economic losses for the pharmaceutical industries, both generic and innovative, of the genuine products. They lose profits and risk acquiring a tarnished image by the misrepresentation inherent in falsified medicines. Health workers, medicine regulatory authorities, and customs and police personnel may also suffer from an increased burden of work, which is hard to sustain in countries with insufficient human resource and financial capacities.

11.4   Pharmacovigilance and SF Medicines

The detection of safety signals and drug alerts in post-marketing medicine surveillance is a vital part of pharmacovigilance activities. It is usually based on spontaneous reports by health professionals and patients themselves of adverse drug events to national centres in many countries.

Although isolated cases of lack of efficacy [87–89, 124, 125] or adverse drug reactions [126–128] have been identified by healthcare professionals, unfortunately we can reasonably assume, especially for countries with limited capacity for surveillance and regulation, that there are many more than we are aware of [91, 114, 129].

Increasing signal detection of adverse reactions or unexpected lack of efficacy because of SF medicines is thus of great importance to enable rapid and appropriate responses to this neglected issue. The WHO international database of Individual Case Safety Reports (ICSRs) 'Vigibase' was retrospectively tested by the Uppsala Monitoring Centre (UMC) in 2013, to evaluate the potential of the database to detect signals related to SF medicines [130]. An algorithm was constructed to identify reporting patterns suggestive of SF medicines in ICSRs. This algorithm used the preferred terms of the Medical Dictionary for Regulatory Activities such as the specific terms 'product quality issue', 'product contamination', or the less specific terms 'Drug effect decreased' and 'Drug ineffective'. Applied to Vigibase, the algorithm yielded a total of 281,000 ICSRs between 2001 and 2013. The vast majority (91%) were reported by five high-income countries. The 147 identified clusters (i.e. groups of ICSRs on a specific product, a year and a country) were assessed by each respective national centre in order to classify the signals as confirmed, potentially, or unlikely related to SF medicines, confirmed as non-related to poor-quality medicines or indecisive. They showed that some events due to SF medicines could be detected through the global pharmacovigilance system but that ICSRs often lack substantial information (e.g. product trade name, batch number, distribution channel) to allow for conclusive classification of many clusters. In a number of countries, prescription is by International Non-proprietary Names and products can be substituted on the basis of their availability. As a result, product trade names are not always reported in ICSRs, impeding investigation. Vigibase has the advantage of large sample size and statistical power to detect signals but suffers from long delays in the process of (i) notification by the reporter, (ii) handling the incoming ICSRs by regional/national centres, and (iii) transferring these reports to the Vigibase, impairing rapid prospective signal detection. In addition, not all low- and middle-income countries (World Bank classification) have yet adhered to the WHO Programme for International Drug Monitoring, and most of those who are official members, adhered to the programme after 2010. This partly explains why almost all the clusters identified in Vigibase were from the wealthiest countries. The methodology developed by the UMC could assist signal detection in national and regional databases of adverse drug reactions or those of pharmaceutical companies. Indeed, in these databases, shorter delays in reporting and more direct access to the original reporter allow faster and in-depth investigation. However, the issue of global under-reporting of ADRs by healthcare professionals is a major impediment towards signal detection of SF medicines through pharmacovigilance databases [131].

Integrating the issue of medicine quality with other methods of pharmacovigilance such as cohort-event monitoring (CEM), a method that was recently implemented by the WHO in its public health programmes in LMICs, is of great interest [132]. CEM usually includes new medicines, but can include older medicines. Patients are interviewed on a regular basis during the treatment course and all events, regardless of their severity or seriousness are recorded, making CEM useful tools to capture problems due to poor storage conditions, substandard or falsified medicines.

Establishing close links between national pharmacovigilance centres, medicine analysis laboratories, and the inspectors of the quality of medical products will be important for ensuring rapid responses to suspected SF medicines [133].

Raising awareness of healthcare providers and patients, and encouraging them to report unexpected lack of effect of medicines or unexpected reactions to the pharmacovigilance centre in the context of SF medicines, would contribute to early signals and to document the extent of the problem of poor-quality medicines.

11.5   Difficulties Faced by Resource-Limited Countries

11.5.1   Regulatory Authority Challenges

The limited capacities of medicine regulatory authorities in LMICs often make investigation of SF medicines and action to address them difficult. Strengthening national MRAs is likely to be a key factor to sustainably improve the quality of medicines.

Corruption, common in many countries, exacerbates the issue of SF medicines [134, 135]. Medicines are diverted by healthcare professionals [136] or from 'to be destroyed' medicine stocks, and then sold in street shops with dubious storage conditions. Corruption of inspectors may also affect conformity at different stages of drug monitoring and quality control procedures [137].

11.5.2   Lack of Accurate, Portable, and Cost-Effective Screening Techniques

What medicines contain and whether their packaging is genuine are vital information to implement interventions against SF medicines. A diversity of new technologies and machines have been developed to identify SF medicines, especially in the field of anti-infectives. The advantages and drawbacks of the main technologies used or under development in the different steps of medicine quality analysis are discussed here. Reviews are available for those looking for more detailed information [138–142].

Basic visual inspection of the packaging using one's own senses is the most inexpensive and rapid way to identify the more crudely produced falsified medicines. Comparing packaging with that of authentic comparators may allow the identification of falsified packaging, but it is often very difficult to obtain the authentic medicines from the legitimate manufacturers for comparison. Observing poor uniformity and conformity of the physical characteristics of the dosage form unit (size, shape, odour, and taste) can raise suspicions at every level of the supply chain, involving minimal training and cost. The International Council of Nurses in partnership with the United States Pharmacopoeia has developed a useful checklist for this purpose [143]. Recently a simplified checklist has been developed to guide non-specialized healthworkers at the frontline to take rapid action upon SF medicines [144]. The German Pharma Health Fund (GPHF)-Minilab, which contains laboratory equipment in two suitcases, that primarily assesses whether the correct API is present in a formulation via colorimetric or chromatographic methods also provides physical inspection schemes for dosage forms and associated packaging material [145].

With increase in availability of technology, there has been an increased sophistication of falsified products by criminals, and only more advanced techniques can detect anomalies of packaging or products that are not apparent to the naked eye. The handheld Counterfeit Detection Device, version 3 (CD3), developed by the US Food and Drug Administration, uses a range of wavelengths of light (from the ultraviolet to the infrared) to reveal differences of the visual features of tablets/capsules and packaging from authentic samples [146]. The CD3 showed high accuracy to detect falsified oral artesunate packaging and tablets [147].

Simple to more advanced techniques have also been developed to detect and quantify APIs, a critical step for medicine quality analysis. Colorimetric tests, designed to create changes in colour when a particular API in a medicine interacts with a specific reagent, provide rapid qualitative API information (semi-quantitative or quantitative information can be further obtained in some cases). Colour reactions on paper analytical cards allow sensitive, cheap (around 0.50 $ per test card), rapid (10 minutes), and user-friendly screening of a wide range of anti-infectives outside the laboratory [148–150].

Developed for resource-limited settings, the GPHF-Minilab is relatively well established in the scientific literature for quality control in the field [151–154]. More than 900 Minilabs have been supplied across 99 countries. Besides the tests described above, the GPHF-Minilab suitcases contain the material to conduct thin-layer chromatography (TLC), a widely used technique for qualitative and semi-quantitative analysis. The GPHF-Minilab provides relatively rapid means for drug quality assessment by moderately trained users. However, it only gives semi-quantitatively API concentration results, thus limiting its use to the identification of grossly substandard medicines. It is recommended to use in conjunction with other more advanced techniques when substandard medicines are suspected [153, 154]. Moreover, it uses destructive techniques, requires sample preparation and reference standard materials that can be difficult to procure in some settings, and is limited to 125 drug compounds, mainly anti-infectives. It also includes one impurity test (DEG/EG) that was added following the recent cough and paracetamol syrup contaminations.

High performance liquid chromatography (HPLC), with the aid of diverse detectors (including mass spectrometry, UV-Vis or fluorescence), is more sensitive, expensive, and sophisticated and often the reference technique used for API content analysis. The gold standard for the exact characterization of chemical composition of a product is mass spectrometry (MS), especially for the determination of unexpected ingredients. However, MS is costly and requires a specific sophisticated laboratory environment and highly experienced staff.

Other spectroscopic technologies provide a spectrum and a unique pattern of the substance, or 'fingerprint', and allow rapid analysis of the medicine, with possibility for many devices to scan through blisters and without using toxic chemicals or flammable solvents. Various techniques such as infrared, near infrared (NIR), nuclear magnetic resonance, and Raman spectroscopy exist, each with its own advantages and drawbacks [138, 155].

New portable (some handheld), battery-powered devices, based on Raman and NIR technology, give fast results and require no extra supplies and minimal end-user training. Unfortunately, the price of many of these devices currently available is still unaffordable in low-resource settings. There has been minimal research on their cost-effectiveness [156]. Another limitation is that they require the creation and regular update of reference libraries of authentic medicines for the comparison of the spectra.

The PharmaCheck, a portable device under development, that uses microfluidic technology, allows quantitative measurements of specific active ingredients [157, 158].

Correct API content is vital but not the only quality requirement for a medicine to be efficacious. When incorrect excipient formulations are used (either in substandard or falsified medicines), this may for example result in failure of oral medicines to dissolve properly in the gastrointestinal tract. In turn, this results in reduced bioavailability of the API in the blood stream and other body compartments, risking decreased efficacy. Reference tests for dissolution assessment, which measures how fast the API is solubilized in liquid media, are costly, time-consuming, and require trained staff. As far as we are aware, the only field-adapted devices that currently could provide data on medicine release is the PharmaCheck device (above) and an unnamed device using capillary electrophoresis currently under development [159].

When a medicine is confirmed as falsified by reference techniques, forensic investigations can be followed in order to give indications as to their origin [140]. Microscopic investigation of the debris, insect parts, and pollen; environmental DNA [160] isotope ratio MS to identify the mineral phases present as excipients and pinpoint their geographical origin [161] and X-ray fluorescence to investigate elemental composition can be performed [162]. However, the process of forensic investigations is rarely conducted because it usually requires a collaborative network of laboratories, and the techniques are costly and/or time-consuming.

11.6 The Way Forward

There are many challenges to ensure that patients gain the benefits from modern pharmaceuticals. Poor-quality medicines negate enormous communal effort to improve global public health. Many urgent actions are needed by nations and the international community to address the issue of SF medicines. These go beyond borders, have global implications, and are far from being exempt from politics. Many human and financial capacity and policy gaps need to be filled.

11.6.1 Need for Rapid and Cost-Affordable Techniques

As described above, a relatively wide range of techniques to identify SF medicines are available. However, there is no clear global vision of which tests are reliable for which medicines at which points in the supply chain. It is unlikely that one single tool will be able to test all aspects of medicine quality throughout distribution systems. Moreover, many devices are too expensive for low-resource countries, not adapted for operations in the field (although new handheld technologies are promising for an initial screening of medicines), have not been extensively tested outside of a research laboratory setting, cannot detect substandard medicines containing reduced amounts of API and require trained users.

As far as we are aware, there is also no accurate and reliable device to distinguish degraded medicines from those which leave the factory as substandard. The issue of degraded medicines is a neglected issue, although its impact may be potentially important, especially in countries where conditions of storage and transport of pharmaceuticals are not always appropriate. Assays to differentiate SF medicines arising due to errors within factories or in supply chains are needed.

Developing and evaluating techniques for the assessment of all aspects of medicine quality is thus a fertile but neglected research field with key implications for public health. The lack of robust evaluations is potentially squandering the effort that has gone into developing these innovative devices.

11.6.2 Law and Regulatory Enforcement

The pharmaceutical market has expanded greatly with increased globalization, and better access to medicines has not necessarily been accompanied by enhanced medicine regulation and the implementation of laws and oversight to prevent the manufacture and trade in SF medicines. Some encouraging examples suggest that efficient regulatory measures can improve the situation. In Laos, in a survey in 2003, 88% of outlets in the private sector where oral artesunate was available sold falsified artesunate [109]. When this survey was repeated using equivalent random sampling methodology in 2012, no falsified oral artesunate was found, showing a significant improvement [58]. Drivers that may have contributed to this change were increased medicine regulation, inspection, and public engagement by the Lao PDR medicine regulator, the Food and Drug Department. The trade and use of genuine oral artesunate monotherapy was reduced concomitantly to these interventions, which may have reduced the financial incentive for the criminal production of falsified artesunate. In addition, the Global Fund provided financial support to enhance access to artemisinin-based combination therapy (ACT) without charge to malaria patients in hospitals and dispensaries in Laos, with good-quality ACTs made available at low cost through specific private healthcare outlets to increase access to quality-assured efficacious antimalarials. Similar findings were reported recently in Cambodia and Tanzania, where no evidence of falsified ACTs was found [59, 60]. The Tanzanian, Lao, and Cambodian regulatory bodies have significantly invested in medicine regulation, education, and communication over the last two decades. This is very likely to have contributed to these promising results. However, we are not aware of prior studies for comparison. It is thus difficult to assess the impact of these interventions for Tanzania and Cambodia. In contrast, there has been clear evidence of severe problems with SF antimalarials in other Asian and African countries.

When criminal laws to prosecute those who manufacture falsified medicines are weak or nonexistent, as in many counties where SF issues are prevalent [163], criminals experience very low risk but are likely to make substantial profits. Penalties tend to be far lower than for heroin or cocaine trafficking. In many countries, medicine laws are often reactive to fatal epidemics of falsified or substandard medicines, as was the case in the USA, when more stringent legislation was implemented following the death of 107 people from diethylene glycol containing elixir in 1937. Attaran proposed a 'Model law on Medicine Crime' [163], covering a wide range of prohibited acts that count as crimes and their penalties. It provides a template for countries to update their laws, focusing strictly on health protection rather than intellectual property and trademark issues.

The lack of international laws and inconsistent definitions of the different types of poor-quality medicines among different nations unfortunately make it very difficult to extradite and prosecute falsifiers or those involved in the global distribution of SF medicines. Global strategic plans are needed. Some commentators advocate for an international convention providing a legal and institutional framework for regulatory action [164, 165].

The Medicrime Convention was adopted in 2011 by the Council of Europe and targeted to member and non-members. Its ratification by Guinea in 2015 allowed the convention to enter into force on the first of January 2016 with the five States ratifying it: Spain, Guinea, Hungary, Republic of Moldova, and Ukraine. By May 13, 2025 the convention had been ratified by a total of 23 countries. However, it has been argued that the convention has been mis-implemented, without public discussion of the draft by the Council of Europe, and with fears that it may impede the availability of generic medicines and criminalize unintentional production of poor-quality medicines when support and regulation are what are needed [166].

11.6.3 Clinical Trials and Medicine Quality

SF medicines may also wrongly find their way into clinical trials. If medicines are not tested for quality and SF products are included, they may harm patients, drive drug resistance in case of anti-infective trials, lead to erroneous conclusions, and be a major waste of time and resources. They may also dilute the power of meta-analyses that underlie many policy recommendations and lead to mistaken policy decisions. For instance, a trial in Africa to test the efficacy of sulfadoxine-pyrimethamine in pregnant women suffering from malaria was planned using four locally available products. One of the brands actually con- tained a reduced amount of the manufacturer's stated amount of sulfadoxine (<90%) [167]. Because medicines may degrade over the course of the trial, regular quality checks are required [168]. In a randomized trial comparing the safety and efficacy of low versus high dose vitamin A supplementation in young Tanzanian infants, within 13 months after the trial started, the 50,000 IU cap- sules, stored under appropriate conditions, had degraded to 32% of the expected amount of vitamin A! Calls have been made for clinical trial guidelines such as CONSORT to include a requirement to determine and state the quality of the medicines used in all clinical trials and to include clear guidance on how to control and guarantee the quality of medicines used throughout the whole length of the study [167]. As far as we are aware, as of 2025, these calls had not been acted upon.

11.6.4   The Need for a Better Global Information Sharing and Collaboration

Inter-regional trade requires inter-regional vigilance and data sharing. Involving all relevant stakeholders in the communication of problems related to SF medicines would help reduce the latency in informing the public when an incident occurs. In 2012, the seizure of 1.4 million packets of falsified medicines in Africa, including artemether-lumefantrine, containing no active ingredients, was shared publicly via Facebook 5 months after it was found, and in the printed press after 11 months [169]! Another recent example showed that sharing of information, on a wider scale, is also crucial. In 2012, 60 people in Pakistan died because of the contamina- tion of dextromethorphan syrups by its toxic enantiomer levometorphan [26]. A few months later in 2013, 44 children were admitted to a hospital, after consuming dextromethorphan syrups on the other side of the world in Paraguay. The imported batch of the culprit API dextromethorphan, produced by an Indian manufacturer, was the same as that causing the deaths in Pakistan. The intervention by WHO that immediately alerted that the cases were related was crucial. The 'product' was found in several other countries in Europe, North Africa, the Middle East, and Latin America.

A large database of pharmaceutical incidents, including falsified, illegally diverted, or stolen pharmaceuticals, has been maintained by the Pharmaceutical Security Institute since 2002. This organization of 37 innovative pharmaceutical manufacturers only provides aggregated data reports [170]. Most data are kept secret by the industry, which is detrimental from a public health perspective, and further discussion with trusted public health stakeholders for data sharing would be helpful [171].

Efforts have been made by the international community for better communication and collaboration. The WHO Medical Product Alert system allows national focal points to report SF medicines in real time and is a valuable source of information and advocacy. Of the 194 WHO member states, 141 were trained in WHO rapid alert reporting by 2018 [172]. However, alerting is not mandatory and only actionable cases are made public. Substandard medicines are under-represented. Evaluation of reporting of SF medicines by the pharmaceutical industry to WHO and medicine regulatory authorities is now included in the 'Access to Medicines Index' [173] and may be a major step forward to encouraging reporting. However, the obligation to disseminate information on medicine quality globally is essential to inform interventions.

Much better cooperation between national customs, medicine regulatory authorities, police, manufacturers, civil society, and other major actors must be reached. The struggle against falsified and substandard medicines cannot be properly addressed without improving the availability and accessibility of quality-assured medicines for the most vulnerable populations globally.

Acknowledgements We are very grateful to the staff of IDDO/WWARN and LOMWRU (Mahosot Hospital, Vientiane, Lao PDR) for their help and for the financial support of the Wellcome Trust.

Conflict of Interest Statement CC and PNN declare that they have no conflict of interest.

References

1. World Health Organisation. WHO member state mechanism on substandard/spurious/falsely-labelled/falsified/counterfeit (SSFFC) medical products. 2017.
2. Newton PN, Amin AA, Bird C, et al. The primacy of public health considerations in defining poor quality medicines. PLoS Med. 2011;8:e1001139.
3. Pisani E, Nistor A, Hasnida A, et al. Identifying market risk for substandard and falsified medicines: an analytic framework based on qualitative research in China, Indonesia, Turkey and Romania. Wellcome Open Res. 4 https://doi.org/10.12688/WELLCOMEOPENRES.15236.1.
4. World Health Organization. WHO: access to HIV medicines severely impacted by COVID-19 as AIDSresponse stalls. https://www.who.int/news/item/06-07-2020-who-access-to-hiv-medicines-severely-impacted-by-covid-19-as-aids-response-stalls. Accessed 24 Nov 2022.
5. Norton S. De materia medica by Pedanius Dioscorides. J Hist Med Allied Sci. 2006;61:218–20.
6. Saunders W. Observations on the superior efficacy of the red Peruvian bark: in the cure of agues and other fevers. Interspersed with occasional remarks on the treatment of other diseases, by the same remedy. Saunders: William; 1782.
7. Newton PN, Green MD, Fernández FM, et al. Counterfeit anti-infective drugs. Lancet Infect Dis. 2006;6:602–13.
8. Croft CJ. Adulteration of quinine. Lancet. 1838;31:292.
9. Moore E. Tests of adulterated quinine. Lancet. 1829:1092.

10. New York Times. Fake consumption cures- doctors call patent and proprietary medicines harmful. The New-York Times 1906; 1906.
11. Geiling EMK. Pathologic effects of elixir of sulfanilamide (diethylene glycol) poisoning. JAMA J Am Med Assoc. 1938;111:919.
12. World Health Organization. Counterfeit drugs—guidelines for the development of measures to combat counterfeit drugs. WHO/EDM/QSM/99.1. Geneva: WHO. https://iris.who.int/handle/10665/65892 Accessed 9 May 2025
13. Grech J, Robertson J, Thomas J, et al. An empirical review of antimalarial quality field surveys: the importance of characterising outcomes. J Pharm Biomed Anal. 2018;147:612–23.
14. Jackson G, Arver S, Banks I, et al. Counterfeit phosphodiesterase type 5 inhibitors pose significant safety risks. Int J Clin Pract. 2010;64:497–504.
15. U.S. Food and Drugs Administration. Drug safety and availability – counterfeit version of Avastin in U.S. Distribution. U.S. Food and Drugs Administration (FDA).
16. SecuringIndustry.com. Pharma boss, facing 30 years in prison, battles US extradition. https://www.securingindustry.com/pharmaceuticals/pharma-boss-facing-30-years-in-prison-battles-us-extradition/s40/a4118/ Accessed 9 May 2025
17. VnExpress. Vietnam's health ministry under scrutiny over cancer drug scam – VnExpress International. https://e.vnexpress.net/news/news/vietnam-s-health-ministry-under-scrutiny-over-cancer-drug-scam-3634997.html Accessed 9 May 2025
18. Busko M. Quality of cardiac drugs in Sub-Saharan Africa: 'a disaster'. Medscape Pharmacists.
19. Jost J, Ratsimbazafy V, Nguyen TT, et al. Quality of antiepileptic drugs in sub-Saharan Africa: a study in Gabon, Kenya, and Madagascar. Epilepsia. 2018;59:1351–61.
20. WHO. Falsified batches of Postinor 2 recently discovered in Nigeria. https://www.who.int/news/item/26-07-2013-medical-product-alert-n-3-2013--falsified-batches-of-postinor-2 Accessed 9 May 2025
21. Monge ME, Dwivedi P, Zhou M, et al. A tiered analytical approach for investigating poor quality emergency contraceptives. PLoS One. 2014;9:e95353.
22. IMPACT. Counterfeit medicines: an update on estimates. https://www.gphf.org/images/downloads/library/whoimpact.pdf Accessed 9 May 2025
23. Ozawa S, Evans DR, Bessias S, et al. Prevalence and estimated economic burden of substandard and falsified medicines in low- and middle-income countries: a systematic review and meta-analysis. JAMA Netw Open. 2018;1:e181662.
24. Infectious Diseases Data Observatory. Medical Product Quality Reports | Infectious Diseases Data Observatory. https://www.iddo.org/mq/research/medical-product-quality-reports. Accessed 7 Oct 2022.
25. Cockburn R, Newton PN, Agyarko EK, et al. The global threat of counterfeit drugs: why Industry and governments must communicate the dangers. PLoS Med. 2005;2:e100.
26. World Health Organization. WHO Global Surveillance and Monitoring System for substandard and falsified medical products. 2017. https://www.who.int/publications/i/item/9789241513425 Accessed 9May2025
27. Jackson G, Patel S, Khan S. Assessing the problem of counterfeit medications in the United Kingdom. Int J Clin Pract. 2012;66:241–50.
28. Tremblay M. Medicines counterfeiting is a complex problem: a review of key challenges across the supply chain. Curr Drug Saf. 2013;8:43–55.
29. Wise J. Record number of fake drugs are seized in crackdown. BMJ. 2013;346:f4204.
30. Irish Medicines Board. Safety notice- Ugrent Product Recall – Durex condoms. https://www.hpra.ie/homepage/medical-devices/safety-information/safety-notices/item?t=/durex-extra-safe-12-pack-condoms-and-durex-fetherlite-12-pack-condoms&id=579af825-9782-6eee-9b55-ff00008c97d0 Accessed 9 July 2018

31. Mackey TK, Cuomo R, Guerra C, et al. After counterfeit Avastin® – what have we learned and what can be done? Nat Rev Clin Oncol. 2015;12:302–8.
32. IRACM. Germany: box of falsified Harvoni uncovered in legal German medicine supply chain. https://www.iracm.com/en/2017/06/germany-box-falsified-harvoni-uncovered-legal-german-medicine-supply-chain/ Accessed 9 July 2018
33. Securing Industry. More fake Harvoni found in Japan. https://www.securingindustry.com/pharmaceuticals/more-fake-harvoni-found-in-japan/s40/a3134/#.W0LmsNUzaUk Accessed 9 May 2025
34. Blossom DB, Kallen AJ, Patel PR, et al. Outbreak of adverse reactions associated with contaminated heparin. N Engl J Med. 2008;359:2674–84.
35. Centers for Disease Control and Prevention. Multistate Meningitis Outbreak – Case Count. http://www.cdc.gov.gate2.inist.fr/hai/outbreaks/meningitis-map-large.html Accessed 9 July 2018
36. Nitrosamine impurities in metformin. Reactions Weekly 1784, 6 (2019). https://doi.org/10.1007/s40278-019-72725-3
37. World Health Organization. WHO Information Note – UPDATE ON NITROSAMINE IMPURITIES. 2019. https://www.who.int/medicines/publications/drugalerts/InformationNoteNitrosamine-impurities_Nov2019.pdf?ua=1 Accessed 26 June 2020
38. US Food and Drug Administration. FDA Updates and Press Announcements on Angiotensin II Receptor Blocker (ARB) Recalls (Valsartan, Losartan, and Irbesartan) | FDA. https://www.fda.gov/drugs/drug-safety-and-availability/fda-updates-and-press-announcements-angiotensin-ii-receptor-blocker-arb-recalls-valsartan-losartan Accessed 9 May 2025
39. INTERPOL. Pharmaceutical crime operations, https://www.interpol.int/Crimes/Illicit-goods/Pharmaceutical-crime-operations. Accessed 24 Nov 2022.
40. Sweileh WM. Substandard and falsified medical products: bibliometric analysis and mapping of scientific research. Glob Health. 2021;17:114. https://doi.org/10.1186/s12992-021-00766-5.
41. Nayyar GML, Breman JG, Herrington JE. The global pandemic of falsified medicines: laboratory and field innovations and policy perspectives. Am J Trop Med Hyg. 2015;92:2–7.
42. Wertheimer AI, Norris J. Safeguarding against substandard/counterfeit drugs: mitigating a macroeconomic pandemic. Res Social Adm Pharm. 2009;5:4–16.
43. Kelesidis T, Falagas ME. Substandard/counterfeit antimicrobial drugs. Clin Microbiol Rev. 2015;28:443–64.
44. Almuzaini T, Choonara I, Sammons H. Substandard and counterfeit medicines: a systematic review of the literature. BMJ Open. 2013;3:e002923.
45. Zabala GA, Bellingham K, Vidhamaly V, et al. Substandard and falsified antibiotics: neglected drivers of antimicrobial resistance? BMJ Glob Health. 2022;7 https://doi.org/10.1136/bmjgh-2022-008587.
46. Bate R, Jin GZ, Mathur A, et al. Poor quality drugs and global trade: a pilot study. https://www.nber.org/papers/w20469 Accessed 9 May 2025
47. Christi Lane LAK. Cambodian ministry of health takes decisive actions in the fight against substandard and counterfeit medicines. Trop Med Surg. 2014;2 https://doi.org/10.4172/2329-9088.1000166.
48. Yoshida N, Khan MH, Tabata H, et al. A cross-sectional investigation of the quality of selected medicines in Cambodia in 2010. BMC Pharmacol Toxicol. 2014;15:13.
49. Yong YL, Plançon A, Lau YH, et al. Collaborative health and enforcement operations on the quality of antimalarials and antibiotics in Southeast Asia. Am J Trop Med Hyg. 2015;92:105–12.
50. Abuga K, Amugune B, Ndwigah S, et al. Quality performance of drugs analyzed in the Drug Analysis and Research Unit (DARU) during the Period 2006–2010. East Cent Afr J Pharm Sci. 16

51. Thoithi G, Abuga K, Nguyo J, et al. Drug quality control in Kenya: observation in drug analysis and research unit during the period 1996-2000. East and Cent Afr J Pharma Sci. 2004;5:28–32.
52. Ahmad K. Antidepressants are sold as antiretrovirals in DR Congo. Lancet. 2004;363:713.
53. Apoola A, Sriskandabalan PS, Wade AA. Self-medication with zidovudine that was not. Lancet. 2001;357:1370.
54. Cohn J, von Schoen-Angerer T, Jambert E, et al. When falsified medicines enter the supply chain: description of an incident in Kenya and lessons learned for rapid response. J Public Health Policy. 2013;34:22–30.
55. Parfitt T. Russia cracks down on counterfeit drugs. Lancet. 2006;368:1481–2.
56. Tabernero P, Fernández FM, Green M, et al. Mind the gaps – the epidemiology of poor-quality anti-malarials in the malarious world – analysis of the World Wide Antimalarial Resistance Network database. Malar J. 2014;13:139.
57. Newton PN, Lee SJ, Goodman C, et al. Guidelines for field surveys of the quality of medicines: a proposal. PLoS Med. 2009;6:e52.
58. Tabernero P, Mayxay M, Culzoni MJ, et al. A repeat random survey of the prevalence of falsified and substandard antimalarials in the Lao PDR: a change for the better. Am J Trop Med Hyg. 2015;92:95–104.
59. Yeung S, Lawford HLS, Tabernero P, et al. Quality of antimalarials at the epicenter of anti-malarial drug resistance: results from an overt and mystery client survey in Cambodia. Am J Trop Med Hyg. 2015;92:39–50.
60. ACT Consortium Drug Quality Project and IMPACT Study Team. Quality of artemisinin-containing antimalarials in Tanzania's private sector – results from a nationally representative outlet survey. Am J Trop Med Hyg. 2015;92:75–86.
61. World Health Organization. WHO | About the WHO Global Malaria Programme. http://www.who.int/malaria/about_us/en/ Accessed 16 July 2018
62. Newton PN, Green MD, Mildenhall DC, et al. Poor quality vital anti-malarials in Africa – an urgent neglected public health priority. Malar J. 2011;10:352.
63. NAFDAC. Welcome to About Ondo State's Blog: NAFDAC raises alarm over circulation of adulterated drugs in Ondo. http://www.aboutondostate.org/2011/10/nafdac-raises-alarm-over-circulation-of.html# ACcessed 12 Jan 2016
64. World Health Organization. Information Exchange System Drug Alert No. 130 8. Falsified batches of Coartem recently circulating in Cameroon.
65. Minilabs Save Lives. https://www.facebook.com/minilab/ Accessed 9 May 2025
66. World Health Organization. Medical Product Alert No. 1/2015 Falsified anti-malarial medicine circulating in West Africa. http://www.who.int/medicines/publications/drugalerts/Artemether-LumefantrineENversion.pdf?ua=1 Accessed 9 May 2025
67. Guo S, Kyaw MP, He L, et al. Quality testing of artemisinin-based antimalarial drugs in Myanmar. Am J Trop Med Hyg. 2017;97:1198–203.
68. Lalani M, Kaur H, Mohammed N, et al. Substandard antimalarials available in Afghanistan: a case for assessing the quality of drugs in resource poor settings. Am J Trop Med Hyg. 2015;92:51–8.
69. Suleman S, Zeleke G, Deti H, et al. Quality of medicines commonly used in the treatment of soil transmitted helminths and giardia in Ethiopia: a nationwide survey. PLoS Negl Trop Dis. 2014;8:e3345.
70. Caillet C, Sichanh C, Syhakhang L, et al. Population awareness of risks related to medicinal product use in Vientiane Capital, Lao PDR: a cross-sectional study for public health improvement in low and middle-income countries. BMC Public Health. 2015;15:1–10.
71. Sanofi-Le Hub. Counterfeit medicines in Asia. https://lehub.sanofi.com/en/access-healthcare/counterfeit-medicines-in-asia/ Accessed 8 Feb 2016
72. Binkowska-Bury M, Januszewicz P, Wolan M, et al. Counterfeit medicines in Poland: opinions of primary healthcare physicians, nurses and lay persons. J Clin Nurs. 2013;22:559–68.

73. Peyraud N, Rafael F, Parker LA, et al. An epidemic of dystonic reactions in central Africa. The Lancet Global Health, Volume 5, Issue 2, e137–e138
74. The Partnership for Safe Medicines. Fake drugs flood Poland. http://www.safemedicines. org/2010/02/fake-drugs-flood-poland.html Accessed 2 Feb 2016
75. Nagaraj A, Tambi S, Biswas G, et al. Counterfeit medication: perception of doctors and medical wholesale distributors in western India. J Int Soc Prev Commun Dent. 2015;5:S7–S11.
76. Agence d'information d'Afrique Centrale. Santé publique: tous debout contre les faux médicaments au Congo. https://www.adiac-congo.com/content/sante-publique-tous-debout-contre-les-faux-medicaments-au-congo-42892 Accessed 9 May 2025
77. OnMedica. OnMedica – News – Fake medicine warning hits cinemas. http://www.onmedica. com/newsArticle.aspx?id=77249860-80b2-46b0-86e9-8088bb08cb9b Accessed 8 Feb 2016
78. IRACM. Le faux médicament, késako? https://www.cespharm.fr/prevention-sante/catalogue/ Le-Faux-medicament-kesako-affiche Accessed 9 May 2025
79. Abdoulaye I, Chastanier H, Azondekon A, et al. Evaluation of public awareness campaigns on counterfeit medicines in Cotonou, Benin. Med Trop (Mars). 2006;66:615–8.
80. Fight The Fakes. https://fightthefakes.org/ Accessed 9 May 2025
81. The Partnership for Safe Medicines. SAFEMEDICINES: Protecting the Safety of America's Drug Supply. https://www.safemedicines.org/ Accessed 9 May 2025
82. The Campaign – MedsWeCanTrust. https://unitaid.org/news-blog/medicines-we-can-trust-campaign-rallies-mekong-governments-and-leaders-to-improve-access-to-quality-medicines/ Accessed 9 May 2025
83. Rozendaal JA. Fake antimalarials circulating in Cambodia. Lancet. 2001;357:890.
84. Newton PN, White NJ, Rozendaal JA, et al. Murder by fake drugs. BMJ. 2002;324:800–1.
85. Renschler JP, Walters KM, Newton PN, et al. Estimated under-five deaths associated with poor-quality antimalarials in sub-Saharan Africa. Am J Trop Med Hyg. 2015;92:119–26.
86. World Health Organization. A study on the public health and socioeconomic impact of substandard and falsified medical products. 2017. http://apps.who.int/bookorders. Accessed 23 Aug 2019
87. Keoluangkhot V, Green MD, Nyadong L, et al. Impaired clinical response in a patient with uncomplicated falciparum malaria who received poor-quality and underdosed intramuscular artemether. Am J Trop Med Hyg. 2008;78:552–5.
88. Nickerson JW, Attaran A, Westerberg BD, et al. Fatal bacterial meningitis possibly associated with substandard ceftriaxone – Uganda, 2013. MMWR Morb Mortal Wkly Rep. 2016;64:1375–7.
89. Newton PN, McGready R, Fernandez F, et al. Manslaughter by fake artesunate in Asia – will Africa be next? PLoS Med. 2006;3:e197.
90. World Health Organization. Substandard and counterfeit medicines.
91. Otte WM, van Diessen E, van Eijsden P, et al. Counterfeit antiepileptic drugs threaten community services in Guinea-Bissau and Nigeria. Lancet Neurol. 2015;14:1075–6.
92. Leslie T, Kaur H, Mohammed N, et al. Epidemic of Plasmodium falciparum malaria involving substandard antimalarial drugs, Pakistan, 2003. Emerg Infect Dis. 2009;15:1753–9.
93. Bate BR. Antimicrobial resistance: how substandard medicines contribute. 2015; 1–4.
94. Pisani E. Antimicrobial resistance: What does medicine quality have to do with it? http:// amr-review.org/sites/default/files/ElizabethPisaniMedicinesQualitypaper.pdf Accessed 9 May 2025
95. Holmes AH, Moore LSP, Sundsfjord A, et al. Understanding the mechanisms and drivers of antimicrobial resistance. The Lancet. 2015;387:176. https://doi.org/10.1016/ S0140-6736(15)00473-0.
96. Newton PN, Caillet C, Guérin P. Antimalarial quality and drug resistance. Expert Rev Anti-Infect Ther. 2016;14:531–3.
97. Taylor RB, Shakoor O, Behrens RH. Drug quality, a contributor to drug resistance? Lancet. 1995;346:122.

98. Okeke IN, Klugman KP, Bhutta ZA, et al. Antimicrobial resistance in developing countries. Part II: Strategies for containment. Lancet Infect Dis. 2005;5:568–80.
99. Okeke IN, Lamikanra A, Edelman R. Socioeconomic and behavioral factors leading to acquired bacterial resistance to antibiotics in developing countries. Emerg Infect Dis. 5:18–27.
100. Green MD. Antimalarial drug resistance and the importance of drug quality monitoring. J Postgrad Med. 52:288–90.
101. White NJ, Pongtavornpinyo W, Maude RJ, et al. Hyperparasitaemia and low dosing are an important source of anti-malarial drug resistance. Malar J. 2009;8:253.
102. Sosa AJ. Antimicrobial resistance in developing countries. New York: Springer; 2009. https://doi.org/10.1007/978-0-387-89370-9.
103. Cavany, S, Nanyonga, S, Hauk, C. et al. The uncertain role of substandard and falsified medicines in the emergence and spread of antimicrobial resistance. Nat Commun. 2023;14:6153. https://doi.org/10.1038/s41467-023-41542-w
104. Hall KA, Newton PN, Green MD, et al. Characterization of counterfeit artesunate antimalarial tablets from Southeast Asia. Am J Trop Med Hyg. 2006;75:804–11.
105. Donald K, Hall S, Seaton C, et al. Is non-therapeutic aspirin use in children a problem in South Africa? S Afr Med J. 2011;101:823–8.
106. Sesay. Fake drugs – a new threat to health-care delivery. Africa Health June/July 1988
107. Wiest J, Schollmayer C, Gresser G, et al. Identification and quantitation of the ingredients in a counterfeit Vietnamese herbal medicine against rheumatic diseases. J Pharm Biomed Anal. 2014;97:24–8.
108. Davies E. Glass particles found in generic atorvastatin. BMJ. 2012;345:e8236.
109. Sengaloundeth S, Green MD, Fernández FM, et al. A stratified random survey of the proportion of poor quality oral artesunate sold at medicine outlets in the Lao PDR – implications for therapeutic failure and drug resistance. Malar J. 2009;8:172.
110. Bowie MD, McKenzie D. Diethylene glycol poisoning in children. S Afr Med J. 1972;46:931–4.
111. Okuonghae HO, Ighogboja IS, Lawson JO, et al. Diethylene glycol poisoning in Nigerian children. Ann Trop Paediatr. 1992;12:235–8.
112. Akuse RM, Eke FU, Ademola AD, et al. Diagnosing renal failure due to diethylene glycol in children in a resource-constrained setting. Pediatr Nephrol. 2012;27:1021–8.
113. Hanif M, Mobarak MR, Ronan A, et al. Fatal renal failure caused by diethylene glycol in paracetamol elixir: the Bangladesh epidemic. BMJ. 1995;311:88–91.
114. O'Brien KL, Selanikio JD, Hecdivert C, et al. Epidemic of pediatric deaths from acute renal failure caused by diethylene glycol poisoning. Acute Renal Failure Investigation Team. JAMA. 1998;279:1175–80.
115. Singh J, Dutta AK, Khare S, et al. Diethylene glycol poisoning in Gurgaon, India, 1998. Bull World Health Organ. 2001;79:88–95.
116. Reuters. Gambia says child deaths linked to cough syrup have risen to 70 I Reuters. https://www.reuters.com/world/africa/gambia-says-child-deaths-linked-to-cough-syrup-have-risen-70-2022-10-14/. Accessed 24 Nov 2022.
117. Reuters. Indonesia bans cough syrup material linked to Gambia child deaths I Reuters. https://www.reuters.com/world/asia-pacific/indonesia-bans-cough-syrup-material-linked-gambia-child-deaths-2022-10-15/. Accessed 24 Nov 2022.
118. World Health Organization. Medical Product Alert No. 4/2015 Adverse reactions caused by Falsified Diazepam in Central Africa. http://www.who.int/medicines/publications/drugalerts/Alert4_2015DiazepamEN.pdf. 2015.
119. Report of the Judicial Inquiry Tribunal. The pathology of negligence. 2012. https://padproject.nd.edu/assets/206307/pathology_of_negligence_pic_drug_inquiry_report_2012.pdf Accessed 12 May 2025
120. Kao SL, Chan CL, Tan B, et al. An unusual outbreak of hypoglycemia. N Engl J Med. 2009;360:734–6.
121. Blackstone EA, Fuhr JP, Pociask S. The health and economic effects of counterfeit drugs. Am Health Drug Benefits. 2014;7:216–24.

122. Ozawa S, Higgins CR, Nwokike JI et al. Modeling the Health and Economic Impact of Substandard and Falsified Medicines: A Review of Existing Models and Approaches. Am J Trop Med Hyg. 2022; 13:14-20. https://doi.org/10.4269/ajtmh.21-1133. PMID: 35895357; PMCID: PMC9294666.

123. Salami RK, Valente de Almeida S, Gheorghe A et al. Health, Economic, and Social Impacts of Substandard and Falsified Medicines in Low- and Middle-Income Countries: A Systematic Review of Methodological Approaches. Am J Trop Med Hyg. 2023; 20;109(2):228-240. doi: 10.4269/ajtmh.22-0525. PMID: 37339762; PMCID: PMC10397424.

124. Kron MA. Substandard primaquine phosphate for US Peace Corps personnel. Lancet. 1996;348:1453–4.

125. Chaccour CJ, Kaur H, Mabey D, et al. Travel and fake artesunate: a risky business. Lancet. 2012;380:1120.

126. Chaubey SK, Sangla KS, Suthaharan EN, et al. Severe hypoglycaemia associated with ingesting counterfeit medication. Med J Aust. 2010;192:716–7.

127. Barber T, Jacyna M. Acute lead intoxication from medications purchased online presenting with recurrent abdominal pain and encephalopathy. J R Soc Med. 2011;104:120–3.

128. Kuramoto N, Yabe D, Kurose T, et al. A case of hypoglycemia due to illegitimate sexual enhancement medication. Diabetes Res Clin Pract. 2015;108:e8–e10.

129. Sun X, Xu X, Zhang X. Counterfeit bevacizumab and endophthalmitis. N Engl J Med. 2011;365:378–9. author reply 379

130. Juhlin K, Karimi G, Andér M, et al. Using VigiBase to identify substandard medicines: detection capacity and key prerequisites. Drug Saf. 2015;38:373–82.

131. Hazell L, Shakir SAW. Under-reporting of adverse drug reactions: a systematic review. Drug Saf. 2006;29:385–96.

132. Pal SN, Duncombe C, Falzon D, et al. WHO strategy for collecting safety data in public health programmes: complementing spontaneous reporting systems. Drug Saf. 2013;36:75–81.

133. Olsson S, Pal SN, Dodoo A. Pharmacovigilance in resource-limited countries. Expert Rev Clin Pharmacol.

134. Ubajaka CF, Obi-Okaro ACEOF, Azumarah MN, Ukegbu AU, et al. Factors associated with drug counterfeit in Nigeria: a twelve year review – ProQuest. Br J Med Med Res. 12

135. Bate R, Mathur A. Corruption and medicine quality in Latin America: a pilot study. BE J Econ Anal Policy. 2018;18 https://doi.org/10.1515/bejeap-2017-0076.

136. CamerNews. Cameroun – Corruption: Pharmaciens, médecins et infirmiers accusés dans le trafic des médicaments de rue – Camernews Camernews. http://www.camernews.com/56348-2/ Accessed 12 Feb 2016

137. Mackey TK, Liang BA. Combating healthcare corruption and fraud with improved global health governance. BMC Int Health Hum Rights. 2012;12:23.

138. Kovacs S, Hawes SE, Maley SN, et al. Technologies for detecting falsified and substandard drugs in low and middle-income countries. PLoS One. 2014;9:e90601.

139. Martino R, Malet-Martino M, Gilard V, et al. Counterfeit drugs: analytical techniques for their identification. Anal Bioanal Chem. 2010;398:77–92.

140. Fernandez FM, Hostetler D, Powell K, et al. Poor quality drugs: grand challenges in high throughput detection, countrywide sampling, and forensics in developing countries. Analyst. 2011;136:3073–82.

141. Kaur H, Green MD, Hostetler DM, et al. Antimalarial drug quality: methods to detect suspect drugs. Therapy. 2010;7:49–57.

142. Vickers S, Bernier M, Zambrzycki S, et al. Field detection devices for screening the quality of medicines: a systematic review. BMJ Glob Health. 2018;3:e000725.

143. International Council of Nurses USP. Tool for Visual Inspection of Medicines. https://www.fip.org/files/fip/counterfeit/VisualInspection/A%20tool%20for%20visual%20inspection%20of%20medicines%20EN.pdf Accessed 12 May 2025

144. Schiavetti B, Wynendaele E, Melotte V, et al. A simplified checklist for the visual inspection of finished pharmaceutical products: a way to empower frontline health workers in the fight against poor-quality medicines. J Pharm Policy Pract. 2020;13:9.
145. The GPHF-Minilab. The GPHF-Minilab – Protection Against Counterfeit Medicines https://www.gphf.org/en/minilab/index.htm. Accessed 13 May 2025.
146. U.S. Food and Drug Administration. FDA Facts: FDA's Counterfeit Detection Device CD-3. https://fr.scribd.com/document/212678912/CD-3-Counterfeit-Detection-Device-FC0413 Accessed 12 May 2025
147. Ranieri N, Tabernero P, Green MD, et al. Evaluation of a new handheld instrument for the detection of counterfeit artesunate by visual fluorescence comparison. Am J Trop Med Hyg. 2014;91:920–4.
148. Weaver AA, Lieberman M. Paper test cards for presumptive testing of very low quality anti-malarial medications. Am J Trop Med Hyg. 2015;92:17–23.
149. Weaver AA, Reiser H, Barstis T, et al. Paper analytical devices for fast field screening of beta lactam antibiotics and antituberculosis pharmaceuticals. Anal Chem. 2013;85:6453–60.
150. Chen H-H, Higgins C, Laing SK, et al. Cost savings of paper analytical devices (PADs) to detect substandard and falsified antibiotics: Kenya case study. Medicine Access @ Point of Care. 2021;5:239920262098030.
151. Strock J, Nguyen M, Sherma J. Transfer of Minilab TLC screening methods to quantitative HPTLC-densitometry for pyrazinamide, ethambutol, isoniazid, and rifampicin in a combination tablet. J Liq Chromatogr Relat Technol. 2015;38:1126–30.
152. Visser BJ, Meerveld-Gerrits J, Kroon D, et al. Assessing the quality of anti-malarial drugs from Gabonese pharmacies using the MiniLab®: a field study. Malar J. 2015;14:273.
153. Risha PG, Msuya Z, Clark M, et al. The use of Minilabs to improve the testing capacity of regulatory authorities in resource limited settings: Tanzanian experience. Health Policy. 2008;87:217–22.
154. Bate R, Hess K. Anti-malarial drug quality in Lagos and Accra – a comparison of various quality assessments. Malar J. 2010;9:157.
155. Kandpal LM, Park E, Tewari J, et al. Spectroscopic techniques for nondestructive quality inspection of pharmaceutical products: a review. J Biosyst Eng. 2015;40:394–408.
156. Caillet C, Vickers S, Zambrzycki S, et al. An evaluation of portable screening devices to assess medicines quality for national medicines regulatory authorities – RETA 8763. 2018. https://www.iddo.org/external-publication/evaluation-portable-screening-devices-assess-medicines-quality-national Accessed 12 May 2025
157. Saving Lives at Birth. PharmaChk: Substandard and Counterfeit Medicines Rapid Detection and Screening Platform.
158. Ho NT, Desai D, Zaman MH. Rapid and specific drug quality testing assay for artemisinin and its derivatives using a luminescent reaction and novel microfluidic technology. Am J Trop Med Hyg. 2015;92:24–30.
159. Chi Z, Zhao S, Cui X et al. Portable and automated analyzer for rapid and high precision in vitro dissolution of drugs. Journal of Pharm Anal. 2021; 4: 490-498. https://doi.org/10.1016/j.jpha.2020.06.001.
160. Perez-Mon C, Hauk C, Roncone A et al. Hide and seek with falsified medicines: Current challenges and physicochemical and biological approaches for tracing the origin of trafficked products. Forensic Sci Int. 2025; 370:112474. doi: 10.1016/j.forsciint.2025.112474. Epub 2025 Apr 15. PMID: 40252581.
161. Roncone A, Kelly SD, Giannioti Z et al. Stable isotope ratio analysis: an emerging tool to trace the origin of falsified medicines, TrAC. 2024; 174:117666. https://doi.org/10.1016/j.trac.2024.117666.
162. Newton PN, Fernández FM, Plançon A, et al. A collaborative epidemiological investigation into the criminal fake artesunate trade in South East Asia. PLoS Med. 2008;5:e32.
163. Attaran A. Stopping murder by medicine: introducing the model law on medicine crime. Am J Trop Med Hyg. 2015;92:127–32.

164. Nayyar GML, Attaran A, Clark JP, et al. Responding to the pandemic of falsified medicines. Am J Trop Med Hyg. 2015;92:113–8.
165. Attaran A, Barry D, Basheer S, et al. How to achieve international action on falsified and substandard medicines. BMJ. 2012;345:e7381.
166. Bate R, Attaran A. A counterfeit drug treaty: great idea, wrong implementation. Lancet. 2010;376:1446–8.
167. Newton PN, Schellenberg D, Ashley EA, et al. Quality assurance of drugs used in clinical trials: proposal for adapting guidelines. BMJ. 2015;350:h602.
168. Idindili B, Masanja H, Urassa H, et al. Randomized controlled safety and efficacy trial of 2 vitamin A supplementation schedules in Tanzanian infants. Am J Clin Nutr. 2007;85:1312–9.
169. Newton PN, Tabernero P, Dwivedi P, et al. Falsified medicines in Africa: all talk, no action. Lancet Glob Health. 2014;2:e509–10.
170. Pharmaceutical Security Institute. Incident Trends | PSI. https://www.psi-inc.org/incident-trends. Accessed 29 Nov 2022.
171. Anon. Fighting fake drugs: the role of WHO and pharma. Lancet. 2011;377:1626.
172. World Health Organization. WHO Global Surveillance and Monitoring System. https://www.who.int/who-global-surveillance-and-monitoring-system. Accessed 29 Nov 2022.
173. Access to Medicines Foundation. Access to Medicine Index. https://accesstomedicinefoundation.org/sectors-and-research/index-ranking. Accessed 24 Nov 2022.

Chapter 12
The Role of Pharmacovigilance Centres in Detecting Medication Errors: Moroccan Experience

Rachida Soulaymani Bencheikh, Loubna Alj, Ghita Benabdallah, and Houda Sefiani

12.1 Background

"To Err Is Human: Building a Safer Health System [1]," the Institute of Medicine's report reveals the alarming results concerning medical errors. In fact, it is estimated that medical errors cause between 44,000 and 98,000 deaths annually in hospitals in the USA, and among them 7,000 were due to medication errors. Even though previous studies on adverse events and on adverse drug events have been made, it is particularly after the Institute of Medicine's report results that patient safety hauled up at the level of health care's high priority.

In fact, the first studies on Adverse Drug Events "ADEs" date back to 1984 with the Harvard Medical Practice Study [2]. Of the 30,195 patients included, 19.4% experienced an ADE and 17.7% of these ADEs were considered preventable.

Harm caused to patient costs a lot to health systems and is estimated between US$ 6 billion to US$ 29 billion per year [3].

In 2002, the 55th World Health Assembly [4], after recognizing that the promotion of patient safety constitutes a priority and a fundamental principle of all health systems, adopted a resolution urging members' state to focus on the question of

R. S. Bencheikh (✉)
Faculté de Médecine et de Pharmacie, Université Mohamed V, Rabat, Morocco

Centre Anti Poison et de Pharmacovigilance du Maroc, Rabat, Morocco

World Health Organization Collaborating Centre for Strengthening Pharmacovigilance Practices, Rabat, Morocco
e-mail: r.soulaymani@pharmacovigilance.ma

L. Alj · G. Benabdallah · H. Sefiani
Centre Anti Poison et de Pharmacovigilance du Maroc, Rabat, Morocco

World Health Organization Collaborating Centre for Strengthening Pharmacovigilance Practices, Rabat, Morocco
e-mail: r.benabdallah@pharmacovigilance.ma; h.sefiani@pharmacovigilance.ma

© Springer Nature Singapore Pte Ltd. 2025
S. R. Ahmad (ed.), *Special Issues in Pharmacovigilance in Resource-Limited Countries*, https://doi.org/10.1007/978-981-96-6154-1_12

patient safety and to pay attention to the problem of monitoring of drugs, medical equipment, and technology.

In October 2004 [5], another major development in realm of patient safety took place with the launching of the World Alliance for Patient Safety "WAPS." The rationale behind such an initiative was mainly to focus on the significant global problem of patient harm and to introduce a concrete health policy designed to prevent harm caused to patients.

In March 2007 [6], the Erice Manifesto highlighted the new vision of Pharmacovigilance focusing on Patient Safety as the main challenge of pharmacovigilance.

Bates, in 2010, highlighted the fact that in developed countries, 1 out of 10 patients is harmed while receiving hospital care [7], and the WAPS pointed out the fact that in developing countries, the probability of patients being harmed in hospitals is higher than in industrialized nations [8].

In fact, the lack of an efficient drug regulatory system leading to an increased number of counterfeit medicines, the poor quality of health care settings, and the low socio economic level are the main contributing factors to ME occurrence in low- and middle-income countries (LMICs) than in developed countries.

From the beginning, Pharmacovigilance Centres have collected ME without being aware of it. Nevertheless, ME are considered part of pharmacovigilance, and therefore, the management of ME should be included in any global national strategy to reduce and prevent harm.

The CAPM has been involved in a WHO/Uppsala Monitoring Centre "UMC" Project funded by the WAPS to extend the role for national pharmacovigilance Centres to include collection of information on adverse events related to ME and to enable international analysis of these data and to disseminate findings internationally. The CAPM undertook three studies to better understand the epidemiology of ME.

The aim of the first study was to assess the ability to collect and identify ME from ADRs reported to the CAPM. It was a retrospective analysis of ADRs reported to the CAPM from 2003 to 2006 and the results showed that 14.6% of ADRs were preventable ADRs [9].

The aim of the second study was to assess the prevalence rate of ADEs and to ascertain those related to medication errors to develop prevention strategies. It was a prospective cohort study performed in 7 Moroccan Intensive Care Units in academic and military hospital of Rabat for a period of three months. The results showed that 7.5% of ADRs were preventable ADRs [10].

The third study was a questionnaire-based analysis sent to pharmacovigilance centres to assess their ability to detect ME and to proceed to building patient safety via their information network. This was an exploratory study conducted in pharmacovigilance centres who were members of the WHO Programme for International Drug Monitoring. The questionnaire asked for information, progress, and improvement made by pharmacovigilance centres in patient safety and ME. The results showed the ability of pharmacovigilance centres to detect and analyze ME, the need to coordinate efforts between countries to optimize ME detection and its analysis, and showed the need to build bridges linking pharmacovigilance centres, patient safety organization, and poison control centres [11].

These studies revealed the contribution of pharmacovigilance centres in improving patient safety and support the fact that pharmacovigilance centres should start to work on ME by collecting them, identifying them, analyzing them, and preventing them.

In order to display these findings, WHO in collaboration with the CAPM, the National Patient Safety Agency, and the UMC have been involved in the Monitoring Medicines Project to expand the role and scope of pharmacovigilance centres to prevent medicine-related adverse events. To this end, a guideline entitled "Reporting and Learning Systems for Medication Errors: The Role of Pharmacovigilance Centres" [12] intended for pharmacovigilance centres, medication safety organizations, and patient safety organizations has been developed to increase the capacity of national pharmacovigilance centres to identify and analyze preventable ME and to stimulate cooperation between national pharmacovigilance centres and the WAPS.

To be able to manage ME, from detecting to implementing risk minimization actions, pharmacovigilance centres should be part of a global national strategy leading to reduce harm from ME. To this end, in each country, basic steps should be followed to be able to manage ME.

- For countries with effective pharmacovigilance centre:

  - ME activities should be included within the daily routine of pharmacovigilance centre, as in a pharmacovigilance centre with integrated vigilances. In the case of a country with an organization dedicated to medication safety, a close collaboration should be built to share ME cases.
  - Pharmacovigilance staff should be trained to detect and analyze ME.

- For countries without pharmacovigilance centres:

  - ME activities should be included within one global integrated pharmacovigilance system dealing with all vigilances (vaccines, medical devices, herbals and adverse events during pregnancy and breastfeeding).
  - Pharmacovigilance staff should be trained to detect and analyze ME.

To build patient safety and improve medication safety, pharmacovigilance centres have a leading role.

12.2   Role of Pharmacovigilance Centres in Detecting Medication Errors

12.2.1   Raising Awareness on Patient Safety and Management of Medication Errors

To reduce the occurrence of ME and improve patient safety, pharmacovigilance centres would have to raise the awareness of pharmacovigilance staff and of health care professionals "HCP" on the concept of patient safety, the culture of patient safety, and the management of medication errors by organizing trainings and sensitization for:

- Pharmacovigilance centres staff:

    - To raise awareness on their ability to detect ME through an improved existing Individual Case Safety Report "ICSR" and by using specific tools to identify a preventable ADR.
    - To raise their awareness on the importance to manage ME.

To reach these objectives, pharmacovigilance centres could be supported by WHO Headquarters and/or WHO collaborating centres for pharmacovigilance.

- Health care professionals:

    - To raise the attention of HCP about their ability in managing Medication Errors "ME" through reported adverse events.
    - To raise awareness on the importance of reporting ADRs and ME.

12.2.2 Identifying ME by Improved Existing ICSR Form

One way to identifying ME through ICSR is to use an improved existing ICSR form. In fact, the use of ICSR is the basis for PV Centres to conduct causality assessment and to optimize detection of ME; individual case safety reporting form should be improved by adding some important items leading to optimize ME detection.

Proposed items to be added in an ICSR form:

- Patient weight, because many doses depend on patient weight.
- Relevant medical history, because of the risk of allergies, renal failure, hepatic failure, hypertension.
- Suspected and concomitant drug, because of the risk of drug-drug interactions, drug-herbal interactions.
- Narrative case, to provide information about circumstances in which ME/ADR occur.
- Relevant laboratory test, to allow detection of drug monitoring errors.
- Information about the process of prescription and dispensation.
- Suspicion or not medication error in order to build the culture of reporting medication errors.

12.2.3 Using Specific Tools to Identify Preventable ADRs: Preventability Method

Another way to identify ME through ICSR is to do preventability assessment by using a preventability method called "The P Method." It is a systematic approach used to detect preventable ADRs among ADRs reported to PV centres [13].

Preventability assessment is performed once causality assessment is done and the adverse event is classified as an adverse drug reaction.

The P Method is not intended to classify ME nor to perform the Root Cause Analysis and is based on the identification of 20 defined preventability criteria. The outcome of the preventability assessment will result in three situations:

- *The event is preventable* when at least one preventability criterion is identified.
- *The event is Non preventable* when none of the preventability criterion is identified.
- *The event is Not assessable* when there is insufficient data for preventability assessment.

A preventable ADR and a non-preventable ADR is not a static condition.
It is closely linked to how drug is used and monitored and depends on:

- Time which means that an ADR is non preventable currently but may be preventable in the future.
- Space which means that an ADR could be non-preventable in a country and may be stated as a preventable ADR in another one.
- Current state of knowledge on mechanism of ADR occurrence which would improve within time.
- Capacity of health services in developing therapeutic protocols and making tools and analysis for reducing the occurrence of ADR (Table 12.1).

12.2.4   Using Specific Tools to Identify Risk/ Contributing Factors

12.2.4.1   Root Cause Analysis

Once an ADR is identified as a preventable ADR, then pharmacovigilance centres may use specific tools to identify contributing factors which lead to medication errors. The Root Cause Analysis is performed [14]. It is an investigatory method designed to identify underlying causes and contributing factors that lead to ME occurrence.

Goals of the Root Cause Analysis are to understand:

- What happened?
- Why did it happen?
- How can we reduce the probability of recurrence?

The Root Cause Analysis is performed using the *Ishikawa diagram* [15]: It is a fish diagram used as a tool to help classify all the possible contributory factors to ME occurrence, which allow us to establish risk minimization actions (Fig. 12.1).

Table 12.1 Preventability criteria in the P method

Factors related to	Preventability criteria	Yes	No	UN	NA
Professional practice "Pr"	1. Incorrect dose?				
	2. Incorrect drug administration route?				
	3. Incorrect drug administration duration?				
	4. Incorrect drug dosage formulation administered?				
	5. Expired drug administered?				
	6. Incorrect storage of drug?				
	7. Drug administration error (timing, rate, frequency, Technique, Preparation, manipulation, mixing)?				
	8. Wrong indication?				
	9. Inappropriate prescription according to characteristics of the patient (age, Sex, pregnancy, other)?				
	10. Inappropriate prescription for patient's clinical condition (renal failure, hepatic failure …), or underlying pathology?				
	11. Documented hypersensitivity to administered drug or drug class?				
	12. Labeled drug-drug interaction?				
	13. Therapeutic duplication? (prescription of 2 medicines or more with similar ingredient)				
	14. Necessary medication not given?				
	15. Withdrawal Syndrome? (due to abrupt discontinuation of treatment)				
	16. Incorrect laboratory or clinical monitoring of medicine?				
Product/drug "Pd"	17. Poor quality drug administered?				
	18. Counterfeit drug administered?				
Patient "Pa"	19. Non compliance?				
	20. Self medication with non OTC drug?				

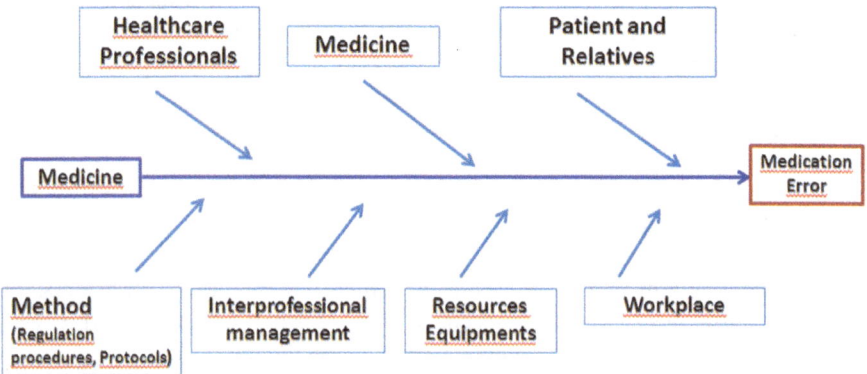

Fig. 12.1 Ishikawa diagram

12.2.5   Setting Up Public Health Risk Minimization Actions (RMA)

Risk minimization measures are public health interventions intended to prevent or reduce the occurrence of adverse reactions associated with the exposure to a medicine or to reduce their severity or impact on the patient should adverse reactions occur [16, 17].

Main objectives of RMA are to limit harm, to prevent its recurrence, and to improve patient safety when a generated and validated signal is validated into an alert.

Planning and implementing RMA and assessing their effectiveness are key elements of risk management.

RMA could be regulatory actions, communicating around the risk or implementation of risk strategies.

12.2.5.1   Regulatory Actions

- Regulatory actions involving Drug Regulatory Authority:

    Dear HCP letters, withdrawal of the product, adding warnings, restrictions as dispensing only in hospital, prescribed only by specific specialist, or contraindicated for children under 18 years old…

- Regulatory actions involving marketing authorization holders who provide additional educational material on medicines and their use: patient information leaflets, guidelines/checklists.

12.2.5.2   Communicating Around the Risk

Targeting the right message to the right population.

The scope of educational tools should be clearly defined, on specific risks and specific steps to be taken by HCP and patient in order to minimize the risk.

Format of tools are specific for each target such as Brochures, checklists, Flyer, bulletins, Posters, patient alert card as well as the use of media and campaign of sensitization.

12.2.5.3   Implementation of Health Strategies

- Implementation of therapeutic protocols requesting HCP to ask systematically specific questions to their patients concerning cases of medication allergies.
- Notification of any adverse events related to a specific medicine.
- Pregnancy prevention program.
- Implementation of pharmacovigilance in health programs.
- Implementation of patient safety.

Any risk minimization action undertaken needs to be assessed to ensure that the risk has been minimized.

- *Assessment by measurement of the direct outcome as*

    Decreased number of ADR/ME.
    Assessment of actions implemented as:
    Testing of educational material of knowledge.
    Surveys.
    Drug utilization studies.

12.2.6   Outlining the Importance of Collaborations Between All Concerned Parties Involved to Prevent ME

Pharmacovigilance centres are tasked with improving patient safety and reducing medication errors. To achieve these objectives, pharmacovigilance centres need to build bridges between all concerned parties to establish effective collaboration leading to strong partnership.

There are four levels of partnership, all dedicated to patient safety:

The first level is embodied by pharmacovigilance centres, poison control centres, and patient safety organizations. They join forces to get an overview of all MEs, to detect them earlier, to generate signals earlier, and to standardize practices.

The second level is represented by patients and healthcare providers. The partnership could not be effective without the *joint engagement* of first and second levels, to report adverse events and MEs to the first level and to inform, train, raise awareness, educate, and prevent MEs to the second level.

The third level is made up of universities, professional organizations, consumer organizations, and the media. The partnership between the first and second levels could not be successful if the third level did not work together to promote, teach, and train healthcare professionals on the concept of patient safety and to educate patients on the importance of their engagement in ME prevention. Partnership with the media is essential to promote, raise awareness, reinforce, and support the concept of patient safety.

The fourth level is formed by the drug regulatory authority, marketing authorization holders, and hospitals. Partnership is fundamental to the implementation of preventive actions decided by the first level, helping to avoid the recurrence of ME.

Collaboration between these four levels of partnership is the key to ME prevention. To achieve these objectives, it is necessary to establish a partnership between poison control centres (PCCs) and Patient Safety Organizations (PSOs), raising awareness among their healthcare professionals on the value of such collaboration. It is also essential to establish a partnership between pharmacovigilance centres, PCCs, PSOs, and medical and pharmacy schools, to concentrate on teaching and training in clinical pharmacology and in practical prescribing principles for undergraduate and postgraduate students and to gain the trust of the media (Fig. 12.2).

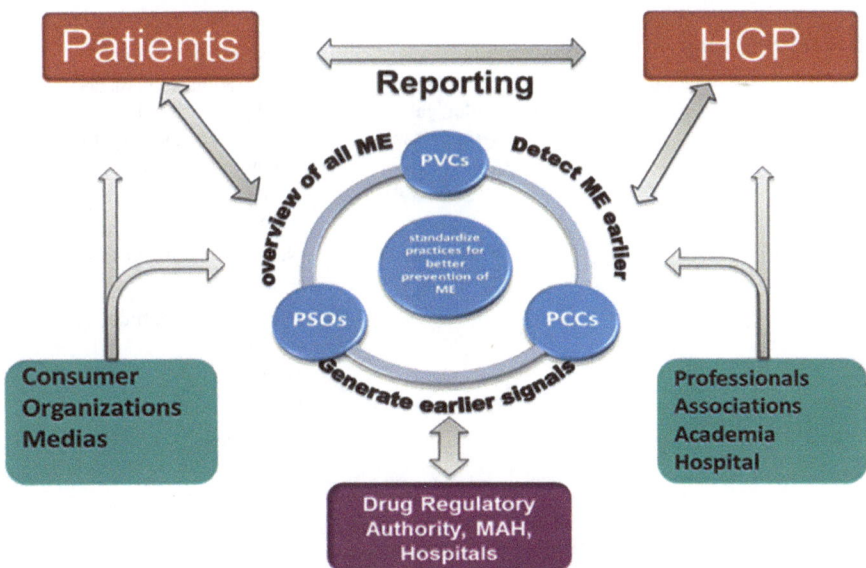

Fig. 12.2 Schematic outline of partnerships between stakeholders engaged in tackling MEs [12]

12.3 Success Stories

12.3.1 Vitamin D

It is well acknowledged that vitamin D is an essential component in the development of strong bones. Deficiency of this vitamin in infants leads to rickets. However, excessive vitamin D leads to nephrocalcinosis and cardiac complications.

Following a study that revealed a high prevalence of rickets, estimated at 60%, in children under 5 years, the Moroccan Program for Preventing Rickets "MPPR" was established since 1972. MPPR recommended two doses of 600,000 IU each—the first dose was scheduled at birth and the second one at six months.

In 2012, the CAPM received 17 ICSRs related to vitamin D in newborns and infants among which 16 experienced nephrocalcinosis. The outcome was fatal for two newborns due to cardiac arrest and terminal renal failure (Table 12.2).

12.3.2 Causality Assessment

Causality assessment has been done, which showed that adverse drug reactions experienced by newborns and infants were probable. The literature review showed that ADRs reported are more related to overdose.

Table 12.2 Description of ICSRs associated with vitamin D

Age	15 days to 6 months
Clinical and biological symptoms	Dehydration, somnolence, vomiting, convulsion, weight loss, tachycardia, hypotonia, hypotrophy, hyperglycemia
Onset date	15 days to 2 months after taking Vitamin D
Explorations	Nephrocalcinosis in 16 cases
Treatment	Rehydration IV
	Diuretics (furosemide) and corticoids
Seriousness	Hospitalization: 17 cases
Outcome	Favorable: 15 cases
	Two fatal outcomes: Cardiac arrest and terminal renal failure

12.3.3   Preventability Assessment

After performing causality assessment, we evaluated the preventability of ADRs reports using the "p method." Preventability assessment revealed that ADRs are due to an incorrect dose of vitamin D prescribed or administered to the pediatric population. Then we considered these ADRs as preventable ADRs and thus as medication errors.

These ADRs was considered as a signal with high priority that should be explored to understand why these cases happened. For that purpose, we conducted the Root Cause Analysis "RCA" to identify underlying causes and contributing factors that lead to vitamin D overdoses occurrence.

12.3.4   RCA/Contributing Factors

The analysis of the overdoses showed that the recommended dose by the MPPR is three times higher than the recommended one by international guidelines. The recommended dose (600,000 IU) was accurate in 1972 due to the high prevalence of rickets at that time. Currently, the incidence of rickets has significantly decreased and then the dose should be changed.

Additionally, the vitamin D 600,000 IU, used as part of this program, is strictly for adult use and the restriction is clearly mentioned in the Patient Package Insert. Moreover, the pediatric formulation of vitamin D is not available in the Moroccan market.

Other contributing factors identified were a lack of awareness of the health care professionals concerning signs of vitamin D overdoses and of patients' relatives concerning the risk of self-medication by giving supplementary doses leading to overdoses.

12.3.5   Risk Minimization Actions

In order to prevent the recurrence of similar cases, the CAPM organized the pharmacovigilance technical committee to discuss these cases in order to propose risk minimization actions to put in place.

12.3.6 RMA Proposed

The CAPM proposed regulatory actions for key pharmacovigilance partners:

• *For the MPPR.*

It was proposed to reduce the recommended dose of vitamin D to 200,000 IU and to send a "Dear Doctor Letter" strengthening preventive measures against the risk of vitamin D overdoses. The content of the "Dear Doctor Letter" would draw up health care professionals attention to give the efficient recommended dose 200.000 UI that means one-third of the vial while waiting for the new formulation, to reduce vitamin D posology when babies are fed with fortified milk with Vitamin D, and to educate consumers and relatives to risks related to vitamin D self-medication.

• *For the Moroccan Health Authorities.*

It was recommended to provide pediatricians with a vitamin D formulation adapted for pediatric population and to add vitamin D 200,000 IU in the list of essential medicines.

• *For Marketing Authorization Holders.*

It was suggested to bring to market as soon as possible the new adapted formulation of vitamin D and to add a Patient Package Insert in Arabic in addition to the French one. It was also suggested to add newborns and infants pictures on the medicine packaging.

12.3.7 RMA Implemented

Among the proposed actions listed, the following were implemented:

• The Moroccan program for preventing rickets adapted its recommendation to 200,000 IU.
• The Moroccan Health authorities gave their approval for a pediatric formulation at 200,000 IU.
• The "Dear Doctor Letter" with preventive measures against the risk of vitamin D overdoses was sent to health care professionals.

12.3.8 Obstacles

In this case, decision making took some time. Indeed, the pediatric formulation of vitamin D was on the market one year after our request. However, after implementation of risk minimizations, we received few cases of vitamin D overdoses from private pediatricians mainly. This was due to the poor dissemination of the new recommendations among pediatricians and general practitioners in the private sector.

12.3.9   Artotec®

Artotec® is a combination of diclofenac and misoprostol used to treat osteoarthritis and rheumatoid in people at high risk for developing stomach or intestinal ulcers. The CAPM received four serious cases related to Artotec® during July 2015. One of the four cases led to a fatal outcome and two cases to life threatening.

Given that abortion is illegal in Morocco, Artotec® is misused as an abortifacient because it contains misoprostol, a prostaglandin that binds to myometrial cells to cause strong myometrial contractions leading to expulsion of tissue [18]. It is important to highlight that misoprostol is considered as a teratogen. Congenital defects following prenatal exposure in early pregnancy to misoprostol include skull defects, bladder exstrophy, arthrogryposis, cranial nerve palsies, facial malformations, terminal transverse limb defects, and Moebius sequence [19].

This signal led to conduct the RCA in order to identify contributing factors that led to Artotec® misuse.

12.3.10   RCA/Contributing Factors

In 2012, the organization "Women on Waves" made a huge campaign among Moroccan women to promote the use of misoprostol for medical abortion that could be done by women themselves outside the hospitals. The organization had a website that described the steps to follow to use misoprostol for abortion. Women experiencing undesired pregnancies who need help can get information about the optimal use of misoprostol for a safe abortion via safe abortion hotline. The campaign allowed women to know about the availability of pills that contain misoprostol which is Artotec®. Consequently sales of the drug dramatically increased. In addition, women could get the drug from pharmacies without prescription, whereas according to the local regulation, Artotec® is a prescription-only medicine. Moreover, the treatment renewal could not be done unless it is explicitly stated by the prescriber.

A survey conducted by the CAPM among some pharmacies in different regions of Morocco to know about the profile of Artotec® prescribers and indication of use revealed that the drug is mainly prescribed by gynecologist and general practitioners for abortion. This outlines the off label use of Artotec® by prescribers in Morocco.

12.3.11   Risk Minimization Actions

Given the high risk of the off label use and misuse of Artotec® on women and their fetus, the CAPM requested for an urgent meeting of the National Commission of Pharmacovigilance.

Our first proposal was to remove the Artotec® from the market. In fact, discussions with the rheumatologists and internal medicine specialists who are the main prescribers of the drug revealed that Artotec® is rarely prescribed. This proposal would have been rejected by the Marketing authorization holder because these ADRs occurred when the drug is used outside the indications for which the Artotec® is authorized. The commission then proposed to restrict Artotec® for hospital use only and to draw up the attention of health care professionals about the teratogenic effects of misoprostol. Finally, in July 2018, after another National Commission of Pharmacovigilance meeting, Artotec® issue was discussed, and it was decided by the Minister of health to remove Artotec® 50 mg and Artotec® 75 mg from the market.

12.3.12   Obstacles

Drugs containing misoprostol including Artotec® are still available and can be bought by online. Sales via the Internet cannot be controlled.

12.4   Hydroxychloroquine/Azithromycin

The WHO defines the COVID-19 pandemic as a "major health crisis of our time." All health systems worldwide have been caught off guard, and several measures have been taken in a hurry, including.

- The use of probabilistic treatments while waiting for the development of new treatments.
- The use of hydroxychloroquine (HCQ)/chloroquine (CQ) in the treatment of COVID-19.

In Morocco, the health authorities have chosen to provide treatment with HCQ/CQ in combination with a macrolide: Azithromycin, to all patients with COVID-19. HCQ is a very old drug with a well-known safety profile and established adverse effects, in which some are serious (QT prolongation, hypokalemia). The state of emergency did not allow specific clinical studies in regards to the off-label use of HCQ for a new indication. Since combination with Azithromycin could potentially increase the risk of QT prolongation in its new dosage, the use of HCQ/CQ required pharmacovigilance monitoring and the implementation of a Risk Management and Minimization Plan in order to establish the safety profile for these products and to support patient management with recommendations for use before, during, and after treatment.

Indeed, the treatment strategy required before starting the HCQ and Azithromycin for all patients to undergo:

- An initial ECG because of the risk of cardiac toxicity.
- A ionogram to check and to correct any existing hypokalemia.
- Avoid the association with hypokalemic antihypertensives, glucocorticoids, or laxatives.

During the treatment, cardiac monitoring in patients at risk has been recommended:

- An ECG 4 hours after treatment initiation.
- A daily ECG during the whole duration of the treatment to check and detect any QT alteration requiring the stop or the modification of the treatment.
- A daily clinical examination to look for symptoms that may suggest a cardiac rhythm disorder (sudden and brief palpitations, syncope).
- An ionogram to check the potassium level. It should be noted that any hypokalemia must be followed by an ECG, a clinical examination and a search for enzyme inhibiting or hypokalemia drugs (diuretics, glucocorticoids).

The CAPM received a cluster of nine cases with hypokalemia and abnormal heart rhythm.

This is the report of one case:

Male patient, 53 years old, asymptomatic with COVID-19 (PCR positive).
Medical history: Thyroidectomy and Arterial Hypertension under:

- Levothyroxine® 175 micrograms.
- Enforce HTC®.

For COVID-19 treatment: Protocol established by the ministry of health:

- Hydroxychloroquine: 200 mg 3 tablets per day for a total of 600 mg per day during 7 days.
- Azithromycin: 500 mg, 1 tablet of 500 mg the first day and 250 mg once a day during 6 days.

The report indicates that the ECG and blood test realized during the third day found out a trouble of the rhythm and a hypokalemia at 2.8 mmol/l. The patient was asymptomatic.

Hydroxychloroquine and Azithromycin were stopped as well as the antihypertensive drug.

Supplementation of potassium was given with ECG monitoring and kalaemia blood analysis.

The outcome was favorable.

Root Cause Analysis (RCA) undertaken highlighted some points:

- The Azithromycin was taken 500 mg during 3 days, instead of 500 mg on Day 1 and 250 mg per day from Day 2 to day 7.
- Drug-drug interaction between Azithromycin, Hydroxychloroquine, and hydrochlorothiazide contained in the antihypertensive medicine Exforge HTC, which

represented an additional risk factor for the hypokalemia. In fact, Exforge HTC contains Valsartan, Amlodipine, and Hydrochlorothiazide.

- The junior doctor did not know that Exforge HCT was containing hydrochloro-thiazide, which is a hypokalemic drug.

Risk minimization actions have been put in place.

12.4.1 Mandatory Measures: Dear Doctor Letter Containing

- List of contributing factors that could increase the risk of cardiovascular ADRs.
- List of torsadogenic drugs, hypokalemic drugs and enzymatic inhibitors.
- Recommendations to reinforce Preventive and corrective actions before treatment.
- List of contraindications.
- In-depth questionnaire to patients before starting treatment to look for risk factors.
- List of a simple and comprehensive explanations to give to patients on how to take medicines.

12.4.2 Communication Measures

- Sensitization on the same recommendations was shared via webinars and scientific publications.

This medication error has been discovered while the patient was asymptomatic.

Thanks to risks minimization measures that have been put in place before and during the treatment that led to discovery of hypokalemia and abnormal heart rhythm.

The role of pharmacovigilance centres in implementing and in putting in place the specific risk minimization actions and a specific risk management plan are essentials during health crisis.

12.5 Lessons Learnt

- Adverse drug reactions can be preventable. Preventability assessment should be routinely performed once a reasonable link between the event and the suspected drug has been validated by causality assessment.
- Detecting medication errors would help pharmacovigilance systems to ensure patient safety and to ensure rational use of drugs within public health programmes.
- The role of Pharmacovigilance centres is essential in implementing specific risk management plan especially during health crisis.

References

1. Khon LT, Corrigan JM, Donaldson MS, editors. To err is human. Building a safer health system. Washington, DC: National Academy Press; 1999.
2. Brennan TA, Leape LL, Laird NM, Hebert L, Localio AR, Lawthers AG, Newhouse JP, Weiler PC, Hiatt HH. Incidence of adverse events and negligence in hospitalized patients. Results of the Harvard Medical practice Study I. TA Brennan, LL Leape .... N Engl J Med. 1991;325(3):210.
3. http://www.who.int/patientsafety/information_centre/reports/Alliance_Forward_Programme_2008.pdf
4. http://www.who.int/patientsafety/about/a59_22-en.pdf?ua=1
5. http://www.who.int/patientsafety/en/brochure_final.pdf?ua=1
6. Anonymous. The Erice Manifesto. For global reform of the safety of medicines in patient care. Drug Saf. 2007;30:187–90.
7. http://www.who.int/features/factfiles/patient_safety/en/
8. http://www.who.int/patientsafety/en/brochure_final.pdf
9. Alj L, Touzani MDW, Benkirane R, Edwards IR, Soulaymani R. Detecting medication errors in pharmacovigilance database. Capacities and limits. Int J Risk Saf Med. 2007;19:187–94.
10. Benkirane RR, Abouqal R, Haimeur CC, EchCherif El Kettani S, Azzouzi AA, Mdaghrialaoui AA, et al. Incidence of adverse drug events and medication errors in intensive care units: a prospective multicenter study. J Patient Saf. 2009;5:16–22.
11. Benabdallah G, Benkirane R, Khattabi A, Edwards IR, Bencheikh RS. The involvement of pharmacovigilance centres in medication errors detection. A questionnaire-based analysis. Int J Risk Saf Med. 2011;23:17–29.
12. Reporting and learning systems for medication errors: the role of pharmacovigilance centres Available at: http://apps.who.int/medicinedocs/documents/s21625en/s21625en.pdf
13. Benkirane R, Soulaymani-Bencheikh R, Khattabi A, Benabdallah G, Alj L, Sefiani H, KhedidjaHedna LO, Olsson S, Pal SN. Assessment of a new instrument for detecting preventable adverse drug reactions. Drug Saf. 2015;38(4):383–93.
14. Massachusetts Medical Society. Patient safety: conducting a root cause analysis of adverse events. Available at http://www.massmed.org/AM/Template.cfm?Section=Patient_Safety_Conducting_a_Root_Cause_Analysis_of_Adverse_Events. Last accessed 28 Feb 2009.
15. Ishikawa K. What is total quality control? The Japanese Way. Englewood Cliffs: Prentice Hall; 1985.
16. http://www.ema.europa.eu/docs/en_GB/document_library/Scientific_guideline/2013/06/WC500144010.pdf
17. https://toolbox.eupati.eu/glossary/risk-minimisation-measures/
18. Lozinski T, Ludwin A, Filipowska J, Zgliczynska M, Wegrzyn P, Kluz T, Ciebiera M. Oxytocin and misoprostol with diclofenac in the preparation for magnetic resonance-guided high-intensity ultrasound treatment of symptomatic uterine fibroids: a prospective cohort study. Ultrasound Med Biol. 2021;47(6):1573–85. https://doi.org/10.1016/j.ultrasmedbio.2021.02.018.
19. Allen R, O'Brien BM. Uses of misoprostol in obstetrics and gynecology. Rev Obstet Gynecol. 2009;2(3):159–68.

Chapter 13
Pharmacovigilance Practices in Indian Systems of Medicine with Additional Highlights of Its Concept in Unani Medicine

Syed Ziaur Rahman, Abdul Latif, Abdur Rauf, and Sumbul Rehman

13.1 Indian Systems of Medicine

India possesses a distinctive characteristic in the form of three prominent acknowl-edged systems of medicine, namely Ayurveda, Siddha, and Unani (ASU). The Ministry of AYUSH, an entity within the Government of India, officially acknowl-edges AYUSH as a recognized system of medicine. AYUSH encompasses Ayurveda, Yoga, Unani, Siddha, Sowa Rigpa, and Homeopathy [1]. The philo-sophical underpinnings, as well as the fundamental principles and approaches to patient care, of these systems exhibit notable distinctions. The pharmaceutical substances formulated and employed inside each of these systems exhibit varia-tions as well.

Ayurvedic and Unani medications are currently available in a variety of formats. They are available in both traditional forms (tablets, powder, decoction, medicated oil, fermented products, and semi-solid preparations such as (Ma'jun)) and modern formulations such as capsules, lotions, syrups, ointments, liniments, creams, gran-ules, and so on [2]. As the world becomes more connected, some worries are being made about the safety of these dosage forms.

Indian Systems of Medicine (ISM) drug manufacture is governed by the Drugs and Cosmetic Act (1940) and its accompanying rules (1945). Many chapters have since been added to these Acts over the years. Drug Technical Advisory Board (DTAB) and Drug Consultative Committee (DCC) to advise the Government and Drug Controller General of India (DCGI) who is in charge of licensing and

S. Z. Rahman (✉)
Department of Pharmacology, Jawaharlal Nehru Medical College, Aligarh Muslim University, Aligarh, India
e-mail: rahmansz@yahoo.com

A. Latif · A. Rauf · S. Rehman
Department of Ilmul Advia, Ajmal Khan Tibbiya College, Aligarh Muslim University, Aligarh, India

© Springer Nature Singapore Pte Ltd. 2025
S. R. Ahmad (ed.), *Special Issues in Pharmacovigilance in Resource-Limited Countries*, https://doi.org/10.1007/978-981-96-6154-1_13

enforcing different laws related to drug manufacturing and dispensing. There are three types of agencies involved in the administration of the Acts and Rules enacted by the parliament. All of these tasks are also the responsibility of the Food and Drug Administration Commissioners at the state level. At the same time, the Good Manufacturing Process (GMP) for ISM has been set, and all agencies that make drugs must follow it.

Unani (also known as Greco-Arab Medicine) and Ayurveda, both of which are widely practiced in the Indian Subcontinent, share an ancient understanding as well as set of guidelines for the safe and effective administration of medication. They both have medications derived from their inherent identities. Some authorities even regard these medical approaches to be holistic in nature. Traditional medicine advocates claim that their remedies are safe and effective without the necessity for modern clinical trials. They insist that their remedies are safe if made according to their traditional formulas. However, if they are not properly prepared, isolated, recognized, and administered, these medications can be extremely dangerous. They say all drugs are made in accordance with a standard format, but in reality, this is not always the case. Also, not all medicines are made to the standards imposed by drug regulatory bodies due to rivalry in the market and a lack of raw materials of sufficient quality. Adverse responses are possible with any medication that deviates from the official pharmacopoeias.

Monitoring for the identification, assessment, understanding, and avoidance of any unpleasant adverse responses to medications that are used or intended to be utilized to change or study physiological system or pathological conditions for the benefit of the recipient constitute pharmacovigilance activities. These medications may be any substance or product, such as botanicals, minerals, etc., used for animals and humans and include those prescribed by ASU practitioners [3].

13.2 Rational Use of ASU Drugs for ADRs Prevention

13.2.1 Concept of Treatment in Unani System of Medicine

According to proponents of Unani Medicine, this branch of medicine takes a "holistic" approach or views the patient's illness in its entirety. When considering the philosophy and principles of Unani Medicine, it is clear that it does not conflict with, viz., *medicatrix naturae*, or the body's innate forces of self-preservation. The goal of Unani medicine is to speed up the body's inherent healing mechanisms so that the sickness can be completely eliminated. *Tabᶜiyat* (similar name for Greek *Physicis* from whence "Physician" originated, also cf. *Tabaêy* and *Tabeeb*), the nature of the body, removes the diseased materials spontaneously through sweating, urination, or defecation.

13.2.2 Rationality in Preparation of Unani Medicine

13.2.2.1 General Measures

The method of drug preparation in Unani medicine is properly justified, including the combination of various medicinal plants, minerals, animal products, etc., method of drug administration, various preservatives used, indications and contraindications of drugs in various circumstances, restriction, avoidance, and abstinence (*Parhez*) of certain foods and diets, the known adverse drug effects, the completion of the drug profile beforehand, and knowledge about the adverse drug-drug or food-drug interaction; guidelines for prescribing in extremes of age or in presence of altered organ function or in presence of pregnancy or lactation, etc. The aforementioned details are often included in numerous Unani formularies and traditional Unani literature. In addition, correctives (*Muslehat*) to drugs have been used for a very long time to minimize some undesirable effects that the basic and adjuvant constituents may generate in combination with single and compound drugs. Before their clinical use, drugs that are toxic in their unprocessed state are refined in a number of ways (*Tadbīr*). Despite the fact that every substance used in traditional systems of medicine may have a side effect (*Muzarrât*), the purpose of the above precautions and reasoning, taken by a knowledgeable and experienced physician, was to avoid ADRs [4].

13.2.2.2 Specific Measures

A distinctive Unani Medicine philosophy is the idea of Temperament (*Mizāj*) of each patient and the categorization of each medicine into 4 degrees of potency (*Ḍarjāt-e Advia*). Furthermore, the Unani Medicine approach incorporates the concept of pharmacotherapy (Ilāj bil advia), according to their temperamental potency, which is categorized into four degrees, as per their efficacy. The higher the degree the higher will be its therapeutic effect. Additionally, Correctives and other Regimental Therapy, referred to as Ilāj bit Tadbir, are utilized to reduce toxicity by considering the temperament of drugs and their impact on minimizing side effects. Moreover, the use of Substitutes (Abdāl-e Advia) is emphasized to enhance efficacy and cost-effectiveness in rational drug management within the Unani Medicine framework.

Concept of Dietotherapy (*Ilāj bil Ġiza*)

To prevent any ADR, certain illnesses are treated using the prescribed methods of dietotherapy, such as by administering particular diets or by controlling the quantity and quality of food. In both health and disease, this method places a high value on nutrition and digestion. When prescribing medication, a doctor specifies a regimen and gives instructions on foods to avoid (*Parhez*). It is believed that a healthy diet will result in good humours (*Akhlā Ṣāliḥa*), whereas an unhealthy diet will result in unhealthy humours (*Akhl Radiyya*). In other words, healthy eating and digestion are thought to produce the proper humour balance (cf. theory of 4 humours of Greek Medicine) and preserve the advancement of health, whereas unhealthy eating and digestion throw off the balance and result in disease. Since incorrect diet and digestion can either worsen the condition or counteract the therapeutic effects of medication, it is obvious that the humoural imbalance can be remedied by medication in conjunction with adequate diet and digestion.

Theory of Temperament

Characterizing pharmacological activity of the drugs, a prominent proponent of Unani System of Medicine (USM), Ibn Sinâ (Avicenna), unlike many other ancient physicians, paid special attention to the individual sensitivity of the organism itself about which he wrote: "Saying that the drug is hot or cold, it does not mean that the drug by its substance is maximally hot or cold or that it is by its substance hotter or colder than human body. No, it means that this drug induces heat or cold in the body, exceeding heat or cold of the human body." According to USM, a drug is also having its own temperament (called *Mizāj-e-advia)* which itself is a compound of four basic elements (*Anasir arba'*), viz., hot, cold, dry, and moist as like Human temperament; according to the basic concepts of Unani medicine, each individual has unique temperament as: Sanguineous (*Damwī*)—hot and dry, Bilious (*Safravi*)—hot and moist, Phlegmatic (*Balġhamī*)—cold and moist, and Melancholic—(*Saudavi*) cold and dry temperament.

A drug used in Unani system has a documented temperament (hot, dry, cold, and moist). The temperament of the drug is measured on a scale of 1 to 4 degree. A drug may have temperament (*Hār* as Hot & Dry, Hot & Moist), (*Bārid* as Cold & Dry, Cold & Moist). This classification of drugs used in USM seems to be based on the clinical observations of its yesteryear physicians. So, whenever a drug is taken by a patient it works along with its different temperament and characteristic (*kaifia't*), undergoes various interactions and metabolism, and produces a therapeutic effect and affects the body's innate heat (*Hararat-e-gharizia*). Thus, if the drug itself is hot in temperament, it will increase body heat and vice versa. Moreover, the drug may be hot for one body and cold for another body. So, the patient is not advised to use one and the same drug for change of nature; it is useless. In other words, stress is laid on the particular temperament of the individual and of drug itself, and the medicines administered go well with the temperament of the patient, thus accelerating the process of recovery and also eliminating the risk of drug reaction [4]. Ibn Sinâ's thesis that only one drug should not be used to treat "one and the same patient" shows that based on his daily observations at patient's bedside, he clearly realized that the body could adapt itself to the drug.

Likewise, Unani Drugs of any origin (plant, animal and mineral) are categorized into four degrees on the basis of their temperament, potentiality (potency), and power of effectiveness (including efficacy) which in its entirety curb ADRs. Higher the degree, higher is the chances of adverse effects. So, drugs are classified into four different groups based on their efficacy, potency, as well as their toxicity. Third and Fourth grade drugs are very efficacious as well as have more toxicity; so they are administered with more caution. However, there are certain substances which are "absolutely toxic" and do not produce any efficacy when administered like Potassium Cyanide and are called as absolute poison (*Simmemutlaq*) in Unani.

All substances that come in contact with the body and react upon it are of three types:

(a) Those which enter into the body undergo metabolism and are able to become a part of body in substantial form (*bil madd'a*) and waste material is excreted out.
(b) Those which enter into the body undergo metabolism and act according to its pharmaceutical effect (*bil kaifiyat*); do not become a part of body in any substantial form (*bil madd'a*) and are excreted out.
(c) Those which enter into the body may or may not undergo metabolism and act according to its unique property (*bil jauhar*).

Substances which are altered (metabolized) by the body but do not produce any appreciable change are:

(i) Nutritive food articles in general which become a part of the body (*ghiza*).
(ii) Semi nutritive substances which are also having some medicinal property (*ghiza-e-d'wai*).

Substances which are altered by the body and also produce changes in it are:

(i) Pharmaceutical drugs in general which help in healing of the body and remove disease (*d'wa*).
(ii) Semi=pharmaceutical substances which are also having some nutritive value (*d'wa-e-ghizai*).

Substances that continue to act even after digestion until they produce destructive changes in the body are poisonous medicines and may be responsible for ADRs.

A drug has a large number of phytochemicals in it that interact and produce a temperament of its own called (*Mizāj-e-advia*) as per USM; therefore, a single chemical constituent is not isolated, as temperament (*Mizāj*) depends upon all constituents. This is also one of the safeguard mechanisms of USM using crude drugs/herbs or their parts as a whole that they provide lesser ADR, as the diversity of phytoconstituents produces an overall healing effect, and it is not just a single molecule approach–drug receptor interaction. If one phytochemical produces the desired therapeutic effect but also causes some adverse drug reactions (ADRs), other phytoconstituents in the herbal formulation may help mitigate or counteract those ADRs.

Concept of Substitution

The practice of using substitutes (Abd al Advia) is based on concise instructions laid out by Unani medicine authors. Only when the intended original medication is unavailable, more harmful than intended, or too expensive for the patient, should a substitute be utilized. Additional limitations on substitution state that no drug can completely replace another medicament. If a medicine is replaced by one with the same properties, the second should be used to replace the original drug for that specific effect. However, a third medicine may be used in place of the second for a different therapeutic effect. It is crucial that the original drug's temperament be replicated in the replacement medication. A hot and dry drug of the first degree should be swapped out with another hot and dry drug of the same grade; the dose may change. A cool and moist temperament medicine should not be used in place of a hot and dry one.

It is then taken into consideration after assessing the patient's temperament and the status of their disease and the temperament of drug alternatives. This is how natural medicine is used in treatment. Each patient is given medication that is appropriate for them. Therefore, this course of treatment results in fewer adverse effects [5]. Additionally, the medicine ought to possess the same temperament as the person to whom it is being prescribed.

Concept of Correctives and Other Regimental Therapy (*Ilāj bit Tadbir*)

When Unani physicians discuss about taking a medicine for any therapeutic effect, they also mention about its toxicity. It is evident from various Unani texts where they have mentioned toxic (*Muzir*) and corrective (*Musleh*) effects of each drug in the literature. So, it becomes quite clear that Unani physicians were well aware that if a drug produces some useful effect, it can be harmful too. Further they have mentioned various measures of correction (*Tadbeer-e-advia*) along with each drug description. As *Termialia belerica* contains tannin and is used in constipation, but it may also cause gastric irritation and may cause dryness on intestinal mucosa by reducing intestinal secretion, so in Unani it is mixed with a small quantity of Ghee (*Roghane-gao*); this process is called *Charb*, thus, reducing the harmful effect. And there are large numbers of such examples as Strychnos processed in milk called as *Kuchla mudabbar*. Maturation (*Munzij*) is done to make the body to remove the morbid matter followed by removal (*Muz'hil*) via diaphoretic, diuretics, and purgatives.

Concept of Environment (*Maholiyat*)

The Unani medical system acknowledges the impact of environmental factors and ecological conditions on people's health. The goal is to get the body's many components, humours, and faculties back in balance. The USM term "six essentials of life"

(*Asbab-e-sitta zarooriya*) refers to the six necessities for maintaining health and preventing sickness (a) atmospheric air, (b) food and drink, (c) rest and activity of body, (d) psychological activity, (e) sleep and wakefulness, (f) elimination and retention, including the avoidance of adverse drug reactions (ADRs), through adequate ecological balance provided by clean water, food, and air.

Traditionally, Unani practitioners have been aware of how medications and herbs affect the environment and surroundings in addition to the way they affect people and animals. The Unani system of medicine has proper guidelines for getting rid of redundant pharmaceuticals, including burying them in soil burning them and lighting them on fire. In the current era, pharmacoenvironmentology is a part of pharmacovigilance that deals with the release of chemicals or medications into the environment after they have been eliminated from people and animals and after therapeutic doses. As a result, it is important to keep an eye on the effects of Unani medications on the environment. Environmental pharmacology and environmental pharmacovigilance are becoming topics of discussion in the current medical system [6–8].

In spite of the above safety measures (as mentioned above in sections i to v), if physicians notice any unknown side effect, they used to write these reactions in their Notebooks (*Bayaz*) or communicate these experiences to their apprentices (like prescription learning and monitoring in today's teaching and learning process). Further in Unani literature, scholars have mentioned toxicity (*Muzir*) and correctives (*Musleh*) with every individual drug description. So, safety measures to be followed are discussed along with adverse effect of each, and these are given in each Unani Pharmacopoeias. Earlier, there were no professional associations of physicians worldwide as prevalent nowadays under different names and different governmental patronage, in order to interact or exchange experiences. These Indian physicians used to practice in their own region or community that has been utilized in the present era by the Government in Pharmacopeia where they have taken reference of authentic classical literature and mentioned them in an authorized book in respective Pharmacopoeia as Unani Pharmacopeia of India. But irrespective of so much safety precautions in USM, there are multiple chances of adverse effects nowadays; the reason lies in misidentification, misuse of drug, adulteration, contamination that affects safety and efficacy of drug and leads to non-uniform therapeutic effects. In other words, there was no Random/Spontaneous or Drug-Oriented ADR Monitoring system.

13.3 Current Perspective in Relation to Herbal Pharmacovigilance

Modern medicine is based mostly on the premise of disease and suffering being healed by providing something to the individual, such as a pill or a potion. However, evidence is mounting that a wide range of seemingly unrelated disorders can be caused by aberrant reactions to ingested elements (such as food) and that just with-holding such materials can result in a cure. Another issue is that symptoms are frequently ambiguous rather than precise and persistent rather than acute. Irritability, sadness, weariness, headache, joint and muscular discomfort, or gastro-intestinal disorders may be rejected as psychological or emotional in nature. Diagnosis is frequently time-consuming and challenging, and it may even require skills that can only be offered by someone who has nurtured an expertise. While adverse reactions are a price of modern therapy, indigenous drugs, which are also known as herbal remedies in developing and developed countries, are still widely used in the community. Consumers contend that because these preparations are "natural," they have no side effects and are safe.

There have been several other high-profile safety concerns with herbs in recent years that have influenced public health, and the need to establish pharmacovigilance systems for herbal medicines is becoming increasingly apparent. Herbal medicine safety monitoring, also known as pharmacovigilance, presents its own set of challenges. The current reporting of adverse effects of herbal medicine is attributed to a wide variety of causes. Herbal medicine's safety and the means by which it is monitored for that safety should be the first and most important considerations. We must address issues to study herbal medicine pharmacovigilance and its effects on safety and efficacy. Calapai et al. (2014) have reported of contact dermatitis as an adverse effect of a selection of topically used herbal medicinal products [9].

Reasons for adverse drug reactions in herbal medicine may be varied; risks associated with parenteral use are greater because all drugs are prepared for internal purpose or for external application. In many nations, the adulteration of herbal remedies with pharmaceutical drugs is a problem. All complementary and alternative medicine (CAM) medications are not prepared according to the standard format mandated by drug regulatory agencies in this era of competitive marketing, unavailability of unfinished quality raw material, substandard, spurious, falsely labelled, falsified, and counterfeit medical products (SSFFCs), etc. [10]

Herbal formulations are being used more frequently by patients and doctors alike. The likelihood of interactions between herbal and conventional medicines or drug-herb interactions are exacerbated by aggressive marketing, intense direct to consumer (DTC) advertising, and the presence of irrational combinations [11]. It is essential to explain their mechanisms and clinical relevance as a consequence. There is also a need to review regulatory loopholes, such as the Traditional Herbal Medicinal Products Directive (THMPD), a European Union directive that provides simplified regulatory process for herbals and the 2001 review of pharmaceutical legislation, in light of their implications for the safety and pharmacovigilance of herbal medicines, regulation of herbal practitioners, over-the-counter (OTC) availability and self-use, authentication of all herbal medicines, quality of herbal medicinal products, uninformed consumers, biased drug information, and sensationalization of adverse drug events.

Many nations are implementing the reporting of adverse drug reactions for prescribed herbal remedies. In the majority of emerging nations, the only method for reporting ADRs is through a spontaneous reporting system. Diverse levels of signal generation and analysis are being carried out. Most nations do a poor job of enforcing the requirement that businesses submit mandatory reports. Both the Register of Chinese Herbal Medicine and the National Institute of Medical Herbalists uses the UK Medicines and Healthcare products Regulatory Agency (MHRA)'s "Yellow Card" system to report ADRs including those associated with herbal medicines. Similar to this, the pharmaceutical industry, UK aromatherapists, European Scientific Cooperative on Phytotherapy (ESCOP), manufacturers of herbal medicines, and traditional healers are all studying and debating ADRs and ADR reporting. Additionally, the "i-Plants project" and "Evamed," a prescription-based electronic system for reporting adverse drug events in complementary medicine, are in use. A strong network of regional Pharmacovigilance centres has been established by the China Food and Drug Administration (CFDA), but the WHO database does not currently contain the reported ADRs.

In current predicament, despite extensive and well-maintained ADR monitoring, there is still very little reporting of adverse drug reactions to herbal medicines. The risks associated with using herbal medicine irrationally are also higher, and the legal status and approval process also differ from country to country. A dedicated drug reaction monitoring system for herbal medicines should be established by the WHO or another organization. However, the WHO Programme for International Drug Monitoring is currently working on a project to monitor the safety of herbal medicines [12]. One step in this direction has been made with the classification of herbal ATC for medicinal uses into a logical hierarchical structure that is compatible with the WHO Drug Dictionary [13]. There are also the WHO Traditional Medicine strategies 2002–2005 and 2004–2007, both of which have a Component 2 that relates to national policies on traditional medicines (TM) and complimentary and alternative medicines (CAM). The WHO urges member states to monitor herbals and TM, and it also recommends their inclusion in national PV systems. In addition, the WHO adopted TM at its 56th World Assembly (WHA56.31) in 2003.

13.4 Paradigms in Relation to Herbal Pharmacovigilance in India

Regarding traditional medicine in India, particularly Ayurveda, Siddha, and Unani (ASU), it was determined that a separate mechanism is required to address them. The number of reported adverse reactions to ASU drugs in the National Pharmacovigilance Programme is insignificant. The widespread belief that ASU medications are safe contributes significantly to this situation. Furthermore, ASU practitioners' lack of understanding of the concept and importance of pharmacovigilance in ASU exacerbated the problem. WHO emphasizes the importance of including traditional medicines in pharmacovigilance systems and in 2004 [12] published guidelines on the safety monitoring of herbal medicines in pharmacovigilance systems. To promote these WHO guidelines, the Ibn Sînâ Academy of Medieval Medicine & Sciences, Aligarh, India, established a special cell in early 2005 called the Centre for Safety & Rational Use of Indian Systems of Medicine (CSRUISM) to improve the use of Indian-originated drugs, particularly Unani Medicine, and their adverse reaction monitoring. CSRUISM receives a large number of ADRs from herbal drugs that were never previously reported. These reactions are evaluated for their causal relationships using the WHO Causality Categories and the Naranjo ADR Probability Scale Evaluation [14].

The "National Symposium on Relevance of Herbal Pharmacovigilance" was held for the first time on November 4, 2006, at the Department of Pharmacology, Jawaharlal Nehru Medical College, Aligarh Muslim University, Aligarh, under the aegis of the Society of Pharmacovigilance, India (SoPI) and CSRUISM of Ibn Sînâ Academy, Aligarh. The National Symposium's report was then turned in, along with suggestions for starting a National Pharmacovigilance Program just for ASU drugs. Recognizing the importance of Pharmacovigilance, the Department of Clinical Pharmacology at Topiwala National Medical College (TNMC) and BYL Nair Hospital in Mumbai organized a "Training program in Pharmacovigilance of Ayurveda Medicine" as part of "Update Ayurveda" in 2006 with the goal of raising awareness about Pharmacovigilance among Ayurveda physicians and developing guidelines for reporting ADR Ayurveda medicines [15]. Likewise, Institute of Post Graduate Teaching & Research in Ayurveda (IPGT & RA), Jamnagar, conducted "National Workshop on Herbal Pharmacovigilance" during third and fourth December 2007. Based on the workshop recommendations, a Pharmacovigilance Cell (PV Cell), the first of its kind in India for ASU drugs, was established, and a Reporting Form for suspected adverse reactions of ASU formulations was developed and distributed among faculty members, research scholars, and physicians, with notification to the Department of AYUSH, Ministry of Health and Family Welfare, Government of India [16].

To properly place pharmacovigilance for ASU drugs in India, the establishment of a National Pharmacovigilance Centre for ASU drugs under the control of the Department of AYUSH, which will centrally monitor the program, is highly commendable [17]. This program aims to provide ADR data for various drugs of herbal, mineral, metallic, animal, and other origins that are available in the country. In this regard, the first National Consultative Meeting of the National Pharmacovigilance Programme for ASU drugs was held on the 29th and 30th of August 2008 at the Department of AYUSH, Ministry of Health and FW, Government of India, New Delhi, where the national draft protocol was technically reviewed and finalized. The finalized draft was then distributed to the meeting's experts for comments and additional input, if any. Based on the feedback received, the final document was released on September 29, 2008, as part of the launch of the National Pharmacovigilance Programme for ASU drugs (NPP-ASU). The NPP-ASU was then coordinated by the National Pharmacovigilance Consultative

Committee for ASU drugs, which was formed by the Department of AYUSH, Ministry of Health, and the Food and Drug Administration, Government of India. The National Pharmacovigilance Programme for ASU drugs was headquartered at Jamnagar's Institute of Postgraduate Teaching and Research in Ayurveda (IPGT & RA). To ensure proper documentation and to regulate, monitor, and control Pharmacovigilance activities, a three-tiered system was implemented: one National Pharmacovigilance Centre (NPC), eight Regional Pharmacovigilance Centres (RPC), and approximately 29 Peripheral Pharmacovigilance Centres (PPC) were established throughout the country. The first training course for coordinators of these centres was held on November 13 and 14, 2008, at the National Pharmacovigilance Training Centre, IPGT & RA, Jamnagar, and since then, many training programs have been held throughout India with the support of WHO in various Ayurvedic and Unani Medical Colleges under the aegis of IPGT & RA. This WHO-sponsored program ran for five years (2008–2013). Prof. K. C. Singhal translated the ADR Terminology of WHO-UMC ADR Monitoring into Hindi to make it easier and more understandable. The Society of Pharmacovigilance India (SoPI) [18] and the Government of India published this Hindi dictionary [16].

On November 20, 2017, the Pharmacovigilance Program of India (PvPI) under the direct control of Indian Pharmacopoeia Commission (IPC), DCGI, Govt. of India had a Memorandum of Understanding (MoU) with Ministry of AYUSH for ASU Drugs Monitoring. This newly initiative called as NCC-PvPI invited AYUSH industry partners, academicians, and regulators as participants and organized a symposium on Pharmacovigilance for Herbal Medicine at IPC Headquarters, Ghaziabad, wherein guest speakers from University of Alberta and other experts of India participated and deliberated. Under this new programme NCC-PvPI, there is One National Centre based at All India Institute of Ayurveda, New Delhi, and Five Intermediary Centres: IPGT & RA, Jamnagar and National Institute of Ayurveda, Jaipur (for Ayurveda), National Institute of Unani Medicine, Bangalore (for Unani), National Institute of Siddha, Chennai (for Siddha) and National Institute of Homeopathy, Kolkata (for Homeopathy).

This program aims at

(i) Inculcating reporting culture among ASU&H stakeholders to facilitate documentation of suspected ADRs ASU & H drugs.
(ii) Inculcating reporting culture among ASU&H stakeholders to facilitate documentation of misleading advertisements for ASU & H drugs.
(iii) Evolving evidence-based recommendations regarding the clinical safety and objectionable advertisements of ASU&H drugs for regulatory actions.

Since its inception, the involved centres are functioning in line with the defined objectives and frequently organising sensitization programmes for various stakeholders across the nation.

13.5   Challenges and Solutions for Monitoring Herbal Medicine in India

If ASU Drugs or any other systems of medicine can provide a cure for certain diseases, then it should be guided that they are used in a prudent manner in order to maximize the likelihood of a successful outcome. Guidelines for the rational use of these traditional medicines, such as the WHO General Guidelines for methodologies on research and evaluation of TM, must be developed. ASU drugs are generally less expensive and may be less toxic. However, the following steps toward quality control methods for ASU drugs are required: the publication of ASU Pharmacopoeias, Formularies, the standardization of ASU drugs, and the establishment of a Traditional Knowledge Digital Library (TKDL). The publication of these official compendiums is governed by the "Indian Pharmacopoeia Commission," Drugs Controller General of India, Government of India, Ghaziabad, while the TKDL project is overseen by the Council of Scientific and Industrial Research (CSIR), Ministry of Science and Technology, Government of India, New Delhi.

The generation of evidence for traditional medicine requires a balance of scientific scepticism and spiritual sensitivity. To evaluate the safety of herbal medicines, various forms of evidence are utilized, including meta-analyses using pharmacoepidemiological methods, individual randomized controlled trials, expert (authority) opinions, statements from credible individuals, sensory or cognitive perceptions, logical inference, clinical experience-based planning, and descriptive studies assessing applicability to both general and diverse populations. However, traditional medicine faces key evidence gaps, particularly in addressing complex, individualized treatments such as those influenced by pharmacogenetics. The following evidence deficiencies in traditional medicine must be addressed: complex, individualized treatments, including pharmacogenetics [19], a lack of standardization, appropriate placebo interventions, ethical limitations on type of comparisons, blinding, and devaluation of information from other sources.

While there has been steady growth in both the number and variety of drugs, there has been little change in the financial resources available for health care services in general. In order to make optimal use of the drug budget and to provide the highest quality, safe, ADR-free health services, rational drug management has become an increasingly important topic. It is therefore critical to study indigenous medicine, including ASU, in relation to drug safety and quality assurance. There is no systematic data on the occurrence of adverse effects associated with traditional medicines. One of the challenges has been the numerous complex issues associated with adverse event detection in traditional products. These include issues with multiple ingredient products, drugs from multiple systems of medicine [20], name misclassification, poor product standardization, a lack of clinical trials [21], variation in manufacturing processes, contamination, adulteration, and misidentification of herbs [22]. There have also been reports of ASU medicines being contaminated with allopathic medicines and chemicals such as NSAIDs, corticosteroids, and so on. Furthermore, many ASU medicines are manufactured for global use, transcending the traditional and cultural contexts for which they were originally intended. Rare adverse events and delayed effects, in particular, may be difficult to detect despite traditional use, undermining the argument that many herbal remedies are safe due to prior traditional use. Currently, the majority of reported adverse events associated with the use of herbal/ traditional products are attributed to either poor product quality or improper use.

Lastly, feedback and promotion of the pharmacovigilance system needs to be strengthened, and there is a need to study chemical and molecular basis of herbal ADRs and other herbal toxicities.

Acknowledgments The authors are thankful to the "Centre for Safety and Rational Use of Indian Systems of Medicine," Ibn Sīnā Academy of Medieval Medicine and Sciences, Aligarh, India, for providing resource materials in writing the above paper.

Conflict of Interest Authors declare that they have no conflict of interest.

References

1. Ministry of AYUSH G of I. National Health Portal: Gateway to authentic health information. http://www.nhp.gov.in/ayush_ms. Accessed 29 Sept 2016.
2. Ravishankar B, Shukla VJ. Indian systems of medicine: a brief profile. Afr J Tradit Complement Altern Med. 2007;4(3):319–37.
3. Chakraverty R, Banerjee A. Emerging issues in pharmacovigilance of herbal medicines in India. Int J Pharm Sci Rev Res. 2013;20(1):40–2.
4. Rahman SZ. Historical perspective of traditional medicine with special reference to ADRs. In: Singhal K, editor. National symposium on relevance of pharmacovigilance for Indian system of medicine. Department of AYUSH, Ministry of Health and Family Welfare, Government of India and Society of Pharmacovigilance; 2006. p. 53–61.
5. Singhal KC, Rahman SZ. Chapter 3: *Abdāl al Advia* (substitution of drugs) – a challenge to pharmacovigilance. In: Gulati ARK, editor. Pharmacovigilance: an update. Delhi: Vallabhbhai Patel Chest Institute, University of Delhi; 2004. p. 22–44.
6. Rahman SZ. Impact of human medicines on environment – a new emerging problem. Popul Envis. 2006;3(2):3–5.
7. Rahman SZ, Khan RA. Environmental pharmacology: a new discipline. Indian J Pharmacol. 2006;38(4):229–30.
8. Rahman SZ, Khan RA, Gupta V, Uddin M. Pharmacoenvironmentology – a component of pharmacovigilance. Environ Health. 2007;6:20.
9. Calapai G, Miroddi M, Minciullo PL, Caputi AP, Gangemi S, Schmidt RJ. Contact dermatitis as an adverse reaction to some topically used European herbal medicinal products. Part 1: *Achillea millefolium–Curcuma longa*. Contact Derm. 2014;71:1–12.
10. Latif A, Rahman S. Adverse events in CAM/TM: a surveillance review. J Pharmacovigil Drug Saf. 2007;5(Conference Special):77.
11. Basalingappa S, Amarnath S, Sharma A. Review article herbal research: current status. Int J Pharm Sci Rev Res. 2014;28(2):111.
12. WHO guidelines on safety monitoring of herbal medicines in pharmacovigilance systems. World Heal Organ Geneva. 2004:82.
13. World Health Organization. The importance of pharmacovigilance – safety monitoring of medicinal products. 2002.
14. Centre for safety & rational use of Indian systems of medicine – a unit of Ibn Sina Academy of Medieval Medicine & Sciences. Newsletter Ibn Sina Academy. 2006;6(1):13–4.

15. Update Ayurveda. Proceeding of pre-conference workshop. Pharmacovigilance of Ayurvedic Medicines. 2006:10.
16. Rahman SZ. History of pharmacovigilance in India. In: Rahman SZ, Shahid M, Gupta A, editors. An introduction to environmental pharmacology. 1st ed. Aligarh: Ibn Sina Academy of Medieval Medicine and Sciences; 2008. p. 227–31.
17. Dept. of AYUSH, Ministry of Health & Family Welfare G of I. Protocol for National Pharmacovigilance Programme for Ayurveda, Siddha and Unani (ASU) Drugs. Jamnagar, Gujarat: National Pharmacovigilance Resource Centre, Institute for Postgraduate Teaching & Research in Ayurveda, Gujarat Ayurveda University.
18. WHO-Adverse Reaction Terminology (WHO-ART), Hindi translation by Prof. K. C. Singhal, Society of Pharmacovigilance India, 2005.
19. Rahman SZ, Kumar A, Singhal K. Pharmacogenetic and pharmacogenomic in the sphere of pharmacovigilance – a review. In: Mathur GP, Mathur S, editors. Current trends in pediatrics. New Delhi; 2005. p. 20–32.
20. Latif A, Rahman SZ. A serious adverse drug interaction of two traditional medicines – a case report. J Pharmacovigil Drug Saf. 2005;2:26–9.
21. Farkhunda J, Singhal KC, Bhargava R, Latif A, Rahman SZ. Clinical trial of an herbal formulation and associated adverse drug reactions in patients of bronchial asthma. J Pharmacovigil Drug Saf. 2005;2:16–9.
22. Rahman SZ, Latif A, Singhal K. Adverse drug reactions of an herbal drug due to misidentification: a case report. Pharmacoepidemiol Drug Saf. 2002;11(Supplement Issue):241.

Chapter 14
Vaccine Safety Issues in Resource-Limited Countries

Daniel Weibel, Robert T. Chen, Osemeke Osokogu, Chioma Ejekam, Rebecca Chandler, Jyoti Joshi, Patrick Zuber, Steven Black, Silvia Perez-Vilar, Esperanca Sevene, Sammy Khagayi, Mandyam Ravi, Bruce Fireman, Laurence Baril, Sonali Kochhar, Jane Gidudu, and Miriam Sturkenboom

14.1 Introduction (History of Vaccine Safety, Northern and Southern Hemisphere)

Robert T. Chen

Immunization against many vaccine preventable diseases (VPD) is highly cost-effective, in terms of both direct morbidity and mortality prevented [1] and broader indirect macroeconomic impact [2]. Considerable resources have been devoted,

D. Weibel (✉) · M. Sturkenboom
Utrecht University Medical Center, Utrecht, The Netherlands

Vaccine monitoring Collaboration for Europe (VAC4EU), Brussels, Belgium
e-mail: d.m.weibel@umcutrecht.nl

R. T. Chen
Brighton Collaboration, Task Force for Global Health, Decatur, GA, USA

O. Osokogu
Erasmus University Medical Center, Rotterdam, The Netherlands

C. Ejekam
University of Lagos, Africa Centre of Excellence for Drug Research, Herbal Medicine Development and Regulatory Science (ACEDHARS), Lagos, Nigeria

R. Chandler
WHO Uppsala Monitoring Centre, (currently with CEPI, London, UK), Uppsala, Sweden

J. Joshi
Center for Disease Dynamics, Economics & Policy, New Delhi, India

Amity Institute of Public Health, Amity University, Noida, India

P. Zuber
WHO, Geneva, Switzerland

S. Black
Global Vaccine Safety Data Network, Auckland, New Zealand

S. Perez-Vilar
Fundación para el Fomento de la Investigación Sanitaria y Biomédica de la Comunitat (FISABIO), Valencia, Spain

E. Sevene
Eduardo Mondlane University, Manhiça Health Research Centre, Maputo, Mozambique

S. Khagayi
Kenya Medical Research Institute, Kisumu, Kenya

INDEPTH Network, Accra, Ghana

M. Ravi
JSS Academy of Higher Education and Research, Mysore, India

B. Fireman
Kaiser Permanente Vaccine Study Center, Oakland, CA, USA

L. Baril
Institut Pasteur de Madagascar, Antananarivo, Madagascar

S. Kochhar
Global Healthcare Consulting, Delhi, India

University of Washington, Seattle, WA, USA

J. Gidudu
Centers for Disease Control and Prevention (CDC), Atlanta, GA, USA

therefore, towards procurement and delivery of existing vaccines (e.g., measles, polio, rotavirus, HPV) [3], development of new vaccines against other known (e.g., malaria, HIV, cervical cancer), and emerging (e.g., COVID-19, Ebola, Zika) pathogens in resource-limited countries (RLCs) and beyond [4, 5]. The decision to immunize a specific individual against a specific VPD, like other medical interventions, ideally requires a careful weighing of risks and benefits. While vaccines have a clinically acceptable safety profile and are generally well tolerated, vaccine-related safety issues can occur either during clinical trials or afterwards at any point during the process from manufacturing to the administration of such vaccines in the "real-world." Therefore, in RLCs, the potential immunization risks expand beyond adverse events following immunizations (AEFI) from the specific vaccine preparation (e.g., anaphylaxis) to those due to poor immunization programme practices such as unsafe injection practices, like reuse of syringe and needles contaminated with pathogens [6, 7], unsafe storage/reconstitution of vaccine [8], unsafe medical waste disposal [9], and overall poor programme monitoring and evaluation [10]. Effective surveillance for AEFIs in RLCs should ideally include this broader scope of immunization risks to enable their eventual control and elimination when possible. This chapter is focusing on pharmacovigilance and pharmacoepidemiological aspects of AEFIs with a focus on RLCs.

There is a complex interaction between the relative number of VPD cases and AEFIs. As seen in Fig. 14.1 [11], prior to vaccine introduction or at relatively low vaccine coverage, the number of VPDs vastly outweigh the number of AEFIs. But

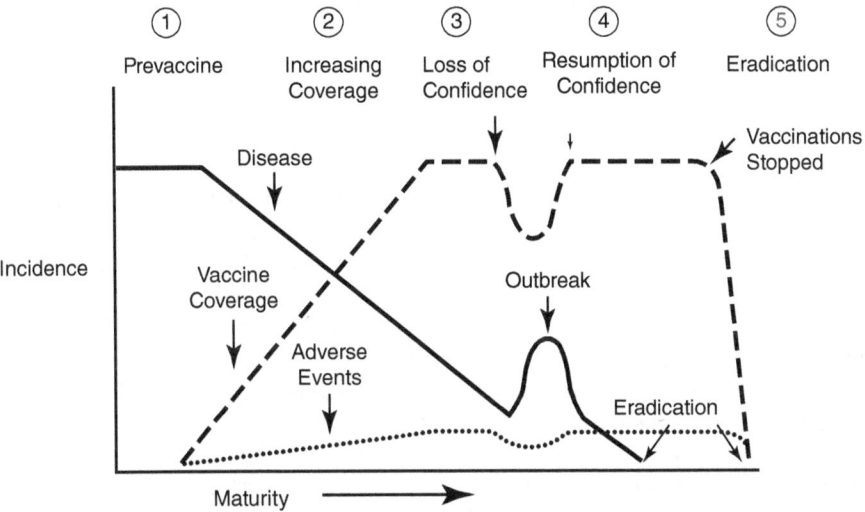

Fig. 14.1 Potential stages in the evolution of immunization program, showing the dynamics of the interaction between vaccine coverage, incidence of targeted vaccine-preventable disease (VPD), and adverse events following immunization (AEFI), as the program matures through the following stages: (1) pre-vaccine, (2) increasing coverage, (3) loss of confidence, (4) resumption of confidence, and (5) VPD eradication. Since few VPDs are eradicable (and thereby allowing their vaccinations to be stopped), most mature immunization programmes are just ahead of stage 3, with high vaccine coverage and AEFIs increasingly prominent relative to disappearing VPDs, a milieu easy for vaccine safety scare and loss of confidence to occur [11]

with sustained high coverage with an efficacious vaccine, the disease is controlled or even essentially eliminated, while AEFIs, both true immunization-related and coincidental events falsely attributed to immunization, increase. This increase in relative prominence of AEFIs and the relative absence of VPDs may become publicized, resulting in a loss of public confidence in the vaccine and consequent resurgence of VPD.

Unfortunately, this "loss of confidence via a vaccine safety scare" paradigm has recurred in multiple national immunization programmes globally since the 1970s. Some of the most prominent examples include fear of neurologic adverse events after whole cell pertussis vaccine in Japan and several European countries [12], fear of autism after measles or thimerosal preservative containing vaccines in the UK [13, 14], fear of neurological disorders after hepatitis B vaccine in France [15], and narcolepsy after influenza vaccine in Scandinavia [16]. While most of these vaccine safety scares have occurred primarily in developed countries, with increasing maturation of immunization programmes and various forms of mass media in RLCs, we are now seeing their eventual spread. The loss of confidence in oral polio vaccine in Nigeria [17] and deaths after pentavalent vaccine in several Asian countries [18] are two such examples.

To better prevent risks from vaccines and detect potential AEFIs, a "life-cycle" approach to vaccine safety has been developed. Such an approach starts from in vitro laboratory-based studies, to toxicology studies in animals, then phased clinical trials in humans, and post- licensure surveillance, all under national regulatory oversight and approval [19, 20]. Since rare AEFIs are unlikely to be detected during pre-licensure clinical trials because of the limited sample sizes of usually 50,000 or less, obtaining accurate vaccine risk estimates usually awaits post-marketing surveillance when millions of doses are administered. Some of the steps and infrastructure needed for this purpose include: (1) hypothesis generation via passive surveillance of AEFIs for detection of potential vaccine safety signals, (2) hypothesis strengthening via standardized case definitions for AEFIs [21] and clinical assessments [22], (3) hypothesis testing in rigorously collected databases of vaccine exposures and clinical outcomes in large populations [23], and importantly (4) communicating these results effectively [24]. As described later in this chapter, various steps are now underway to create similar vaccine safety capacity in RLCs [25].

The currently limited vaccine safety capacity in RLCs will soon need to meet a new test. Historically, the relatively high cost of newly licensed vaccines usually meant decades-long delay before their price fall enough for widespread use in most RLCs [26]. While this time delay was bad for VPD prevention, one silver lining was that the safety profile of these vaccines was usually well characterized via developed vaccine safety surveillance systems in high-income countries before the vaccines were introduced to RLCs. This paradigm largely recurred during COVID-19 [27]. The Global Alliance on Vaccines and Immunizations (GAVI) and other similar initiatives seek to reduce/eliminate the time delay in introducing new vaccines to RLCs [28]. But, up until now, these countries have not usually been *first users* of new vaccines with the need to help define the safety profile of the new vaccine [29]. But with vaccines in development for typhoid, cholera, etc., this paradigm is likely to change and new vaccines are being first introduced in RLCs [30–33]. Some of these vaccines have entered the registration process, while others are in phase 2b/3 trials [34–37].

There is nascent recognition by major funders of immunization programmes of the need to bolster the capacity for AEFI surveillance and assess/validate new safety signals in RLCs [38]. The projects in RLCs described in this chapter will also hopefully suggest a way forward to meet this new need.

14.2   Examples of Vaccine Safety Issues in Resource-Limited Countries

Osemeke Osokogu and Chioma Ejekam

A systematic review of malaria, tuberculosis, and HIV clinical trials was conducted to assess the nature and consistency of safety data reporting [39]. The results showed that out of 107 trials conducted in adults where the vaccine was administered via the skin, pain (93 [87%]), erythema (81 [76%]), and induration (69 [65%]) were the most commonly reported local adverse events. In 109 publications that reported trials in adults irrespective of administration site, the most commonly reported systemic AEFI were headache (91 [84%]), fever (90 [83%]), myalgia (74 [65%]), nausea (72 [65%]), and malaise (71 [62%]). Also, MenAfriVac®, a meningococcal A conjugate vaccine, was linked to paralysis in African children [31]. Although most centres involved in clinical trials of this vaccine reported pain mostly at injection site with no hospitalizations and death, there were reports of serious adverse events such as exanthematous pustulosis, angioedema, bronchospasm, and severe vomiting [40].

Regarding vaccine safety issues occurring after clinical trials, available literature and field experience suggest that the most common issues in RLCs are immunization error-related reactions, coincidental events, and sometimes, vaccine quality or product defect-related reactions. However, transparency in reporting and confidentiality issue remain, and consequently underreporting may be an issue since such information can undermine public confidence or suggest lapses in the service quality or delivery system. Public access to this type of information requires balancing safeguards to avoid breaches of proprietary information and public trust and confidence [41]. From a National programme perspective, safety issues are often related to challenged risk-benefit logic, limited data for a response, and limited resources to address reported safety issues. Also, anti-vaccination groups can coalesce on specific issues and preempt a more reasoned response.

Generally, incompletely understood medical conditions such as autism and multiple sclerosis are more likely to be wrongly attributed to vaccines. In the absence of adequate capacity to quickly confirm or reject a causal association for such AEFI, loss of public confidence in a vaccine may occur. Although the WHO has emphasized the need for vaccine PV specifically, there is still no global collation of vaccine safety data to support the effective analysis of new and serious vaccine-safety issues. In addition, in many countries particularly in the RLCs, there is little communication and data exchange between the national immunization programme and the regulatory agency responsible for PV [42].

Still, there are recently reported specific vaccine safety concerns in RLCs including Yellow fever vaccine-related acute neurotropic disease and acute viscerotropic disease and hypersensitivity reactions following AEFI surveillance in multiple African countries following vaccination campaign [43]. In many African countries, muscle weakness and paralysis have been documented following vaccination with oral polio vaccines (OPV). In 2003, five states in northern Nigeria ordered a boycott of the oral polio vaccine (OPV) because OPV have been believed to cause sterility and being ineffective, as polio persists among partially immunized children [44, 45]. Consequently, polio reappeared in more than 15 formerly polio-free African countries and rumors and misconceptions regarding OPV threatened to derail the polio eradication efforts in India [46].

In India, pentavalent vaccine produced by the Serum Institute of India was linked to serious adverse events including infant deaths.

In Sri Lanka, in April 2008, 25 serious adverse reactions including 5 deaths lead to the withdrawal of pentavalent vaccine [47].

More recently, the introduction of Measles-Rubella (MR) vaccine in campaign mode for children 9-month- to 15-year-old in February 2017 in 5 Indian states has suffered from rumors on social media (WhatsApp) about complications such as autism and subacute sclerosing panencephalitis (SSPE) following vaccination and in certain segments concern about vaccine causing sterility. In fact, in some districts in southern India even among the educated where a good number of children already received multiple doses of measles, the general opinion (even of pediatricians) was to avoid vaccines on these protected children (Media reports: WhatsApp rumours about vaccinations hamper India's drive to halt measles and rubella, the government plans to extend the campaign by a week to achieve targets (https://scroll.in/pulse/830129/rumours-about-measles-rubella-vaccine-hit-coverage   Accessed March 18, 2018) and states seek to allay fears over measles-rubella vaccine (http://www.thehindu.com/news/national/States-seek-to-allay-fears-over-measles-rubella-vaccine/article17110296.ece Accessed March 18, 2018).

Acceptability of human papilloma virus (HPV) vaccine has been marred with safety issues including syncope, anaphylaxis, venous thrombotic episodes, adverse pregnancy outcomes, Guillain-Barre syndrome, stroke, multiple sclerosis, and macrophagic myofaciitis (MMF). In South Africa, there is currently a debate about its safety concerns especially the recent case HPVL1 gene DNA fragment in HPV vaccine and its interaction with aluminum salts [48]. In Kenya, a possible link between tetanus toxoid and sterility was reported in October 2014 [49]. Important to note is that these signals and perceived issues have been addressed and are followed closely by the WHO.

Confidence in vaccines needs to be fostered globally. Pivotal is the stimulation of information sharing and education about vaccination programmes within the population through trusted resources. People need to gain trust in visible national safety monitoring and surveillance procedures and systems. Capacity building and investments need to be directed and sustained towards pharmacovigilance in RLC.

14.3   Passive Reporting Systems in Resource-Limited Countries: The COVID-19 Pandemic as a Catalyst for Progress

Rebecca Chandler

The WHO Programme of International Drug Monitoring (PIDM) began in 1968 when the 16th World Health Assembly called for the "a systematic collection of information on serious adverse drug reactions during the development and particularly after medicines have been made available for public use" in response to the thalidomide disaster. The aim of the WHO PIDM is to ensure that early signs of previously unknown medicines-related safety problems are identified and that information about them is shared so that action to protect patients may be taken by individual countries where necessary.

Beginning with only 10 countries at its inception, the PIDM has grown to include over 180 members in 2025. Ref: About the WHO Programme for International Drug Monitoring | UMC (who-umc.org)

The Uppsala Monitoring Centre (UMC) in Sweden has provided technical and operational support to the PIDM since 1978. At its heart is VigiBase, the WHO international database of suspected adverse reactions from medical products. Member countries submit reports of suspected adverse reactions after both medicines and vaccines into VigiBase. Members of the PIDM have access to an entire suite of pharmacovigilance tools to support their work, including a data management system, VigiFlow, and a data analysis tool, VigiLyze. VigiLyze can support both qualitative and quantitative approaches to signal detection at a national level as well as facilitate signal management with the ability to explore for similar reports at both regional and global levels.

Prior to the COVID-19 pandemic, there was evidence of disparity of sharing of reports of AEFI (Adverse Events Following Immunization) with VigiBase between high and low resource countries. A snapshot taken on 1 May 2017 revealed a total of 14,873,497 individual case safety reports (ICSRs) included in VigiBase; 1,052,290 ICSRs (35.1%) described suspected ADRs for products under the ATC code J07 "Vaccines." By continent, 57.6% of all vaccine reports come from the Americas, 29.0% from Europe, 6.4% from Oceania, 5.8% from Asia, and only 1.3% from Africa. Vaccine reports had largely been received from the United States and Canada, the larger European countries including the UK, Italy, Germany, and France, as well as Australia and New Zealand. Contribution of vaccine reports from RLC was low.

This disparity was especially obvious in a comparison of reporting after introduction of a new vaccine between high- and low-resource settings. MenAfriVac, the meningococcal A conjugate vaccine which was developed in a collaborative effort between the Meningitis Vaccine Project (a partnership between the WHO and PATH) and the Serum Institute of India, was directly introduced into "meningitis belt" of Africa in 2010. By the end of 2013, 12 countries had introduced the vaccine, vaccinating over 150 million eligible people. However, within VigiBase, there are only a total of 210 reports on MenAfriVac, received from only four countries. For the sake of comparison, a new meningococcal b vaccine, Bexsero, which was licensed by the European Medicines Agency in 2013, was introduced into the routine childhood vaccination programme in the UK in September 2015; thus far, there have been a total of 1108 reports for this vaccine from the UK alone.

A publication in the MMWR was reported on "Progress in Immunization Safety Monitoring — Worldwide, 2010–2019." This publication demonstrated that only a minority of countries was combining AEFI data from national immunization programs and national regulatory authorities into a single national data source for the purpose of safety surveillance, and these countries were primarily high-income countries. The authors noted a primary challenge to sharing AEFI data to be "the licensing and operation of AEFI data management and surveillance systems, particularly from data management software developers" [50].

In response to the COVID-19 pandemic, the WHO and UMC worked together to improve capture of AEFI reports from national immunization programmes into VigiBase. Adaptations to VigiFlow were developed to facilitate the management and analysis of AEFI reports by national immunization programmes, and VigiMobile was developed to support the collection of reports of AEFI by immunization field workers. Ref: VigiMobile for AEFI I UMC (who-umc.org) Evidence to support an argument of the positive impact of this work is recent reporting rates for COVID-19 vaccines into VigiBase with increasing proportions of total reports from Asia and Africa. As of 6 November 2023, there were a total of 5,212,324 reports for COVID-19 vaccines, 45% from Europe, 36% from the Americas, 11% from Asia, 4% from Oceania, and 4% from Africa. Ref: https://www.vigiaccess.org/ Accessed 6 November 2023.

Despite the progress in data collection and sharing, the generation of evidence of safety from these regions remains limited. Safety signals for the COVID-19 vaccines have been limited to those identified in high-income countries. No signals of thrombotic thrombocytopenia syndrome with the Vaxzevria or the Covishield adenoviral platformed vaccines have been identified or communicated in LMICs, where the majority of these vaccines have been used. Furthermore, no safety signals have been communicated for any of the other vaccines approved by the WHO which were not used in either the USA or Europe. Only two safety signals identified in VigiBase have been communicated through the WHO Pharmaceuticals Newsletter: myocarditis and hearing loss/tinnitus. Ref: WHO Pharmaceuticals Newsletter—N°4, 2021. 2021. https://www.who.int/publications/i/item/who-pharmaceuticals-newsletter%2D%2D-n-4-2021 (Accessed May 16, 2022); WHO Pharmaceuticals Newsletter—N°1, 2022. 2022. https://apps.who.int/iris/handle/10665/351326 (Accessed May 16, 2022).

One very important initiative to advance analysis of data contained within passive reporting systems in Africa had a very successful pilot during the COVID-19 pandemic: The African-Union Smart Safety Surveillance (3S) project (See Chap. 20). Four countries, Ethiopia, Ghana, Nigeria, and South Africa, participated in a pilot of data sharing and joint signal management. The programme has to expand with additional countries and to include in its surveillance other products used for public health priorities. Central to this work will be further development of AfriVigilance data platform. Ref: African Union Smart Safety Surveillance (AU-3S) I AUDA-NEPAD (Accessed 9 November 2023).

Data sharing and collaboration in signal management will continue to be key success factors in optimizing the potential from passive surveillance systems in RLC.

14.4   Signal Validation and Causality Assessment in Resource-Limited Countries

Jyoti Joshi

Allegations that vaccines or vaccination are/is linked to suspected adverse events must be assessed and communicated rapidly and effectively. Timely investigation of adverse events and collection of evidence are critical components of AEFI surveillance and vaccine pharmacovigilance. Post-licensure AEFI surveillance at the national level is essential for continuous monitoring of the safety of marketed vaccines [51]. Vaccines are markedly different from drugs and consequently vaccine pharmacovigilance demands specific causality assessment and signal detection methods. In 2013, the WHO issued a new Causality Assessment Protocol (CAP), which comprises four components: (a) the eligibility criteria for application of the tool, (b) a data review checklist, (c) a causality assessment algorithm, and (d) classification of adverse event.

These assessments can reveal increased frequencies or severity of known vaccine product-related reactions, identify vaccine quality issues or immunization programme-related weaknesses, and bring to light previously unknown adverse events not detected during clinical trials. The use of this protocol will standardize the identification and assessment of vaccine safety signals in a standardized manner [52]. An example is given by Joshi et al. with the rapid onset of optic neuritis after measles vaccination [53]. A recent review highlighted little information on the actual use of the algorithm in both high- and low-income countries [54].

Many countries among World Health Organization (WHO) members have national or local AEFI surveillance programmes in place. In India, the national AEFI surveillance system is managed by the Universal Immunization Programme (UIP) and covering the largest birth cohort in the world with 26 million births annually. Initiated in 1985, the surveillance system is focusing on reporting and investigation serious AEFIs [55]. It gained momentum in 2012, following the establishment of National AEFI Secretariat for the National AEFI Committee at Immunization Technical Support Unit, Ministry of Health and Family Welfare [56]. The National AEFI guidelines were first published in 2005, revised in 2010 and recently in 2015. According to the latest version of Operational Guidelines for AEFI Surveillance, all reported serious and severe AEFIs need to be assessed for causality using the WHO and the Council for International Organizations of Medical Sciences (CIOMS) consensus Causality Assessment Protocol (CAP) that was revised in 2013 [52, 57].

With annual estimated 2.4 to 3.0 million cases and 72,000 deaths in under-5 children attributed to disease caused by the Haemophilus-type B (Hib) bacteria, the introduction of Hib containing pentavalent vaccine provided immense public health benefits. However, its introduction in 2011 was followed by reports of infant deaths following vaccine use. The programme however could face these challenges head on due to investments made to build strong AEFI networks. All field AEFI reports were rapidly investigated (Central AEFI team reports http://www.mohfw.nic.in/index1.php ?lang=1&level=4&sublinkid=3928&lid=2421 Accessed on 26 February 2017), and detailed case by case assessments were conducted by applying the global causality assessment criteria to determine a cause-effect association with the vaccine. None was found (Media report: Kashmir Times; Central team says Pentavalent Vaccine safe http://www.greaterkashmir.com/news/news/central-team-says-pentavalent-vaccine-safe/157079.html). Though at the time, many neighboring countries (WHO Web page: Pentavalent vaccine in Asian Countries http://www.who.int/vaccine_safety/ committee/topics/pentavalent_vaccine/Jul_2013/en/) suspended pentavalent use under pressure of allegations about its safety. India built reliable systems for AEFI surveillance, a functional National AEFI committee supported techno-managerially by an AEFI Secretariat in the Ministry of Health and Family Welfare (Immunization Technical Support Unit, AEFI Secretariat India http://www.itsu.org.in/aefi-program-1)

close coordination with the district and state level ensuring availability of detailed hospital and clinical case records to trained experts for making scientific assessments using the CAP. Medical specialists (i.e., pediatrics, infectious diseases, public heath, forensic medicine, pathology, microbiology, vaccinology, community medicine, and pharmacology) conducted the causality assessments of the reported serious AEFI cases. Results of all such assessments done so far are available help to enable the use of surveillance data to inform vaccine safety policy issues [58]. Moreover, all cluster reports (2 or more AEFI reports) were rapidly assessed for signal validation. These assessments were pivotal to maintain the pentavalent vaccine programmes to combat bacterial meningitis and childhood pneumonia, the largest killer of Indian children.

Causality Assessment is an important and critical final step that informs the feedback and communication to the reporter (health professional), immunization program, and the target community. Vaccine confidence and trust of a community in a vaccination programme is sustained with simple, timely, and comprehensive communication of the findings of the AEFI investigation and causality assessment. This is especially critical for clusters of events, program error, and previously unknown "new" events.

In India, the AEFI surveillance programme works closely with other vaccine pharmacovigilance partners including Central Drugs Standards and Control Organization (CDSCO), Indian Pharmacopoeia Commission (IPC), Central Drug Laboratory (CDL), other immunization partners such as WHO and UNICEF (See Chap. 3). It is not surprising thus that during the NRA assessment 2017, vaccine pharmacovigilance was assessed as the most mature function in the country [59]. New vaccine introductions demand greater investments in capacity building of existing health staff and community regarding the benefits and potential adverse events reported with vaccines. Communication tools such as Communication Guidelines (Immunization Technical Support Unit, AEFI Secretariat India http://www.itsu.org.in/aefi-program-1) for Health workers have been developed and implemented to interact confidently with the community about AEFIs, while simultaneously efforts have been made to build capacity of policy makers for timely response to the media about AEFIs by providing guidance in the form of a Media Response Protocol.

Researchers appointed by the programme continued to assess and evaluate community concerns and signals generated from reported AEFIs and generated evidence for policy decisions. As an example, a community cohort study on deaths and hospitalizations following UIP vaccines was established in two Indian states after concerns about reported AEFIs following pentavalent vaccine. Additional research projects are being undertaken to understand barriers and facilitators for AEFI reporting in the health system and develop a multi-site active AEFI surveillance system for India through a pilot research project (Internal communication to National AEFI Committee (2013–2016)).

Efforts are on for greater convergence between vaccine pharmacovigilance stakeholders including CDSCO, PvPI and AEFI surveillance programme especially at district and state level (Requirement at state and district level for Immunization and Patient Safety Associates (SISPA and DISPA) in Pharmacovigilance Programme of India http://governmentjobsindia.net/2017/04/

requirement-in-indian-pharmacopoeia-commission-ipc-apr-2017/ and http://ipc.nic.in/writereaddata/mainlinkFile/File753.pdf) and use of IT tools are needed to ensure vaccine safety issues are handled rapidly and transparently by informing and involving those most affected and those concerned with public health in effective ways.

Vaccine hesitancy persists as a global concern with a spectrum from those who believe, those who doubt, and those who are not aware or troubled by the volume of information on vaccines. Experts have recommended [60] a framework for understanding the factors that affect hesitancy, which will help prepare strategies to address these gaps. Vaccine confidence is generated through open and transparent research and communication through collaborations. This will ensure higher vaccine uptake rates and inform the public and other stakeholders of the benefits and risks of vaccines, the way vaccine safety is constantly assessed, assured, and communicated [57].

14.5 From Minimal to Enhanced Pharmacovigilance Capacity in Resource-Limited Countries

Patrick Zuber

Post-licensure monitoring of vaccines is one of the two regulatory functions that WHO recommends all countries to perform (together with licensing activities) [61]. Ensuring minimal capacity for vaccine safety is a strategic objective of the WHO Global vaccine safety blueprint (the Blueprint) [62, 63]. Minimal capacity (Table) encompasses a set of tools and procedures with defined roles and responsibilities to ensure that any safety concern following immunization is detected, reported, and investigated for appropriate and timely response to prevent reoccurrence. It is accompanied by managerial elements that enable the system to function and develop through regular monitoring and evaluation and continuous quality improvement. It also requires a commitment from national authorities—vaccine regulators and immunization programme in particular—to share information internationally for global public health benefit. Countries have the possibility of self-assessing progress with their system or to request support from WHO and its partners for external evaluation.

In recent years, attention to vaccine safety monitoring has progressed tremendously, and, according to WHO/UNICEF, by 2015 there were at least 84 of 194 member states that met a reporting threshold for adverse events following immunization (AEFI) of at least 10 per 100,000 surviving infant [64]. Progress has been quite significant in countries that manufacture vaccines and their neighbors from Asia and Latin America. Establishing sustainable AEFI monitoring is a complex endeavor as it often requires a behavioral shift to counter possible negative perceptions associated with reporting untoward events and immunization errors. As exemplified by progress from China, such systems can be established over the course of a decade, provided political will and capacity-building are adequate [65].

Enhanced pharmacovigilance is required when vaccine safety signals require further investigation [61] or when newly available vaccines are deployed and their safety profiles need to be further characterized in order to assess possible rare events that would not have been identified during clinical development, or possible risks among particular sub-populations such as people with disabilities, immune-deficiencies, or for vaccines administered during pregnancy. In recent year, several products have become available that will be used essentially in low- and middle-income countries. Introduction of a meningitis A conjugate vaccine in the Meningitis Belt countries illustrates how enhanced safety monitoring detected adverse events of interest more reliably than passive reporting infrastructure reassuring all stakeholders about the safe profile of this particular product [31, 66, 67] including for pregnant women and their off springs [68]. Likewise, the deployment of rotavirus vaccines worldwide, including newer products, requires that the risk of intussusception be assessed in different large populations, as was the case in Latin America [69].

In some instances, hypothesis testing of a particular vaccine-outcome association might require collaboration across multiple countries. This is the case in particular for rare events that require thorough clinical ascertainment. To that effect, international collaborative models have been proposed [29], piloted during the 2009 influenza pandemic response [70, 71], and a demonstration project involving 16 countries from all WHO regions was recently completed [72]. Such networks and enhancement of information systems that allow verifying health outcomes while ascertaining immunization status need to be further developed in order to ensure that safety concerns can properly be addressed and verified regardless of where a particular product is being utilized [73] (Table 14.1).

Table 14.1 Elements of minimal capacity for vaccine pharmacovigilance at country level[a]

Structural elements	Dedicated vaccine pharmacovigilance capacity (with designated staff for this purpose and stable basic funding)
	National reporting form for AEFI
	National AEFI database
	Access to AEFI expert review committee (ARC)
	Strategy for risk communication
	Harmonized methods and tools for the monitoring and investigation of AEFI
Managerial elements	Regulatory framework in place that defines the provisions for monitoring and management of AEFI
	Clear lines of accountability identified for the conduct of vaccine safety work
	Institutional development plan (including performance indicators and periodic evaluation/revision)
	Commitment to sharing information on vaccine safety with other countries

[a]Adapted from the WHO Global vaccine safety blueprint[i]

14.6 Background Rates and the Concept of Ecological Studies

Steven Black

The evaluation of vaccine safety in resource-limited settings has relied upon passive surveillance exclusively; this was usually sufficient to identify vaccine safety or programmatic concerns. In this setting, reporting of adverse events was encouraged, and in some countries, an expert committee would review problematic cases. Recently, however, the dynamics of vaccine introductions have changed, and this trend is likely to continue. One rotavirus vaccine was first introduced in Mexico [74], and a meningococcal A conjugate vaccine was introduced and used exclusively used in developing countries in Africa [75]. Additionally, vaccines targeting malaria [76], cholera [77], shigella, and dengue [78] are likely to be introduced in developing countries. Some of these vaccines, such as the malaria vaccine or shigella vaccine, utilize new technologies and adjuvants that have not been utilized earlier. In response to the COVID pandemic, many vaccines have been developed and implemented outside of Europe and North America for which only limited vaccine safety information is available. Without large population experience with new vaccines in the post-licensure setting, it is possible that rare safety concerns may exists or that even in the absence of a real concern, a vaccine safety scare could derail a successful vaccine program. To address these issues, it will be necessary to develop infrastructure in early introducing countries that not only allow for passive reporting of events, but also allow for rapid assessment of potential concerns and if necessary performance of epidemiologic causality assessment studies [73]. Although not available in all countries, infrastructure exists in many developing countries likely to be early introducers of vaccine for the performance of these types of analyses. Here we will explore the utility and experience with two techniques—assessment of background rates and the performance of observational studies—that can meet this need.

When presented with a potential vaccine safety issue or scare, there is a need for a rapid response to address public concern and to prevent loss of confidence and unwarranted damage to a vaccine program. Such concerns may arise out of passive surveillance but also out of the press or single case reports. When faced with this situation for a specific outcome, it would be useful to refer to experience in other countries regarding this outcome. However, for a newly introduced vaccine, this is not likely to be possible. In the absence of this possibility, one approach is to try and rapidly assess the number of observed cases of the events versus the number of events one would expect to occur by change alone unrelated to vaccination—the background rate. In one example in Austria, a case of sudden death was observed following receipt of HPV vaccine. This outcome, while dramatic and tragic, unfortunately occurs sporadically in the population without vaccination. In this example, vaccine safety experts were able to estimate the number of such deaths that would occur by change alone in vaccinees and show that actually the observed number was lower than one would have expected as a background rate [79]. In another example in Finland, cases of narcolepsy were observed to occur following receipt of 2009 pandemic H1N1 influenza vaccine and the number of cases that were observed was higher than one would have expected based upon the known background rate [16]. This then led to further epidemiologic evaluations as discussed below.

Prior to the introduction of the 2009 H1N1 vaccine, an international collaboration was established to develop such rates to address potential safety concerns. Some of estimated background rates of events of potential concern were quite high. For example, using background rates, one would anticipate that within 6 weeks of a vaccine, one would see 160,000 spontaneous abortions per ten million pregnant women, and 21.5 cases of Guillain-Barre syndrome and 575 cases of sudden death within 1 h of vaccination per ten million population [80]. Clearly awareness of the expected number of events would be very useful in responding to a potential safety concern regarding cases of these events. The evaluation of George Wak and colleagues of meningococcal A conjugate vaccine in pregnant women in Ghana provide a demonstration of the feasibility of this approach in developing countries. In this study, background rates of events in an epidemiologic surveillance network were used to assess the safety of this new vaccine [68].

An issue has been the lack of availability of background rates of events in developing countries and a lack of understanding of how such rates can be estimated. One approach has been to utilize hospital registries or databases to estimate such rates. Since most safety events of potential concern are serious, one can rely on hospital utilization information to determine the background rate of such an event. Although this is much facilitated if access to electronic databases is available, it is also feasible through accessing survey data available in the INDEPTH [81] epidemiologic sites or through a rapid review of paper hospitalization logs. Optimally, if countries that were going to be known early introducers of a new vaccine were identified well before the vaccine introduction, such infrastructure and data were tabulated for the pre-introduction period.

Having reviewed passive reporting data and compared the number of expected events against the expected number from available background rate, it is still possible that a legitimate safety concern still remains. In this situation, it is necessary to perform an epidemiologic study to assess causality. To do this, it is necessary to identify cases of the event of concern in an unbiased manner from hospital registries or other logs and then identify an appropriate analytic approach to evaluate the relative and attributable risk of the events following vaccination. For example, following the availability of COVID-19 vaccines in Africa, GAVI has funded hospital-based surveillance in eight low-income countries in Africa. Within this project, potential cases of pre-specified AESIs are identified from hospital logs and then the patients are reviewed against Brighton Collaboration case definitions for each AESI. In this project, validated cases are then evaluated in a self-control risk internal analysis. While a detailed discussion of other approaches is beyond the scope of this chapter, these can include cohort, case-control, case-coverage, self-controlled case series, and case-crossover studies. Each of these approaches, if performed appropriately, can yield an estimation of the absolute and attributable risk of vaccination. For each assessment method, it is necessary to define an "exposed" time period or risk window following receipt of vaccination. For adverse events whose pathophysiology is well understood, this may be trivial. Often, however, one has to make a choice uninformed by such knowledge. In this case, arbitrary windows, such as 48 h for local or systemic reactions, 30 days for other events following a killed vaccine, or up to 6 weeks for events following a live vaccine, are used. Other logistic issues include the potential for different schedules or different vaccine formulations to be used during the study period, and the lack of denominator data for the population being evaluated. If a defined denominator is lacking, the self-controlled case series approach is ideal, as it does not require a denominator.

14.7   Hypothesis-Testing of Vaccine Safety Concerns in R esource-Limited Countries: Hospital-Based Sentinel Network Approach

Silvia Perez-Vilar

An ideal active vaccine safety monitoring approach should provide timely and reliable data useful for both signal refinement and confirmation. If the vaccine is used in large populations, particularly if they represent a significant fraction of the total population of that age cohort, and if the events being investigated are rare and serious, simple active systems that do not require population denominators are a good option to perform analytical hypothesis-testing studies to confirm (or refute) the associations between signaling events and vaccines, particularly in resource-poor environments. In such circumstances, an active surveillance hospital-based sentinel network integrated into an international active surveillance collaborative effort could be implemented at low cost and with no additional local infrastructure in almost every country [29, 82, 83]. The international hospital-based collaborative investigation of Guillain Barré syndrome following the 2009 (H1N1) influenza vaccination [70, 71], the WHO-sponsored multi-country proof-of-concept investigation of the association of immune thrombocytopenic purpura and aseptic meningitis with measles-mumps-containing vaccines [83–85], and the investigation of the association between intussusception and rotavirus vaccines in Mexico and Brazil [69] are examples of the successful application of this approach.

The main analytical method used for the proof-of-concept studies described above is the self-controlled case series (SCCS) method, chosen because of its cost-efficiency, flexibility, and applicability in countries where population denominator information may be unreliable or not available [86–88]. In SCCS studies, only individuals with the event of interest need to be investigated [86–88]. The rate of occurrence of the event is compared between predefined "risk" and "non-risk" periods around the time of the vaccination of interest (exposure) [86–88]. Because only cases are needed for analysis, population denominators are not required [29, 70,

71]. Also, given that the risk of occurrence of the event is compared between two time periods within the same individual, time-fixed confounders are intrinsically adjusted for, and the possibility of bias is decreased (Whitaker et al. 2006). The hospital-based approach could also be used for investigations performed with study designs other than the SCCS methodology [29, 82], such as the case-crossover design [89], case-time-control design [90], case-control design, or the test-negative case-control method [91]. A requirement for these hospital-based approaches is the reliable and independent determination of the exposure status of cases (or, if a case-control approach is used, of both cases and controls). Because the events of interest are usually rare and their diagnosis may require complex diagnostic capabilities, participating hospitals are usually national or regional reference centres, which do not often have direct access to the vaccination status of patients. Therefore, prior to study initiation, the candidate hospitals must provide evidence of capacity to gain access to vaccination records and to reliably link outcomes and exposures at the individual level.

14.8 The Testing of a Hypothesis of a Vaccine Safety Concern in Resource-Limited Countries: INDEPTH Sites

Esperanca Sevene and Sammy Khagayi

The gap between the vaccine registration and the availability of vaccine in resource-limited countries (RLCs) is expected to reduce; there is a concern regarding safety monitoring post-licensure. Historically the safety profile was already well described before the introduction of the vaccine in RLCs [92].

To address the need to monitor and assess the safety of newly introduced vaccines as well as older vaccines in RLC, new methods and tools for active surveillance are required. Countries that already have an established infrastructure for epidemiological studies can offer a useful platform and optimize use of resources. The International Network for the Demographic Evaluation of Populations and Their Health (INDEPTH) is an example of this platform. INDEPTH centers exist in a wide geographic area including south Asia and Africa where vaccines are likely to be introduced and offer unique access to both household individual and clinic based health and demographic data, much of which is linked at the individual level with unique identifiers [93]. The INDEPTH centers perform a biannual socio-demographic data collection and some of the centers also collect clinical data on a daily basis [94, 95].

The socio-demographic data collected in the centres comprises household and individual characteristics, household socio-economic assets, vital data, migration, individual health history and cause of death, among others. Information on vaccination is also collected including date of vaccination, dosage, product information (brand name, batch, and expiry date). This information could be retrieved from the infant vaccination card where data on date of birth and birth weight is also available.

Mortality data, including verbal autopsies, are routinely collected at INDEPTH centres. Field workers are also trained in social and verbal autopsy data collection techniques, an important tool in collecting data on all-cause/cause-specific mortality. These data can be used to adjust for observational studies of vaccination and mortality. This in addition to other data collected from health facilities linked to the household data can be used to capture other alternative outcome data.

Some of the INDEPTH centres have established morbidity surveillance platforms that register any out-patient or in-patient visit to the health facilities within the area [94, 95]. The information includes date of visit, clinical history, physical examinations, laboratory results, and medications prescribed. This information is registered in a database with a unique identifier from health and demographic surveillance system (HDSS).

To investigate a vaccine safety concern, a start point should be previously defined and that could be a vaccine or an event. The introduction of a new vaccine could be an example of starting point. The programme could then design a safety monitoring plan to assess any death or visit to the health facility after the administration of the new vaccine. The database on regular surveillance will have information on exposure to a new vaccine or deaths after vaccination, while the database of morbidity surveillance will have information on events post vaccination. Specific events of interest should also be assessed (e.g., convulsion after measles vaccine). The database on morbidity surveillance will then identify the infants with convulsions, and exposure date can then be found in the regular surveillance data. Using the electronic databases and unique identifiers, record linkage between the different source of data is possible and access to other patient information [94, 95]. Alternatively the unique identifier can be used to get to the household, visit the individual, and collect additional information regarding confounder factors and to confirm both the event and exposure information.

Different study designs can be incorporated in the HDSS. For vaccine safety, cohort studies (exposure based) and self-controlled designs (case based) are mostly used [96, 97]. Each design has requirements in terms of case identification and validation, follow-up, exposure, and co-variate data. Cohort studies require that the study population be defined and followed over time. During the follow-up time, all outcomes of interest, the exposure, and co-variates need to be assessed. In the HDSS, a cohort is already established and data can be retrospectively assessed reducing costs of the safety monitoring.

The morbidity surveillance can give information for the case-based studies. In this design, the control (moments) serve to provide the exposure distribution in the population that gives rise to the cases. This distribution can be obtained in various ways: controls could be other subjects in the cohort who are in follow-up at the time the case occurs (case control study), but the case itself can also provide control moments (case-crossover), until the moment it becomes a case. The case control and case crossover studies require that exposure is accurately assessed at the index date only and therefore require less information than the full dynamic cohort study.

A hybrid design is the self-controlled case series. This design uses only the cases (as in case crossover); however, in this design, cases are followed over a specific period of time and their follow-up time is classified according to exposure. This requires adequate assessment of the index date (onset of disease) and the ability to classify exposure during follow-up time for the cases. The case cross-over and self-controlled case series studies inherently control for confounding factors that remain stable within one person; however, they both require data on time varying confounding factors. The cohort and case control designs require collection of data on all covariates (stable and time varying) [88, 98, 99]. Each design has strengths and limitations and different requirements in terms of data. Selection of the best design should be made according to the HDSS data available and the requirements of the safety concern to be addressed.

The population dynamics requires a regular surveillance (two or three times a year) and this makes the HDSS an expensive platform. Most centres are reducing the surveillance rounds to one or two per year and missing data could become a problem. The quality of data collected should be regularly verified, and data cleaning process should be part of the maintenance of the platform. Vaccine safety has specificities that are not part of the routine data collection in the HDSS, and communication between the immunization programme team and the HDSS team should be critical for the success of the implementation of a vaccine safety monitoring programme.

14.9 The Testing of a Hypothesis of a Vaccine Safety Concern in India

Mandyam Ravi

All adverse events following immunization lead to death or hospitalization or where the vaccine quality is suspect need to be investigated [56]. The initial report (case reporting) needs to be given to the medical officer (MO) in charge of the primary health centre in rural areas and to the District Immunization officer (DIO) in urban areas within 48 h of the incident. From here a preliminary case investigation report is sent to the Assistant Commissioner of the Universal Immunization programme and state expanded program of immunization officer within 7 days. Generally, reports are also sent to the Indian Academy of Pediatrics and the company manufacturing the vaccine. Each state has a state/regional expert committee, which will submit a final case investigation to the Government of India. If the AEFI committee decides to investigate the vaccine quality, then the incriminated vial of vaccine and diluents should be collected and sent under cold chain requirement to Central Drug Laboratory Kasauli for laboratory investigation. On completion of the investigation, the DIO should provide feedback on the outcome of the investigation to the MO of the Primary health centre (PHC) and health assistant (HA) with appropriate corrective measures. Recently GSK has also started a portal for reporting AEFI. The JSS University in association with the WHO Programme for International Drug Monitoring has been conducting training programmes which include AEFI monitoring and reporting training.

The Government of India (GOI) introduced pentavalent vaccine (HIB+DwPT+HepB) vaccine in a few states in 2011. Following this, there were 14 deaths in Kerala from December 2011 to March 2013 (more than 2.5 million doses were given). There was considerable media hype and a group of people including doctors actively lobbied against the pentavalent vaccine, quoting incidents from Vietnam and Bhutan. A team from the GOI visited Kerala and concluded, after detailed study of the cases, that there was no causal relationship to the vaccine. The national AEFI committee met in August 2013 where it endorsed the findings of its causality subcommittee that the AEFI deaths reported in Kerala were not causally associated with Pentavalent vaccine [100]. The programme was not stopped, and upscaling went on as per original schedule. A paper published in 2018 demonstrated an increase in reports of sudden unexplained deaths within 72 h of administering Pentavalent vaccine compared to DTP vaccine. This received wide publicity in the media but did not impact immunization programmes as an expert team investigated all these events constituted by Government of India and were found to be not vaccine product related [101–104]. Pentavalent vaccine under the country's expanded program of immunization has now been rolled out in many more states.

Several media and other reports relate some infant deaths to the oral polio vaccine within the National Pulse Polio programme, one of the most successful mass immunization programmes worldwide. There were some instances of mass hysteria; however, medical professionals effectively controlled these at the local level without being escalated to the GOI. A mass scale Measles Rubella vaccine programme took place in February 2017 with only three reported serious adverse events all classified as coincidental after investigation [56].

Mass COVID 19 vaccine was introduced in India, one of the largest mass vaccination programmes in the world. The AEFI reporting system was therefore revamped by the Ministry of Health and Family Welfare (MOHFW) India, a causality assessment Special Group, was made with multiple specialties being represented, i.e., physicians, neurologists, cardiologists, pulomonologists, and obstetrician-gynecologists. This group presented their results to the National AEFI committee that would then give the final approval. Two hundred and fifty-four cases of reported serious AEFIs following COVID 19 vaccination were thus analyzed. Seventy-eighty were found to have a consistent causal association to the vaccination, 31 vaccine product related, and 47 anxiety related (https://main.mohfw.gov.in/sites/default/files/NACM_approved_cases_english_merge_0.pdf). All AEFIs were not captured by this system; however, an independent study by Armed Forces Medical Services in health care workers found that all AEFIs reported were nonserious subsiding in 1–2 days (higher incidence of reported adverse events following immunization (AEFI) after first dose of COVID-19 vaccine among previously infected health care workers Medical Journal Armed Forces India Volume 77, Supplement 2, July 2021, Pages S505–S507).

14.10   Active Vaccine Safety Surveillance in the United States

Bruce Fireman

This section is describing the US vaccine monitoring system. The Vaccine Safety Datalink (VSD) is the global role model for active post-licensure vaccine safety surveillance and is thus included in this chapter to illustrate a high capacity system.

Clinical trials for new vaccines are powered to detect efficacy and/or immunogenicity of the vaccine, against the targeted pathogen. Although safety data are required for licensure, the studies generally cannot say much about rare adverse events potentially causally linked to the vaccine. For that reason, post-licensure studies of larger populations are crucial to detect rare adverse events, or events arising in special populations. Post-licensure safety studies may be needed for new vaccines, new indications for vaccines, and even for older vaccines for which there is limited data.

In the USA, the Food and Drug Administration (FDA) often mandates post-licensure safety studies (Phase IV), supported by the manufacturer. These studies may focus on specific worrisome outcomes (from clinical trials or post-licensure VAERS or case report), or may contain analyses that screen for a broad range of potential adverse events. In addition, as part of the FDA's sentinel system [105], Post-licensure Rapid Immunization Safety Monitoring programme (PRISM) uses claims data from medical insurers and delivery systems with very large populations, to support vaccine safety surveillance.

CDC's Immunization Safety Office (ISO) and FDA are charged with ensuring the safety of vaccines in the USA, and in a collaborative effort, they support the Vaccine Adverse Events Reporting System (VAERS), a passive online reporting system. Inference about vaccine safety from data yielded by passive reporting, however, can be fraught with issues of confounding, so in order to bolster vaccine safety surveillance, ISO created the VSD [23], a system of large linked databases with epidemiologists specializing in vaccine safety at each of multiple sites. VSD maintains ongoing surveillance of many vaccines through the Rapid Cycle Analysis (RCA), utilizing weekly updates of vaccine-outcome data from the sites. The group strives to design appropriate analyses to examine vaccine safety while carefully adjusting for various sources of bias in observational studies.

Both VSD and FDA's Sentinel use a number of study designs for vaccine safety surveillance. FDA's Sentinel PRISM has a listing of multiple methods on their website (FDA "Mini Sentinel, Statistical Methods" from http://www.minisentinel.org/methods/methods_development/default.aspx.). Standard cohort and case control designs for epidemiologic studies of observational data are often utilized in VSD and PRISM as well [106]. Because of underlying differences between vaccinated and unvaccinated individuals that may not be measured [107–109], some vaccine safety studies use vaccinated individuals only, comparing risk during post-vaccination intervals when adverse events are biologically plausible versus risk during comparison time intervals. Several methods utilize the risk interval (RI), the brief period of time following exposure (vaccination) during which an adverse event may be causally related, and compare the rate of outcome events during with the RI with rates in an earlier or later control interval. A risk interval study can be conditioned on the individual, making this a "self-controlled" study which controls better for factors that are stable over time. These self-controlled vaccine safety studies generally use only individuals who are vaccinated and have had events and make their inferences from the timing of the events in relation to the vaccinations [110, 111]. A variant of the cohort study that only uses vaccinated individuals is the case-centered design [110]. This method has the advantages of adjusting for seasonality, and in making use of population-based immunization patterns which allows calculation of the risk difference and attributable risk which is not possible when only the vaccination of cases is known.

14.11 The Safety Surveillance of the Malaria Vaccine as an Example

Laurence Baril

Malaria, a mosquito-borne disease, sickens millions of people and kills hundreds of thousand each year. Malaria impacts social and economic development of many low-income countries. *Plasmodium falciparum* is recognized as the major cause of severe morbidity and mortality. Current vector-control measures (such as insecticide impregnated bed-nets and insecticide indoor spray) combined with curative measures (such as access to rapid diagnostic test and treatment using artemisinin-based combination) are not sufficient to control the disease. Other interventions to reduce the malaria burden are tested on the field. Even partially efficacious, a vaccine was identified as adding a major benefit to malaria fight (Weekly Epidemiological Record n°4, 29 January 2016).

The first malaria vaccine, named Mosquirix®, was developed for young children (aged 6 weeks to 17 months) living in sub-Saharan African, the most affected population. In July 2015, a positive scientific opinion was given by the Committee for Medicinal Products for Human Use of the European Medicines Agency (EMA) in the context of cooperation with the World Health Organization (WHO) in accordance with Article 58 of Regulation (EC) No 726/2004 (http://www.ema.europa.eu/ema/index.jsp?curl=pages/news_and_events/news/2015/07/news_detail_002376.jsp&mid=WC0b01ac058004d5c1).

Mosquirix® is a recombinant, adjuvanted vaccine against *Plasmodium falciparum* and Hepatitis B (RTS,S/ASO1$_E$) to target the pre-erythrocytic stage of *P. falciparum* [112]. Based on several clinical trials including a pivotal Phase III, the clinical safety profile showed that the most common solicited adverse events (AEs) in infants (6–12 weeks) were pain and fever with only a few Grade 3 reaction and a higher risk of febrile convulsions in the older age groups (5–17 months) [112–114].

The Pharmacovigilance Risk Assessment Committee (PRAC) from EMA endorsed the Risk Management Plan (RMP).

Febrile convulsion was an identified risk. Meningitis, potential immune-mediated diseases, hypersensitivity (including anaphylaxis), malaria rebound, and behavioral changes regarding usage of other malaria preventive measures were classified as potential risks in the RMP. Together with risk minimization measures mentioned in the product information notice, several post-licensure (Phase IV) studies, monitoring incidence rates of events of special interest through comparison of the incidence rates, assessed prospectively from start of vaccination to pre-vaccination period incidence rates.

Following the CHMP position, in October 2015, two independent WHO advisory groups (the Strategic Advisory Group of Experts (SAGE) on immunization and the Malaria Policy Advisory Committee (MPAC)) recommended a pilot implementation of Mosquirix® in three settings in sub-Saharan Africa and in children 5–17 months old (i.e., in Ghana, Kenya, and Malawi) (http://www.who.int/mediacentre/news/releases/2015/sage/en/). In April 2017, WHO regional office for Africa announced that implementation will start in Ghana, Kenya, and Malawi (http://www.afro.who.int/en/media-centre/pressreleases/item/9533-ghana-kenya-and-malawi-to-take-part-in-who-malaria-vaccine-pilot-programme.html). The African Vaccine Regulatory Forum (AVAREF) together with the national regulatory authorities are working together to enable the appropriate safety monitoring. In addition, safety studies will be conducted to address the RMP. Results should be available by 2020.

14.12 Safety Surveillance of Immunization in Pregnancy

Sonali Kochhar

Immunization of pregnant individuals induces vaccine-specific immune responses in them and helps to prevent and/or minimize vaccine-preventable infectious diseases-related severe illness, death, and adverse pregnancy outcomes including spontaneous abortions, stillbirth, and preterm birth [115]. It would also provide benefit to the fetus and neonate through transplacental transfer of maternal vaccine-induced immune globulin (IgG) antibodies and provide protection from the targeted pathogen to the infant during their first months of life, when they are vulnerable to severe disease but too young to get vaccinated [116]. The immunization also has the additional benefit of preventing infection in the mother with reduced risk of transmission of infection to the infants 115. Immunization in pregnancy helps to reduce maternal, neonatal, and under-five childhood mortality and morbidity [117]. Immunization in pregnancy is especially important for vaccine-preventable diseases for which there are no other options for protecting young infants, e.g., tetanus, pertussis, and influenza. Tetanus vaccination for pregnant individuals has been administered for decades, and influenza and pertussis vaccines are being increasingly recommended as a part of immunization in pregnancy programmes [62, 63, 118]. It is globally recommended that pregnant individuals be vaccinated against COVID-19. Respiratory syncytial virus (RSV) vaccines have been recently implemented in high-income countries as a single dose to be administered during weeks 32–36 of pregnancy to protect infants from birth to 6 months of age from lower respiratory tract disease (LRTD) and severe LRTD caused by RSV (FDA Approves First Vaccine for Pregnant Individuals to Prevent RSV in Infants. August 21, 2023. Accessed on 6 Dec 2024 at https://www.fda.gov/news-events/press-announcements/ fda-approves-first-vaccine-pregnant-individuals-prevent-rsv-infants.) Examples of candidate vaccines under development for use in pregnancy include Group B streptococcus, Lassa fever, and *cytomegalovirus* vaccines [119]. Live attenuated vaccines (e.g., varicella and measles-mumps-rubella (MMR) vaccines) are contraindicated during pregnancy due to the theoretical risk of the live attenuated virus in the vaccine crossing the placenta and resulting in viral infection of the fetus.

Introduction of these vaccines comes with tremendous public health benefit, specifically for pregnant individuals and infants living in low and middle-income countries (LMIC). However, there are many barriers when it comes to immunization of pregnant individuals. These include the fear of adverse pregnancy outcomes and of vaccine-transmitted infection occurring in the mothers and their infants. These concerns are also raised with the use of the same vaccines (e.g., influenza and pertussis vaccines) in childhood and adult immunization programmes. A vaccine found to be safe for pregnant individuals and infants would likely be well accepted by the general public for other target groups. There is a need for a thorough assessment of the safety of vaccines during pregnancy [120], given the potential for numerous confounding events associated with pregnancy in women, the fetus, and the neonates [115].

The key challenge for safety monitoring of vaccination in pregnancy is that the follow-up for obstetric and neonatal outcomes needs to be done for several months post-vaccination (in the pregnant individual) and post-birth (in the neonate). Long-term maternal and infant follow-up is costly and logistically very challenging in developing countries with limited infrastructure. The maternal and neonatal follow-up duration depends on the vaccine properties (e.g., inclusion of an adjuvant) and the population being studied. It is important to distinguish between vaccine-related and pregnancy-related outcomes. Complications like congenital malformations, stillbirth and obstetric, and neonatal complications are not uncommon even in "low risk" pregnancies. It is important to distinguish adverse events related to the vaccines from the background rates of adverse maternal and neonatal outcomes in that population [121]. Depending on the vaccine, the safety parameters to be followed up on could include growth of the neonate and development outcomes (these are not necessary for all vaccines) [115].

It is critical to know background rates for common adverse events in the study population. This would help with safety monitoring, e.g., miscarriage occurs in 10–15% of all pregnancies and preterm births occur in 4–16% of pregnancies (WHO. Preterm birth. 10 May 2023. Accessed on 6 Dec 2024 at https://www.who. int/news-room/fact-sheets/detail/preterm-birth). The background rates are often not known in LMICs and need to be collected in the target populations [115]. It is important to utilize standard definitions of key obstetric and neonatal outcomes of vaccination in pregnancy [115]. The standard definitions for key events are required for defining, identifying, capturing, reporting, and analyzing AEFI and would lead to a common understanding of key events related to vaccination in pregnancy worldwide. It is key to ensure applicability and usefulness of definitions for data analysis in all settings. It would lead to data comparability, pooling, and consistent analysis within and across safety studies and surveillance systems, This has been addressed through the Global Alignment of Immunization safety Assessment in pregnancy (GAIA) project, which was set up in response to the call of the World Health Organization for a globally harmonized approach to actively monitor the safety of immunization in pregnancy programmes with a specific focus on LMIC needs and requirements [115]. In the GAIA project, experts from 13 organizations collaborated with over 200 volunteers to respond to this need. They developed a core set of 26 globally standardized case definitions of selected key obstetric and neonatal outcomes (https://www.sciencedirect.com/journal/vaccine/vol/35/issue/48/part/PA; https://www.sciencedirect.com/journal/vaccine/vol/34/issue/49), a glossary of enabling terms critical to the case definitions, concept definitions and ontology of over 3000 terms, a preliminary map of disease codes across coding terminologies, including MedDRA (Medical Dictionary for Regulatory Activities) and ICD (*International Classification of Diseases) and a*n online tool for automated case classification (single case or batch cases classification) of events according to the standardized case definitions. Two guidelines for harmonized data collection, analysis, and presentation of safety data were developed [115]. The GAIA outputs have been developed based on a standard global consensus process with key public health institutes, regulatory organizations, investigators, vaccine manufacturers, and academia and are increasingly being utilized in the field of immunization in pregnancy and maternal and child health by stakeholders such as investigators, regulators, and industry for clinical research and epidemiological and safety studies [115, 122].

There is a need to develop a validated developmental assessment for newborns [121] and to develop a systematic approach to classifying adverse events to be able to assess causality. It would be useful to develop a framework for defining adverse events (AE) as maternal or infant (e.g., intrauterine growth restriction-complication of pregnancy is a maternal AE and small for gestational age (SGA) is an infant AE). The severity scales for grading the severity of adverse outcomes should be based on pregnancy-specific physiologic and laboratory values.

The Pharmacovigilance Plan for Assessing Safety of Immunization in Pregnancy could include

regular assessment of passively reported adverse events (e.g., through VAERS or the Global Individual Case Safety Reports Database System (VigiBase) which is a WHO global database to which member countries of the WHO Programme for International Drug Monitoring submit reports). The issues associated with this are lack of denominator data, lack of control groups, recall bias associated with retrospective reporting, low reporting of AEFI by healthcare providers, selective reporting of adverse events (AE), incomplete data on AE, lack of specific evidence for the diagnosis submitted in many reports, and lack of utilization of standardized case definitions to enable comparability of data. Analyses of spontaneous AE reports may provide a potential signal for higher than expected rates of AE or previously unrecognized AE. Individual reports can usually not be used to determine causal relationships [123].

Signals coming from spontaneous AE reports could warrant additional clinical and epidemiological investigations and further confirmation in controlled studies. Especially in HIC, the association of rare adverse events or patterns of adverse events can be studied by pharmaco-epidemiological studies using large electronic health record databases and timely answers provided [123]. The studies are limited by the quality of the information contained in the electronic databases, as these observational data are not collected for research purposes. The combined use of multiple healthcare databases for the conduct of active surveillance studies for vaccine safety is being increasingly done, especially in HIC. There are issues associated with this including the different underlying healthcare systems, type of information collected, medical event coding systems, vaccines/drugs information collected, lack of harmonized case definitions, and the language and programs selected for data management and analyses. Several HIC have developed active surveillance systems for AEFI for analyses of the association between a vaccine and one or more pre-specified adverse health outcomes, e.g., CDC's Vaccine Safety Datalink (VSD) and the US FDA's Post-Licensure Rapid Immunization Safety Monitoring (PRISM) programme [123]. Rapid cycle analysis (where weekly, the VSD analyzes their data to determine if the rate of predefined adverse events of special interest (AESI) following a specific vaccine is higher than the AESI rates in a comparison group) help signal to CDC if additional follow-up analyses are needed. Statistical methods have been used to conduct reliable and timely vaccine safety studies on VSD data, including tree-scan, case centered, group sequential, and sequential concurrent comparator analysis. VSD data has been effectively used to show the safety of immunization during pregnancy with COVID-19, Tdap, influenza, inadvertent HPV vaccination, etc. (CDC. About the Vaccine Safety Datalink (VSD). Accessed on 6 Dec 2024 at https://www.cdc.gov/vaccine-safety-systems/vsd/index.html; [124]).

Some LMIC have surveillance systems in place to collect population health data, including maternal health information, e.g., through health and demographic surveillance systems (HDSS). As these databases generally contain aggregated data, studies or analysis is not possible at the individual level. Households are visited regularly and this could serve as a platform to collect data on the safety of immunization in pregnancy.

Pregnancy registries may be set up and used to collect immunization in pregnancy safety data. They are used commonly in HICs, including the CDC COVID-19 Vaccine Pregnancy Registry from Jan 2021 to Aug 2023 (CDC. COVID-19 Vaccine Pregnancy Registry. Accessed on 6 Dec 2024 at https://www.cdc.gov/vaccine-safety-systems/monitoring/covid-preg-reg.html). Their use in LMIC has been limited and is slowly being expanded [115, 125]. These are prospective observational studies, which actively collect information on the exposure of pregnant women to different vaccines, and the outcome (e.g., rates of spontaneous abortion, premature delivery, congenital malformations) [121]. Pregnant women are enrolled before the outcome of pregnancy is known. Registries that capture specific types of disease could be of relevance to specific vaccines. The advantages of Pregnancy Registries are that a single registry can collect data on many pregnancy outcomes, can provide margins of reassurance regarding the lack of risk when a precise measure is impossible, is possible to monitor for suspected risks raised by preclinical studies, clinical trials, or post marketing reports, and can identify factors that affect the risk of adverse outcomes, such as dose, timing of exposure, or maternal characteristics and serve as hypothesis-generating tools.

One potential approach for monitoring the safety of immunization in pregnancy in LMIC is the use of a network of health centers or hospitals within a country or in several countries using case-only analytic methods. This would help to overcome the difficulty of obtaining denominator data to calculate rates of adverse events. Landscape analysis could be used to identify sentinel surveillance sites in countries to study the safety of vaccines given to pregnant individuals [123].

The development of robust systems for vaccination in pregnancy safety monitoring, surveillance, reporting, and response is needed to advance vaccination in pregnancy research and post-marketing surveillance in LMICs.

14.13   Capacity Building and Training in Resource-Limited Countries

Daniel Weibel and Miriam Sturkenboom

Capacity building and training is crucial to enable resource-limited countries to build up and sustain successfully the surveillance and monitoring of vaccine effects (i.e., coverage, safety, effectiveness, and benefit/risk evaluations). Only a local functioning pharmacovigilance vaccine surveillance and response system can securely sustain vaccination programmes and the introduction of new vaccines. Much effort is being done to build capacity and train people within the pharmacovigilance spontaneous reporting systems. It is however critical that these efforts go beyond spontaneous reporting and surveillance, including enhanced capacity of hypothesis testing and active surveillance capabilities. Only enhanced capacity systems will be able to assess potential adverse events and respond timely and locally to vaccine safety scares in the public [19, 25, 29].

Capacity building and training needs to target pharmacovigilance and pharmacoepidemiologic procedures, methods, and skills. Pharmacovigilance needs to cover all processes and steps from safety signal detection, validation/verification, hypothesis testing, and communication. Pharmacoepidemiologic methods and practices for data collection and management, setting up of studies (i.e., study protocols, statistical analysis plans), analysis, and dissemination of results need to be trained.

Next to epidemiologists, data managers, database specialists, and biostatisticians need to be included in capacity building that is targeting on improving the health system in its totality in a RLCs.

WHO's Global Vaccine Safety Blueprint and the succeeding Global Vaccine Safety Initiative are addressing explicitly the strategic goal of building enhanced pharmacovigilance capacity and infrastructure in place to respond to safety concerns rapidly, as they occur. One example of activities is the establishment of a sentinel hospital network including RLCs and build capacity through that [62, 63, 83, 85].

Vaccine pharmacovigilance in RLCs has started to build up in the last 10 years. The process towards enhanced active surveillance is slowed down through health system development in general. While access to vaccination is increasingly secured, and vaccination coverage is increasing, there is a lack of information about the vaccinated subjects in accessible digital data format. Linkable vaccination and medical event registries and health record databases need to be established, like in developed countries, much of the progress in active surveillance has been made upon secondary use of routine care health data, which exist to a lesser degree in RLCs. Initially a landscape analysis of existing data and surveillance systems is needed to build on existing capacity, infrastructure, initiatives, and activities in RLCs such as demographic and health surveillance centers or reference hospital networks. There is enormous potential for capacity building and leveraging international expertise to strengthen pharmacovigilance systems in RLCs.

A 2012 review of pharmacovigilance in Africa showed that financial and other logistic support from WHO and other donors [US Agency for International Development (USAID), Global Fund and other initiatives] has enabled capacity building and training of personnel in pharmacovigilance in the past 15 years. In addition, the establishment of a WHO Collaborating Centre for Advocacy and Training in Accra, Ghana, has been a major step towards consolidating the establishment of pharmacovigilance in Africa [126]. Since 2009 this center is providing pharmacovigilance training, focusing on passive surveillance in African countries. Additionally, the WHO is also building capacity in sub-Saharan Africa through the Global Training Network (GTN) and the through the WHO Uppsala Monitoring Centre with courses on Adverse Events Following Immunization (passive surveillance). PIASA (Pharmaceutical industry Association of South Africa) organized pharmacovigilance trainings in South Africa with a focus on premarketing clinical safety research or post marketing AEFI reporting, single case assessments, and communication of AEFIs. Since 2014 the African Society of Pharmacovigilance Conference (ASoP) is teaching "Pharmacovigilance in Africa: Successes, best practices, innovations, and lessons learned." The past 15 years have allowed for passive surveillance training to grow; however, there is hardly any training on active surveillance or "enhanced" capacity in Africa. In the EU, the Eu2P programme was developed through funding from the Innovative Medicines Initiative. It is currently offering an innovative web-based education and training in pharmacovigilance and pharmacoepidemiology. Eu2P online education and training has been designed and is reviewed by a partnership of seven EU universities associated with two regulatory agencies and fifteen industry partners (see Chap. 16). Additionally, Chen et al. provide an overview and discussion of capacity building activities and related challenges taking a "lifecycle" approach for northern hemisphere and RLCs [19].

14.14 Perspective and Future: Needs, Investments, and Potentials

Jane Gidudu

Remarkable resources have been devoted towards procurement and delivery of vaccines into routine immunization programmes [3]. As new vaccines are targeted for highly endemic diseases such as malaria, dengue, HPV, switch from trivalent OPV to bivalent OPV [127], occurring mostly in RLCs, has added an urgency to establish functional post-marketing surveillance systems to monitor the adverse events following immunization (AEFI). Resources and expertise to establish these systems are limited worldwide most prominently in RLC, and the global community must include vaccine safety activities in their priorities and commitment to ensure monitoring systems are available at country level, regional and global levels to obtain public confidence in immunization programmes [128]. Besides, vaccine safety has remained a low priority for countries for too long with key players lacking long-term commitments for funding vaccine safety activities.

The future of vaccine safety will rely on establishing global platforms with a proactive focus on the following suggested priority areas for the next 3–5 years to strengthen capacity to monitor, characterize, and communicate emerging vaccine safety data and to appropriately adapt vaccine safety policy. These are organized into three main categories: passive surveillance, active or enhanced surveillance, and programmatic aspects of vaccine safety activities in support of WHO's Global Vaccine Safety Initiative [128] according to 5 stages from pre-vaccine introduction to vaccine eradication [19]. Some studies below are referenced as examples and acknowledging some will be quite challenging to implement in RLC where countries are already strained by the vaccine supply chains [129, 130].

Passive surveillance

- Establishing effective, sustainable spontaneous surveillance, and vaccine safety response systems
- Incorporating AEFI surveillance into existing surveillance systems
- Identifying and responding to vaccine safety and hesitancy issues in a timely manner
- Utilizing evidence to support risk communication
- Utilizing prior integrated passive surveillance systems to detect vaccine safety signals or concerns (e.g., assessment of meningococcal vaccine in Bukina Faso [31], rotavirus in Mexico [69], and GBS [29].

Active surveillance

- Establishing effective, sustainable active surveillance and vaccine safety response systems. Enhanced surveillance coupled with sound epidemiologic studies for vaccine safety from local to global levels helps provide the best evidence for decision making [41] and develop consortiums as platforms for conducting multi-center studies [29]
  Programmatic aspects

- Supporting WHO in strengthening country level vaccine safety capacity [128]
- Conducting a wide range of vaccine safety operations research including obtaining background rates for outcomes of interest for safety, vaccine hesitancy studies: overall programme evaluation. Building strong public and private collaborations and partnerships on vaccine safety
- Developing evidence-based guidance for addressing AEFI or recovery
- Supporting new vaccine delivery methods: evaluating immunization programme practices such as unsafe injection practices
- Evaluating the impact of adverse events following immunization on vaccine preventable diseases [131]

Establishing key global public and private partnerships and platforms with expertise and interest in vaccine safety activities is key to attaining WHOs goals, as summed up by Gavi's model: *"By bringing the key stakeholders in global immunisation together around one mission, Gavi combines the technical expertise of the development community with the business know-how of the private sector"* (http://www.gavi.org/our-alliance/operating-model/, Accessed December 31, 2024). This is key to attaining WHOs goals of attaining minimum vaccine safety capacity especially in RLCs. While there are several approaches available or in the works to address vaccine safety concerns [29], there is a compelling need for more targeted and effective approaches such as incorporating vaccine safety into strategic and funding considerations in achieving sustainable programmes and monitoring the safety of vaccines. Future efforts could be directed at leveraging efforts and resources to existing global public and private partnerships and platforms.

References

1. McGovern ME, Canning D. Vaccination and all-cause child mortality from 1985 to 2011: global evidence from the Demographic and Health Surveys. Am J Epidemiol. 2015;182(9):791–8.
2. Bloom DE. Valuing vaccines: deficiencies and remedies. Vaccine. 2015;33(Suppl 2):B29–33.
3. Feikin DR, Flannery B, Hamel MJ, Stack M, Hansen PM. Vaccines for children in low- and middle-income countries. In: Black RE, Laxminarayan R, Temmerman M, Walker N, editors. Reproductive, maternal, newborn, and child health: disease control priorities, vol. 2. 3rd ed. Washington: World Health Organization; 2016.
4. Barocchi MA, Rappuoli R. Delivering vaccines to the people who need them most. Philos Trans R Soc Lond Ser B Biol Sci. 2015;370(1671):20140150.
5. Poland GA, Whitaker JA, Poland CM, Ovsyannikova IG, Kennedy RB. Vaccinology in the third millennium: scientific and social challenges. Curr Opin Virol. 2016;17:116–25.

6. Gyawali S, Rathore DS, Shankar PR, Kumar KV. Strategies and challenges for safe injection practice in developing countries. J Pharmacol Pharmacother. 2013;4(1):8–12.
7. Hauri AM, Armstrong GL, Hutin YJ. The global burden of disease attributable to contaminated injections given in health care settings. Int J STD AIDS. 2004;15(1):7–16.
8. Drain PK, Nelson CM, Lloyd JS. Single-dose versus multi-dose vaccine vials for immunization programmes in developing countries. Bull World Health Organ. 2003;81(10):726–31.
9. Altaf A, Mujeeb SA. Unsafe disposal of medical waste: a threat to the community and environment. J Pak Med Assoc. 2002;52(6):232–3.
10. Ronveaux O, Rickert D, Hadler S, Groom H, Lloyd J, Bchir A, Birmingham M. The immunization data quality audit: verifying the quality and consistency of immunization monitoring systems. Bull World Health Organ. 2005;83(7):503–10.
11. Chen RT, Rastogi SC, Mullen JR, Hayes SW, Cochi SL, Donlon JA, Wassilak SG. The vaccine adverse event reporting system (VAERS). Vaccine. 1994;12(6):542–50.
12. Gangarosa EJ, Galazka AM, Wolfe CR, Phillips LM, Gangarosa RE, Miller E, Chen RT. Impact of anti-vaccine movements on pertussis control: the untold story. Lancet. 1998;351(9099):356–61.
13. Stratton K, Gable A, McCormick MC. Immunization safety review: thimerosal-containing vaccines and neurodevelopmental disorders. Washington: National Academy Press; 2001.
14. Stratton K, Gable A, Shetty P, McCormick M. Immunization safety review: measles-mumps-rubella vaccine and autism. Washington: National Academy Press; 2001.
15. Stratton K, Almario D, McCormick MC. Immunization safety review: hepatitis B vaccine and demyelinating neurological disorders. Washington: National Academies Press; 2002.
16. Nohynek H, Jokinen J, Partinen M, Vaarala O, Kirjavainen T, Sundman J, Himanen SL, Hublin C, Julkunen I, Olsen P, Saarenpaa-Heikkila O, Kilpi T. AS03 adjuvanted AH1N1 vaccine associated with an abrupt increase in the incidence of childhood narcolepsy in Finland. PLoS One. 2012;7(3):e33536.
17. Aylward B, Tangermann R. The global polio eradication initiative: lessons learned and prospects for success. Vaccine. 2011;29(Suppl 4):D80–5.
18. GACVS. Global Advisory Committee on vaccine safety, 12–13 June 2013. Wkly Epidemiol Rec. 2013;88(29):301–12.
19. Chen RT, Shimabukuro TT, Martin DB, Zuber PL, Weibel DM, Sturkenboom M. Enhancing vaccine safety capacity globally: a lifecycle perspective. Am J Prev Med. 2015;49(6 Suppl 4):S364–76.
20. Salmon DA, Pavia A, Gellin B. Editors' introduction: vaccine safety throughout the product life cycle. Pediatrics. 2011;127(Suppl 1):S1–4.
21. Bonhoeffer J, Kohl K, Chen R, Duclos P, Heijbel H, Heininger U, Jefferson T, Loupi E. The Brighton collaboration: addressing the need for standardized case definitions of adverse events following immunization (AEFI). Vaccine. 2002;21(3–4):298–302.
22. LaRussa PS, Edwards KM, Dekker CL, Klein NP, Halsey NA, Marchant C, Baxter R, Engler RJ, Kissner J, Slade BA. Understanding the role of human variation in vaccine adverse events: the clinical immunization safety assessment network. Pediatrics. 2011;127(Suppl 1):S65–73.
23. McNeil MM, Gee J, Weintraub ES, Belongia EA, Lee GM, Glanz JM, Nordin JD, Klein NP, Baxter R, Naleway AL, Jackson LA, Omer SB, Jacobsen SJ, DeStefano F. The vaccine safety datalink: successes and challenges monitoring vaccine safety. Vaccine. 2014;32(42):5390–8.
24. Ball LK, Evans G, Bostrom A. Risky business: challenges in vaccine risk communication. Pediatrics. 1998;101(3 Pt 1):453–8.
25. Maure CG, Dodoo AN, Bonhoeffer J, Zuber PL. The global vaccine safety initiative: enhancing vaccine pharmacovigilance capacity at country level. Bull World Health Organ. 2014;92(9):695–6.
26. Kane MA. Global implementation of human papillomavirus (HPV) vaccine: lessons from hepatitis B vaccine. Gynecol Oncol. 2010;117(2 Suppl):S32–5.
27. Rebecca E, Chandler Madhava Ram, Balakrishnan Daniel, Brasseur Philip, Bryan Emmanuelle, Espie Katharina, Hartmann Corinne, Jouquelet-Royer James, Milligan Linda, Nesbitt Shanthi, Pal Alexander, Precioso Paulo, Takey Robert T, Chen (2024) (2024)

Collaboration within the global vaccine safety surveillance ecosystem during the COVID-19 pandemic: lessons learnt and key recommendations from the COVAX Vaccine Safety Working Group BMJ Global Health 9(3) e014544-10.1136/bmjgh-2023-014544

28. Kaddar M, Lydon P, Levine R. Financial challenges of immunization: a look at GAVI. Bull World Health Organ. 2004;82(9):697–702.
29. Izurieta HS, Zuber P, Bonhoeffer J, Chen RT, Sankohg O, Laserson KF, Sturkenboom M, Loucq C, Weibel D, Dodd C, Black S. Roadmap for the international collaborative epidemiologic monitoring of safety and effectiveness of new high priority vaccines. Vaccine. 2013;31(35):3623–7.
30. Lydon P, Levine R, Makinen M, Brenzel L, Mitchell V, Milstien JB, Kamara L, Landry S. Introducing new vaccines in the poorest countries: what did we learn from the GAVI experience with financial sustainability? Vaccine. 2008;26(51):6706–16.
31. Ouandaogo CR, Yameogo TM, Diomande FV, Sawadogo C, Ouedraogo B, Ouedraogo-Traore R, Pezzoli L, Djingarey MH, Mbakuliyemo N, Zuber PL. Adverse events following immunization during mass vaccination campaigns at first introduction of a meningococcal A conjugate vaccine in Burkina Faso, 2010. Vaccine. 2012;30(Suppl 2):B46–51.
32. Pitisuttithum P, Bouckenooghe A. The first licensed dengue vaccine: an important tool for integrated preventive strategies against dengue virus infection. Expert Rev Vaccines. 2016;15(7):795–8.
33. Tate JE, Arora R, Bhan MK, Yewale V, Parashar UD, Kang G. Rotavirus disease and vaccines in India: a tremendous public health opportunity. Vaccine. 2014;32(Suppl 1):vii–xii.
34. Hoft DF, Blazevic A, Selimovic A, Turan A, Tennant J, Abate G, Fulkerson J, Zak DE, Walker R, McClain B, Sadoff J, Scott J, Shepherd B, Ishmukhamedov J, Hokey DA, Dheenadhayalan V, Shankar S, Amon L, Navarro G, Podyminogin R, Aderem A, Barker L, Brennan M, Wallis RS, Gershon AA, Gershon MD, Steinberg S. Safety and immunogenicity of the recombinant BCG vaccine AERAS-422 in healthy BCG-naive adults: a randomized, active-controlled, first-in-human phase 1 trial. EBioMedicine. 2016;7:278–86.
35. Lopez P, Lanata CF, Zambrano B, Cortes M, Andrade T, Amemiya I, Terrones C, Gil AI, Verastegui H, Marquez V, Crevat D, Jezorwski J, Noriega F. Immunogenicity and safety of yellow fever vaccine (Stamaril) when administered concomitantly with a tetravalent dengue vaccine candidate in healthy toddlers at 12–13 months of age in Colombia and Peru: a randomized trial. Pediatr Infect Dis J. 2016;35(10):1140–7.
36. Rerks-Ngarm S, Pitisuttithum P, Nitayaphan S, Kaewkungwal J, Chiu J, Paris R, Premsri N, Namwat C, de Souza M, Adams E, Benenson M, Gurunathan S, Tartaglia J, McNeil JG, Francis DP, Stablein D, Birx DL, Chunsuttiwat S, Khamboonruang C, Thongcharoen P, Robb ML, Michael NL, Kunasol P, Kim JH. Vaccination with ALVAC and AIDSVAX to prevent HIV-1 infection in Thailand. N Engl J Med. 2009;361(23):2209–20.
37. White MT, Verity R, Griffin JT, Asante KP, Owusu-Agyei S, Greenwood B, Drakeley C, Gesase S, Lusingu J, Ansong D, Adjei S, Agbenyega T, Ogutu B, Otieno L, Otieno W, Agnandji ST, Lell B, Kremsner P, Hoffman I, Martinson F, Kamthunzu P, Tinto H, Valea I, Sorgho H, Oneko M, Otieno K, Hamel MJ, Salim N, Mtoro A, Abdulla S, Aide P, Sacarlal J, Aponte JJ, Njuguna P, Marsh K, Bejon P, Riley EM, Ghani AC. Immunogenicity of the RTS,S/AS01 malaria vaccine and implications for duration of vaccine efficacy: secondary analysis of data from a phase 3 randomised controlled trial. Lancet Infect Dis. 2015;15(12):1450–8.
38. Bollyky T, Stergachis A. Drug and vaccine safety in global health: a report to the safety and surveillance working group; 2014.
39. Tamminga C, Kavanaugh M, Fedders C, Maiolatesi S, Abraham N, Bonhoeffer J, Heininger U, Vasquez CS, Moorthy VS, Epstein JE. A systematic review of safety data reporting in clinical trials of vaccines against malaria, tuberculosis, and human immunodeficiency virus. Vaccine. 2013;31(35):3628–35.
40. Steffen C, Tokplonou E, Jaillard P, Dia R, Alladji MNDB, Gessner B. A field based evaluation of adverse events following MenAfriVac® vaccine delivered in a controlled temperature chain (CTC) approach in Benin. Pan Afr Med J. 2014;18:344.

41. Asturias EJ, Wharton M, Pless R, MacDonald NE, Chen RT, Andrews N, Salisbury D, Dodoo AN, Hartigan-Go K, Zuber PLF. Contributions and challenges for worldwide vaccine safety: The Global Advisory Committee on Vaccine Safety at 15 years. Vaccine. 2016;34:3342.
42. Olsson S, Pal SN, Dodoo A. Pharmacovigilance in resource-limited countries. Expert Rev Clin Pharmacol. 2015;8(4):449–60.
43. World Health Organization. Yellow fever vaccine safety during mass immunization campaign in sub-Saharan Africa; 2013. Retrieved 5th July, 2016, from http://www.who.int/vaccine_safety/committee/topics/yellow_fever/Jun_2013/en/.
44. Jegede AS. What led to the Nigerian boycott of the polio vaccination campaign? PLoS Med. 2007;4(3):e73.
45. Nzolo D, Aloni MN, Ngamasata TM, Luemba BM, Marfeza SB, Ekila MB, Nsibu CN, Tona NL. Adverse events following immunization with oral poliovirus in Kinshasa, Democratic Republic of Congo: preliminary results. Pathog Glob Health. 2013;107:381.
46. Chaturvedi S, Dasgupta R, Adhish V, Ganguly KK, Rai S, Sushant L, Srabasti S, Arora NK. Deconstructing social resistance to pulse polio campaign in two North Indian districts. Indian Pediatr. 2009;46(11):963–74.
47. Dodoo ANO, Renner L, van Grootheest AC, Labadie J, Antwi-Agyei KO, Hayibor S, Addison J, Pappoe V, Appiah-Danquah A. Safety monitoring of a new pentavalent vaccine in the expanded programme on immunisation in Ghana. Drug Saf. 2007;30(4):347–56.
48. Health Impact News. South Africa debates safety of HPV vaccine; 2017.
49. London School of Hygiene & Tropical Medicine. The state of vaccine confidence; 2015.
50. Salman O, Topf K, Chandler R, Conklin L. Progress in immunization safety monitoring — Worldwide, 2010–2019. MMWR Morb Mortal Wkly Rep. 2021;70:547–51.
51. Giannattasio A, Mariano M, Romano R, Chiatto F, Liguoro I, Borgia G, Guarino A, Lo Vecchio A. Sustained low influenza vaccination in health care workers after H1N1 pandemic: a cross sectional study in an Italian health care setting for at-risk patients. BMC Infect Dis. 2015;15:329.
52. WHO. Causality assessment of an adverse event following immunization (AEFI). User manual for the revised WHO classification. W. Press; 2013.
53. Joshi J, Seth A, Aneja S, Singh AK, Aggarwal MK, Gupta N. Rapid onset optic neuritis following measles vaccine in India: case report. Vaccine Rep. 2016;6:86–8.
54. Tafuri S, Gallone MS, Calabrese G, Germinario C. Adverse events following immunization: is this time for the use of WHO causality assessment? Expert Rev Vaccines. 2015;14(5):625–7.
55. Chitkara AJ, Thacker N, Vashishtha VM, Bansal CP, Gupta SG. Adverse event following immunization (AEFI) surveillance in India: position paper of Indian academy of pediatrics, 2013. Indian Pediatr. 2013;50(8):739–41.
56. Ministry of Health and Family Welfare Government of India. Adverse events following immunization surveillance and response operations guidelines guidelines; 2015.
57. Tozzi AE, Asturias EJ, Balakrishnan MR, Halsey NA, Law B, Zuber PL. Assessment of causality of individual adverse events following immunization (AEFI): a WHO tool for global use. Vaccine. 2013;31(44):5041–6.
58. Singh AK, Wagner AL, Joshi J, Carlson BF, Aneja S, Boulton ML. Application of the revised WHO causality assessment protocol for adverse events following immunization in India. Vaccine. 2017;35(33):4197–202.
59. Government of India Ministry of Health and Family Welfare. 2017. Press release from the Press Information Bureau dated 17 Feb 2017, from http://www.searo.who.int/india/mediacentre/events/2017/press_release_nra_who_assessment.pdf?ua=1. Accessed 22 Oct 2017.
60. Peretti-Watel P, Larson HJ, Ward JK, Schulz WS, Verger P. Vaccine hesitancy: clarifying a theoretical framework for an ambiguous notion. PLoS Curr. 2015;7. https://doi.org/10.1371/currents.outbreaks.6844c80ff9f5b273f34c91f71b7fc289.
61. Belgharbi L, Dellepiane N, Wood DJ. Regulation of vaccines in developing countries. In: Plotkin SA, Orenstein WA, Offit PA, editors. Vaccines. Elsevier; 2013. p. 1454–63.
62. WHO. Global vaccine safety blueprint; 2012.
63. WHO. Vaccines against influenza and pertussis WHO position papers; 2012.

64. Strategic Advisory Group of Experts on Immunization (SAGE). Global vaccine action plan; 2017.
65. Guo B, Page A, Wang H, Taylor R, McIntyre P. Systematic review of reporting rates of adverse events following immunization: an international comparison of post-marketing surveillance programs with reference to China. Vaccine. 2013;31(4):603–17.
66. Diomande FV, Yameogo TM, Vannice KS, Preziosi MP, Viviani S, Ouandaogo CR, Keita M, Djingarey MH, Mbakuliyemo N, Akanmori BD, Sow SO, Zuber PL. Lessons learned from enhancing vaccine pharmacovigilance activities during PsA-TT introduction in African countries, 2010–2013. Clin Infect Dis. 2015;61(Suppl 5):S459–66.
67. Vannice KS, Keita M, Sow SO, Durbin AP, Omer SB, Moulton LH, Yameogo TM, Zuber PL, Onwuchekwa U, Sacko M, Diomande FV, Halsey NA. Active surveillance for adverse events after a mass vaccination campaign with a group a meningococcal conjugate vaccine (PsA-TT) in Mali. Clin Infect Dis. 2015;61(Suppl 5):S493–500.
68. Wak G, Williams J, Oduro A, Maure C, Zuber PL, Black S. The safety of PsA-TT in pregnancy: an assessment performed within the Navrongo Health and Demographic Surveillance Site in Ghana. Clin Infect Dis. 2015;61(Suppl 5):S489–92.
69. Patel MM, Lopez-Collada VR, Bulhoes MM, De Oliveira LH, Bautista Marquez A, Flannery B, Esparza-Aguilar M, Montenegro Renoiner EI, Luna-Cruz ME, Sato HK, Hernandez-Hernandez Ldel C, Toledo-Cortina G, Ceron-Rodriguez M, Osnaya-Romero N, Martinez-Alcazar M, Aguinaga-Villasenor RG, Plascencia-Hernandez A, Fojaco-Gonzalez F, Hernandez-Peredo Rezk G, Gutierrez-Ramirez SF, Dorame-Castillo R, Tinajero-Pizano R, Mercado-Villegas B, Barbosa MR, Maluf EM, Ferreira LB, de Carvalho FM, dos Santos AR, Cesar ED, de Oliveira ME, Silva CL, de Los Angeles M, Cortes CR, Matus J, Tate PG, Parashar UD. Intussusception risk and health benefits of rotavirus vaccination in Mexico and Brazil. N Engl J Med. 2011;364(24):2283–92.
70. Dodd CN, Romio SA, Black S, Vellozzi C, Andrews N, Sturkenboom M, Zuber P, Hua W, Bonhoeffer J, Buttery J, Crawford N, Deceuninck G, de Vries C, De Wals P, Garman P, Gimeno MV, Heijbel H, Hur K, Hviid A, Kelman J, Kilpi T, Chuang SK, Macartney K, Rett M, Lopez-Callada VR, Salmon D, Sanchez FG, Sanz N, Silverman B, Storsaeter J, Thirugnanam U, van der Maas N, Yih K, Zhang T, Izurieta H. International collaboration to assess the risk of Guillain Barre Syndrome following Influenza (H1N1) 2009 monovalent vaccines. Vaccine. 2013;31:4448.
71. Dodd CN, Romio SA, Black S, Vellozzi C, Andrews N, Sturkenboom M, Zuber P, Hua W, Bonhoeffer J, Buttery J, Crawford N, Deceuninck G, de Vries C, De Wals P, Gutierrez-Gimeno MV, Heijbel H, Hughes H, Hur K, Hviid A, Kelman J, Kilpi T, Chuang SK, Macartney K, Rett M, Lopez-Callada VR, Salmon D, Gimenez-Sanchez F, Sanz N, Silverman B, Storsaeter J, Thirugnanam U, van der Maas N, Yih K, Zhang T, Izurieta H, H. N. G. B. S. C. Global. International collaboration to assess the risk of Guillain Barre Syndrome following Influenza A (H1N1) 2009 monovalent vaccines. Vaccine. 2013;31(40):4448–58.
72. GACVS. Wkly Epid Rec, 15–16 June. 2016;91:341–348.
73. Amarasinghe A, Black S, Bonhoeffer J, Carvalho SMD, Dodoo A, Eskola J, Larson H, Shin S, Olsson S, Balakrishnan MR, Bellah A, Lambach P, Maure C, Wood D, Zuber P, Akanmori B, Bravo P, Pombo M, Langar H, Pfeifer D, Guichard S, Diorditsa S, Hossain MS, Sato Y. Effective vaccine safety systems in all countries: a challenge for more equitable access to immunization. Vaccine. 2013;31(Supplement 2(0)):B108–14.
74. Velazquez FR, Colindres RE, Grajales C, Hernandez MT, Mercadillo MG, Torres FJ, Cervantes-Apolinar M, DeAntonio-Suarez R, Ortega-Barria E, Blum M, Breuer T, Verstraeten T. Postmarketing surveillance of intussusception following mass introduction of the attenuated human rotavirus vaccine in Mexico. Pediatr Infect Dis J. 2012;31(7):736–44.
75. Kristiansen PA, Diomande F, Ba AK, Sanou I, Ouedraogo AS, Ouedraogo R, Sangare L, Kandolo D, Ake F, Saga IM, Clark TA, Misegades L, Martin SW, Thomas JD, Tiendrebeogo SR, Hassan-King M, Djingarey MH, Messonnier NE, Preziosi MP, Laforce FM, Caugant

DA. Impact of the serogroup A meningococcal conjugate vaccine, MenAfriVac, on carriage and herd immunity. Clin Infect Dis. 2013;56(3):354–63.

76. Agnandji ST, Lell B, Fernandes JF, Abossolo BP, Methogo BG, Kabwende AL, Adegnika AA, Mordmuller B, Issifou S, Kremsner PG, Sacarlal J, Aide P, Lanaspa M, Aponte JJ, Machevo S, Acacio S, Bulo H, Sigauque B, Macete E, Alonso P, Abdulla S, Salim N, Minja R, Mpina M, Ahmed S, Ali AM, Mtoro AT, Hamad AS, Mutani P, Tanner M, Tinto H, D'Alessandro U, Sorgho H, Valea I, Bihoun B, Guiraud I, Kabore B, Sombie O, Guiguemde RT, Ouedraogo JB, Hamel MJ, Kariuki S, Oneko M, Odero C, Otieno K, Awino N, McMorrow M, Muturi-Kioi V, Laserson KF, Slutsker L, Otieno W, Otieno L, Otsyula N, Gondi S, Otieno A, Owira V, Oguk E, Odongo G, Woods JB, Ogutu B, Njuguna P, Chilengi R, Akoo P, Kerubo C, Maingi C, Lang T, Olotu A, Bejon P, Marsh K, Mwambingu G, Owusu-Agyei S, Asante KP, Osei-Kwakye K, Boahen O, Dosoo D, Asante I, Adjei G, Kwara E, Chandramohan D, Greenwood B, Lusingu J, Gesase S, Malabeja A, Abdul O, Mahende C, Liheluka E, Malle L, Lemnge M, Theander TG, Drakeley C, Ansong D, Agbenyega T, Adjei S, Boateng HO, Rettig T, Bawa J, Sylverken J, Sambian D, Sarfo A, Agyekum A, Martinson F, Hoffman I, Mvalo T, Kamthunzi P, Nkomo R, Tembo T, Tegha G, Tsidya M, Kilembe J, Chawinga C, Ballou WR, Cohen J, Guerra Y, Jongert E, Lapierre D, Leach A, Lievens M, Ofori-Anyinam O, Olivier A, Vekemans J, Carter T, Kaslow D, Leboulleux D, Loucq C, Radford A, Savarese B, Schellenberg D, Sillman M, Vansadia P. A phase 3 trial of RTS,S/AS01 malaria vaccine in African infants. N Engl J Med. 2012;367(24):2284–95.

77. Mahalanabis D, Lopez AL, Sur D, Deen J, Manna B, Kanungo S, von Seidlein L, Carbis R, Han SH, Shin SH, Attridge S, Rao R, Holmgren J, Clemens J, Bhattacharya SK. A randomized, placebo-controlled trial of the bivalent killed, whole-cell, oral cholera vaccine in adults and children in a cholera endemic area in Kolkata, India. PLoS One. 2008;3(6):e2323.

78. Monath TP. Dengue: the risk to developed and developing countries. Proc Natl Acad Sci USA. 1994;91(7):2395–400.

79. Siegrist CA, Lewis EM, Eskola J, Evans SJ, Black SB. Human papilloma virus immunization in adolescent and young adults: a cohort study to illustrate what events might be mistaken for adverse reactions. Pediatr Infect Dis J. 2007;26(11):979–84.

80. Black S, Eskola J, Siegrist CA, Halsey N, Macdonald N, Law B, Miller E, Andrews N, Stowe J, Salmon D, Vannice K, Izurieta HS, Akhtar A, Gold M, Oselka G, Zuber P, Pfeifer D, Vellozzi C. Importance of background rates of disease in assessment of vaccine safety during mass immunisation with pandemic H1N1 influenza vaccines. Lancet. 2009;374(9707):2115–22.

81. Sankoh O, Byass P. The INDEPTH network: filling vital gaps in global epidemiology. Int J Epidemiol. 2012;41(3):579–88.

82. Izurieta HS, Moro PL, Chen RT. Hospital-based collaboration for epidemiological investigation of vaccine safety: a potential solution for low and middle-income countries? Vaccine. 2018;36(3):345–6.

83. Perez-Vilar S, Weibel D, Sturkenboom M, Black S, Maure C, Castro JL, Bravo-Alcantara P, Dodd CN, Romio SA, de Ridder M, Nakato S, Molina-Leon HF, Elango V, Zuber PLF. Enhancing global vaccine pharmacovigilance: proof-of-concept study on aseptic meningitis and immune thrombocytopenic purpura following measles-mumps containing vaccination. Vaccine. 2018;36(3):363–70.

84. Bravo-Alcántara P, Pérez-Vilar S, Molina-León HF, Sturkenboom M, Black S, Zuber P, Maure C, Castro JL, L. A. N. F. V. Pharmacovigilance. Building capacity for active surveillance of vaccine adverse events in the Americas: a hospital-based multi-country network. Vaccine. 2018;36(3):363–70.

85. Guillard-Maure C, Elango V, Black S, Perez-Vilar S, Castro JL, Bravo-Alcantara P, Molina-Leon HF, Weibel D, Sturkenboom M, Zuber PLF, W. H. O. G. V. S.-M. C. Collaboration. Operational lessons learned in conducting a multi-country collaboration for vaccine safety signal verification and hypothesis testing: the global vaccine safety multi country collaboration initiative. Vaccine. 2018;36(3):355–62.

86. Hua W, Sun G, Dodd CN, Romio SA, Whitaker HJ, Izurieta HS, Black S, Sturkenboom MC, Davis RL, Deceuninck G, Andrews NJ. A simulation study to compare three self-controlled case series approaches: correction for violation of assumption and evaluation of bias. Pharmacoepidemiol Drug Saf. 2013;22(8):819–25.

87. Weldeselassie YG, Whitaker HJ, Farrington CP. Use of the self-controlled case-series method in vaccine safety studies: review and recommendations for best practice. Epidemiol Infect. 2011;139(12):1805–17.

88. Whitaker HJ, Farrington CP, Spiessens B, Musonda P. Tutorial in biostatistics: the self-controlled case series method. Stat Med. 2006;25(10):1768–97.

89. Maclure M, Fireman B, Nelson JC, Hua W, Shoaibi A, Paredes A, Madigan D. When should case-only designs be used for safety monitoring of medical products? Pharmacoepidemiol Drug Saf. 2012;21(Suppl 1):50–61.

90. Schneeweiss S, Sturmer T, Maclure M. Case-crossover and case-time-control designs as alternatives in pharmacoepidemiologic research. Pharmacoepidemiol Drug Saf. 1997;6(Suppl 3):S51–9.

91. De Serres G, Skowronski DM, Wu XW, Ambrose CS. The test-negative design: validity, accuracy and precision of vaccine efficacy estimates compared to the gold standard of randomised placebo-controlled clinical trials. Euro Surveill. 2013;18(37):20585.

92. Graham JE, Borda-Rodriguez A, Huzair F, Zinck E. Capacity for a global vaccine safety system: the perspective of national regulatory authorities. Vaccine. 2012;30:4953.

93. INDEPTH N. Population and health in developing countries: population, health, and survival at indepth sites; 2000.

94. Odhiambo FO, Laserson KF, Sewe M, Hamel MJ, Feikin DR, Adazu K, Ogwang S, Obor D, Amek N, Bayoh N, Ombok M, Lindblade K, Desai M, ter Kuile F, Phillips-Howard P, van Eijk AM, Rosen D, Hightower A, Ofware P, Muttai H, Nahlen B, DeCock K, Slutsker L, Breiman RF, Vulule JM. Profile: the KEMRI/CDC health and demographic surveillance system—Western Kenya. Int J Epidemiol. 2012;41(4):977–87.

95. Sacoor C, Nhacolo A, Nhalungo D, Aponte JJ, Bassat Q, Augusto O, Mandomando I, Sacarlal J, Lauchande N, Sigauque B, Alonso P, Macete E, Munguambe K, Guinovart C, Aide P, Menendez C, Acacio S, Quelhas D, Sevene E, Nhampossa T. Profile: Manhica Health Research Centre (Manhica HDSS). Int J Epidemiol. 2013;42(5):1309–18.

96. Harmark L, van Grootheest AC. Pharmacovigilance: methods, recent developments and future perspectives. Eur J Clin Pharmacol. 2008;64(8):743–52.

97. Noren GN, Edwards IR. Modern methods of pharmacovigilance: detecting adverse effects of drugs. Clin Med (Lond). 2009;9(5):486–9.

98. Greenland S. A unified approach to the analysis of case-distribution (case-only) studies. Stat Med. 1999;18(1):1–15.

99. Lu CY. Observational studies: a review of study designs, challenges and strategies to reduce confounding. Int J Clin Pract. 2009;63(5):691–7.

100. GAVI. GAVI alliance annual progress report 2013; 2013.

101. IANS. Infant deaths doubled after getting pentavalent vaccine than DPT: study. Business Standard; 2018.

102. Puliyel J, Kaur J, Puliyel A, Visnubhatla S. Deaths reported after pentavalent vaccine compared with death reported after diphtheria-tetanus-pertussis vaccine: an exploratory analysis. Med J DY Patil Vidyapeeth. 2018;11:99–105.

103. Puliyel J, Phadke A. Deaths following pentavalent vaccine and the revised AEFI classification. Indian J Med Ethics. 2017;2(4):300.

104. Service EN. More children died after getting pentavalent vaccine than DPT, says study. The New Indian Express. 4th Nov 2018.

105. Platt R, Carnahan RM, Brown JS, Chrischilles E, Curtis LH, Hennessy S, Nelson JC, Racoosin JA, Robb M, Schneeweiss S, Toh S, Weiner MG. The U.S. Food and Drug Administration's Mini-Sentinel program: status and direction. Pharmacoepidemiol Drug Saf. 2012;21(Suppl 1):1–8.

106. Rothman KJ. Modern epidemiology. Philadelphia: Wolters Kluwer Health/Lippincott Williams & Wilkins; 2008.
107. Baxter R, Lee J, Fireman B. Evidence of bias in studies of influenza vaccine effectiveness in elderly patients. J Infect Dis. 2010;201(2):186–9.
108. Fireman B, Lee J, Lewis N, Bembom O, van der Laan M, Baxter R. Influenza vaccination and mortality: differentiating vaccine effects from bias. Am J Epidemiol. 2009;170(5):650–6.
109. Jackson LA, Jackson ML, Nelson JC, Neuzil KM, Weiss NS. Evidence of bias in estimates of influenza vaccine effectiveness in seniors. Int J Epidemiol. 2006;35(2):337–44.
110. Baker MA, Lieu TA, Li L, Hua W, Qiang Y, Kawai AT, Fireman BH, Martin DB, Nguyen MD. A vaccine study design selection framework for the postlicensure rapid immunization safety monitoring program. Am J Epidemiol. 2015;181(8):608–18.
111. Chen RT, Glanz JM, Vellozzi C. Pharmacoepidemiologic studies of vaccine safety. In: Pharmacoepidemiology. Wiley-Blackwell; 2012.
112. Agnandji ST, Lell B, Soulanoudjingar SS, Fernandes JF, Abossolo BP, Conzelmann C, Methogo BG, Doucka Y, Flamen A, Mordmuller B, Issifou S, Kremsner PG, Sacarlal J, Aide P, Lanaspa M, Aponte JJ, Nhamuave A, Quelhas D, Bassat Q, Mandjate S, Macete E, Alonso P, Abdulla S, Salim N, Juma O, Shomari M, Shubis K, Machera F, Hamad AS, Minja R, Mtoro A, Sykes A, Ahmed S, Urassa AM, Ali AM, Mwangoka G, Tanner M, Tinto H, D'Alessandro U, Sorgho H, Valea I, Tahita MC, Kabore W, Ouedraogo S, Sandrine Y, Guiguemde RT, Ouedraogo JB, Hamel MJ, Kariuki S, Odero C, Oneko M, Otieno K, Awino N, Omoto J, Williamson J, Muturi-Kioi V, Laserson KF, Slutsker L, Otieno W, Otieno L, Nekoye O, Gondi S, Otieno A, Ogutu B, Wasuna R, Owira V, Jones D, Onyango AA, Njuguna P, Chilengi R, Akoo P, Kerubo C, Gitaka J, Maingi C, Lang T, Olotu A, Tsofa B, Bejon P, Peshu N, Marsh K, Owusu-Agyei S, Asante KP, Osei-Kwakye K, Boahen O, Ayamba S, Kayan K, Owusu-Ofori R, Dosoo D, Asante I, Adjei G, Chandramohan D, Greenwood B, Lusingu J, Gesase S, Malabeja A, Abdul O, Kilavo H, Mahende C, Liheluka E, Lemnge M, Theander T, Drakeley C, Ansong D, Agbenyega T, Adjei S, Boateng HO, Rettig T, Bawa J, Sylverken J, Sambian D, Agyekum A, Owusu L, Martinson F, Hoffman I, Mvalo T, Kamthunzi P, Nkomo R, Msika A, Jumbe A, Chome N, Nyakuipa D, Chintedza J, Ballou WR, Bruls M, Cohen J, Guerra Y, Jongert E, Lapierre D, Leach A, Lievens M, Ofori-Anyinam O, Vekemans J, Carter T, Leboulleux D, Loucq C, Radford A, Savarese B, Schellenberg D, Sillman M, Vansadia P. First results of phase 3 trial of RTS,S/AS01 malaria vaccine in African children. N Engl J Med. 2011;365(20):1863–75.
113. RTS, S Clinical Trials Partnership. Efficacy and safety of the RTS,S/AS01 malaria vaccine during 18 months after vaccination: a phase 3 randomized, controlled trial in children and young infants at 11 African sites. PLoS Med. 2014;11(7):e1001685.
114. Rts SCTP. Efficacy and safety of RTS,S/AS01 malaria vaccine with or without a booster dose in infants and children in Africa: final results of a phase 3, individually randomised, controlled trial. Lancet. 2015;386(9988):31–45.
115. Kochhar S, Bonhoeffer J, Jones CE, Munoz FM, Honrado A, Bauwens J, Sobanjo-Ter Meulen A, Hirschfeld S. Immunization in pregnancy clinical research in low- and middle-income countries – study design, regulatory and safety considerations. Vaccine. 2017;35:6575.
116. Swamy GK, Heine RP. Vaccinations for pregnant women. Obstet Gynecol. 2015;125(1):212–26.
117. Beigi RH, Fortner KB, Munoz FM, Roberts J, Gordon JL, Han HH, Glenn G, Dormitzer PR, Gu XX, Read JS, Edwards K, Patel SM, Swamy GK. Maternal immunization: opportunities for scientific advancement. Clin Infect Dis. 2014;59(Suppl 7):S408–14.
118. GACVS. Safety of immunization during pregnancy- a review of the evidence; 2014.
119. Kochhar S, Bauwens J, Bonhoeffer J; GAIA Project Participants. Electronic address: http://www.gaia-consortium.net/. Safety assessment of immunization in pregnancy. Vaccine. 2017 Dec 4;35(48 Pt A):6469-6471. doi: 10.1016/j.vaccine.2017.09.033. Epub 2017 Oct 12. PMID: 29031696; PMCID: PMC5714434.

120. Bonhoeffer J, Kochhar S, Hirschfeld S, Heath PT, Jones CE, Bauwens J, Honrado A, Heininger U, Munoz FM, Eckert L, Steinhoff M, Black S, Padula M, Sturkenboom M, Buttery J, Pless R, Zuber P. Global alignment of immunization safety assessment in pregnancy–the GAIA project. Vaccine. 2016;34:5993.
121. Kochhar S, Okomo U, Nkereuwem O, Shaum A, Gidudu JF, Bittaye M, Fofana S, Marena M, Kaira MJ, Kampmann B, Longley AT (2023) Establishing vaccine pregnancy registries and active surveillance studies in low-and middle-income countries: Experience from an observational cohort surveillance project in The Gambia Vaccine 41(44) 6453-6455 10.1016/j.vaccine.2023.09.038
122. Kochhar S, Edwards KM, Ropero Alvarez AM, Moro PL, Ortiz JR. Introduction of New Vaccines for Immunization in Pregnancy- Programmatic, Regulatory and Safety Considerations. Vaccine 2019, 37:25, 3267-3277. https://doi.org/10.1016/j.vaccine.2019.04.075
123. Kochhar S, Excler JL, Bok K, Gurwith M, McNeil MM, Seligman SJ, Khuri-Bulos N, Klug B, Laderoute M, Robertson JS, Singh V, Chen RT; Brighton Collaboration Viral Vector Vaccines Safety Working Group (V3SWG). Defining the interval for monitoring potential adverse events following immunization (AEFIs) after receipt of live viral vectored vaccines. Vaccine. 2019 Sep 10;37(38):5796-5802. doi: 10.1016/j.vaccine.2018.08.085. Epub 2018 Nov 26. PMID: 30497831; PMCID: PMC6535369.
124. Kharbanda EO, Haapala J, Lipkind HS, DeSilva MB, Zhu J, Vesco KK, Daley MF, Donahue JG, Getahun D, Hambidge SJ, Irving SA, Klein NP, Nelson JC, Weintraub ES, Williams JTB, Vazquez-Benitez G. COVID-19 Booster Vaccination in Early Pregnancy and Surveillance for Spontaneous Abortion. JAMA Netw Open. 2023 May 1;6(5):e2314350. https://doi.org/10.1001/jamanetworkopen.2023.14350. PMID: 37204791; PMCID: PMC10199343.
125. WHO. Revised guidance on the choice of pertussis vaccines. World Health Organization. Weekly Epidemiologic Record 2014;89(30).
126. Isah AO, Pal SN, Olsson S, Dodoo A, Bencheikh RS. Specific features of medicines safety and pharmacovigilance in Africa. Ther Adv Drug Saf. 2012;3(1):25–34.
127. US CDC. 2016–2010 CDC's strategic framework for global immunization framework; 2016.
128. WHO. GAVI annual report 2013–2014; 2015.
129. Kaufmann JR, Miller R, Cheyne J. Vaccine supply chains need to be better funded and strengthened, or lives will be at risk. Health Aff (Millwood). 2011;30(6):1113–21.
130. Shen AK, Fields R, McQuestion M. The future of routine immunization in the developing world: challenges and opportunities. Glob Health Sci Pract. 2014;2(4):381–94.
131. Li X, Wiesen E, Diorditsa S, Toda K, Duong TH, Nguyen LH, Nguyen VC, Nguyen TH. Impact of adverse events following immunization in Viet Nam in 2013 on chronic hepatitis B infection. Vaccine. 2016;34(6):869–73.

Chapter 15
Risk Perception and Communication in the Developing World

Bruce Hugman

15.1 Introduction

Few generalizations can be made about how any individual or community will perceive risk,[1] and very few reliable guidelines can be offered from a distance about exactly how to communicate risk to any particular audience in any specific situation. What we can say with certainty is that everyone views all kinds of risk in varying and inconsistent ways that are unique to them in their social and cultural context; though we can list the multiple variables, including cognition, emotion, socioeconomic status, and culture, we cannot be sure which ones will exercise the greatest power at any one moment or in any one circumstance, though affect (emotion) is

---

[1] In this chapter, 'risk' is understood to be: the possibility (chance, odds) of something bad happening or something good not happening. It is customarily conflated with the word 'hazard'. There is a risk of injury or death when riding a motorcycle, a risk that increases substantially for riders not wearing a crash-helmet; while TB can be successfully treated, the risks of untreated TB are serious, and there is a risk of medication not working if patients do not adhere strictly to their regimen or if they are suffering from a multi-resistant strain. The risks of life range from small, domestic hazards (e.g. a burn from hot cooking oil) to radical global hazards (e.g. pandemics, war or climate change). Risk as a phenomenon is universal, unavoidable and cannot easily be categorised; its management by individuals or communities is complex. See also 'Risk,' page 12.

In the preparation of this chapter, a number of colleagues and friends round the world contributed their wisdom and insight on the issues. Their specific input is indicated by the mention of their country in the text rather than by a formal reference. Their names and countries appear in the acknowledgements at the end of the chapter.

B. Hugman (✉)
Independent Communications Specialist; formerly consultant to Uppsala Monitoring Centre, Oxford, UK
e-mail: brucehugman@hotmail.com; bruce3594@gmail.com

S. R. Ahmad (ed.), *Special Issues in Pharmacovigilance in Resource-Limited Countries*, https://doi.org/10.1007/978-981-96-6154-1_15

a strong influence in almost all spontaneous reactions to risk. We also know that communications about risk that have any chance of reaching anyone must be tailored precisely to their individuality, their state of mind and emotions and their readiness; that information and statistics may play a small, if any, part in how people assess risk and in the decisions they make.

Perception[2] of risk may have little relationship to the statistical reality of risk: people dread some risks that are very rare, for example, while taking for granted common, everyday, sometimes serious risks. If you ask even two friends what they regard as the greatest risks in their lives or the most serious threats to their safety, or what they think are the most effective methods of communicating safety information, they are likely to come up with very different ideas; if you put the same questions to people from diverse countries around the world, the differences and variations will be huge. There will also be great differences in the methods that will successfully influence individuals or communities in different places to change their behaviour, attitudes or values.

It is rather obvious that, if your daily life exposes you to the risk of disease, starvation, abduction, abuse of one kind or another or death, your hierarchy of risk looks very different from that of someone living in a stable, prosperous and safe environment.[3] This is true for governments as well as citizens. For hundreds of millions of people in the developing world, daily risks belong to the former, radical survival category, excluding most of the comparatively smaller daily preoccupations of the developed world.[4] Nevertheless, for those facing less palpable danger in richer societies, important, major or relatively subtle risks, such as road deaths, chronic diseases or harm from medicines, may be ignored or invisible and not given the prominence they deserve. Even very large numbers of repeated dispersed deaths (road accidents, smoking, cardio-vascular disease, adverse drug reactions) fail to grab public attention when there are other infrequent events which involve multiple

---

[2] Some psychologists use 'perception' to refer to direct physiological responses to stimuli, and 'judgement' for the processing of those and associated cognitive and emotional elements. In this chapter, 'perception' is used to encompass both kinds of response and the effects shown in opinion and behaviour.

[3] This is poignantly illustrated by a story from a British citizen who gave house-room to a Syrian refugee: 'One day I got in a tizz about how to fit a new curtain rail in my bay window. "In my country, people worry about whether a barrel bomb will hit their house. In England, you are worried about your curtains," Yasser said, laughing at his own joke. "We all have our problems".' Pidd H. 'Would he disapprove of my single heathen lifestyle?': me and my Syrian refugee lodger. Guardian. 9 Jan 2016. http://www.theguardian.com/world/2016/jan/09/my-syrian-refugee-lodger-helen-pidd. Accessed 15 July 2020.

[4] The frequency and seriousness of risks in the developed world are changing: extreme weather events (and, recently, wildfires) and terrorist acts, for example, are bringing new hazards and causes for anxiety. While terrorist acts are extremely rare and the numbers of dead and injured they cause are comparatively very low, terrorism is perceived as a particularly dreadful and destabilising threat. That threat is far greater in the developing world and those at risk far more numerous.

simultaneous deaths (mass shootings, ferry or aeroplane disasters, industrial accidents, epidemics).

A colleague from Bhutan reports that the risks perceived as most serious in that country are natural disasters (earthquake and flood), loss of crops and animals, and accidents on poor roads. In Uganda and Ethiopia, there is anxiety about violent crime, robbery, car jacking; in Georgia about peace, unemployment, poverty, crime and hunger; in Nigeria food poisoning, toxic chemicals, HIV, other STDs and epidemics; in Sierre Leone, not surprisingly, Ebola remains a major social anxiety.

Swedish anthropologist Åsa Boholm [1] quotes Rappaport [2] in characterizing the complexity of understanding risk perception: 'Comparative cross-national and cross-cultural risk perceptions studies need to address questions about how risk is embedded in the social fabric and take into account 'conceptions of morality, equity, justice and honour; religious doctrine; ideas concerning sovereignty; property and rights and duties; and aesthetic values and what constitutes quality in life' (p. 51). Much of this chapter will be concerned with these issues and their implications for practice.

Reflection The perception that there are threats to safety and health is universal; but risk perception is as complex as people themselves, infinitely variable and unique in its manifestation in individuals and communities.

Pharmacovigilance
In this chapter, we use the term 'pharmacovigilance' in its widest, modern sense: a concern with the safety of patients and citizens in relation to the use of vaccines, allopathic and traditional medicines, devices and other interventions, and in particular, with identifying any kind of adverse effects or associated problems. This goes well beyond the founding task of reporting and analysing adverse drug reactions (ADRs). It extends to study of the multiple ways in which patients may be harmed by medicines and medical treatment, including intrinsic pharmaceutical ingredients and quality, errors of all kinds (e.g. misdiagnosis, prescribing and dispensing mistakes), patient behaviour and the use and impact of communication. It embraces public health programmes as well as individual therapy. The collection of data about safety must lead to action and communication that reduces risk, leads to good decisions and enhances individual and community health. Positive results are achieved only through successfully influencing politicians, regulators, health workers, patients and the public at large through effective communication. That can come about only through the most intimate knowledge of target audiences, their perceptions, preferences, cultural context and a host of other variables. This is the primary focus of the first part of this chapter; in the second part, it moves on to consideration of risk communication principles and methods.

15.2   Hoping for the Best

A common feature of human psychology everywhere is what is known as the 'optimism bias' [3]: this is the self-serving belief that one is at less risk than others, with the expectation of less risk for oneself and more risk for others. 'It won't happen to me', relates to a persistent tendency to overestimate the chance of positive outcomes and underestimate negative ones in many (maybe all) aspects of life. This is echoed by the amusing and statistically implausible fact that most drivers of motor vehicles assess themselves as better than average, often much better [4]. Some smokers and criminals display this tendency, believing that they will not be caught, respectively, by cancer or the arm of the law. The Dunning-Kruger effect [5] refers to those with low cognitive abilities or competence whose lack of *metacognition* (reflective self-awareness and analysis) gives them a sense of illusory superiority over others irrespective of the evidence of the real world.[5] (This widespread psychologically buoyant approach to life, however, will not show up in the feelings of those who are vulnerable, anxious or depressed and some other groups, who might be characterized as having a pessimistic bias; they are more likely to be cautious and risk-averse with a tendency to expect the worst. There is a gender difference too, with men tending to overestimate their competence and women more likely to underestimate theirs [6].)

National average levels of optimism bias and self-positivity seem to differ from country to country.[6] These, in turn, have their differential effects on individuals within particular cultures. There is evidence that people feel different levels of optimism about the immediate locality, their nation and the world as a whole [7]. One study from 2003 [8] suggested that Chinese were more pessimistic than their American peers. That may have changed in the last decade or so, but the point at issue is that

---

[5] The reverse effect is that competent people assume that tasks that are simple for them are also simple for everyone else; in Dunning and Kruger's words: 'the miscalibration of the incompetent stems from an error about the self, whereas the miscalibration of the highly competent stems from an error about others'. The miscalibration of the highly competent has immense implications for the practice of risk communication (and, indeed, for politics and many other major aspects of national life).

[6] The World Economic Forum has published a fascinating review of the accuracy of national populations' perception of the world in relation to the data (murder, teenage pregnancies, terror attacks, wealth, health and much more), based on Ipsos MORI's 2017 'Perils of Perception' survey. All countries have a tendency to believe things are worse than they are, with South Africa the most pessimistic and Scandinavian countries the least. The survey also tests many other aspects of perceptual accuracy. An understanding of national norms in relation to perception of the world is an essential component of communication that has any chance of being seen as credible; while there will be much secondary variation, there will also be a prevailing ethos. World Economic Forum article at: McKenna J. Most people around the world are overly pessimistic. World Economic Forum. 14 Dec 2017. https://www.weforum.org/agenda/2017/12/you're-probably-too-pessimistic/. Accessed 15 July 2020. Slides of the Ipsos MORI survey at: Ipsos. The Slides. http://perils.ipsos.com/slides/. Accessed 15 July 2020.

social values and elements of context matter, can be investigated, and need to be a part of any review of risk perception in any given society and must be factored into risk communication. Those who feel that everything will work out well are likely to take more risks and are less likely to pay attention to cautionary risk communications and to plan fewer measures to manage risk. (Degree of optimism varies not only across the world, but within countries, according to the object of consideration: for example, when considering family, hometown, region, nation or the world [9].)

The optimism bias is one element in the risk-taking behaviour of young people who, almost universally, especially young men, in almost all cultures, are likely to be further along the scale of recklessness than their elders or females of any age [10]. Such recklessness is associated with an innate feeling of invulnerability that is not always compromised even when things go badly wrong. This is just one indicator of the great challenge of risk communication: this characteristic alone will almost certainly make people deaf to evidence of danger or to even passionate pleas for changed behaviour. In most countries of the world, reckless driving is a major social problem, even where the annual toll of injuries and deaths [11] outruns the fatalities from some major illnesses and certainly those from domestic terrorist attacks. Only in countries like Sweden, where traffic law is (some might say) draconian, where enforcement is frequent and strict, and penalties are painful and inconvenient, do we see a major element of social behaviour being dramatically modified. In those countries where there has been strict enforcement of seat-belt and motorcycle helmet laws, behaviour has also changed almost universally, risk reduced and lives saved.

In countries where there are laws but lax enforcement, and where police are amenable to the influence of a few bank notes being slipped to them, behaviour does not change and, neither, of course, does perception of risk change: the perceived risk is being caught without a helmet and the financial penalty of evading arrest, not of dying from head-injuries. The evidence of this blindness to serious risk is provided by the multitudes of motorcycle drivers who place a helmet on their heads but do not secure the chin-strap: they are alert to the need to placate police and so manage that risk but are seemingly unaware that an unsecured or loosely secured helmet may offer no protection at all in an accident or even increase the risk of serious injury. (Wearing cycle helmets, on the other hand, probably does not unequivocally save lives [12] and there is some evidence to suggest that cyclists wearing helmets may be at greater risk of injury than those who aren't [13]. The risks to cyclists are more to do with road conditions and the behaviour of vehicle drivers. This is a fine example of the way in which so-called 'common sense' can lead to error or misdirection, in spite of evidence.)

15.3 Perverse Perceptions

There is a paradoxical effect of enforcing safety measures: being safely strapped into their cars, drivers will feel safer (which, in respect of impact injuries and death, indeed they are) but may, as a consequence, take greater risks in other aspects of driving like speeding, texting or playing with their GPS. A smoker's habit may be reinforced by a symptomless chest X-ray. A clean bill of health in HIV or STD tests may prompt in a promiscuous individual a feeling of invulnerability to sexual infection: 'It hasn't happened to me and it won't'. There is some evidence that the success of antiretroviral treatments for HIV leads infected patients and others to take greater risks in their sexual behaviour [14].

The decline of one kind of risk and the rise of a consequential one is a common phenomenon. Perhaps one of the most significant and alarming is the aftermath of the astonishing decline in the global impact of infectious diseases during the era of vaccines and antimicrobials: first, the rise of anti-vaccine movements; second, the abuse and over-use of antibiotics and the rise in untreatable resistance. In many countries, hardly a patient leaves a clinic or hospital without antibiotics almost irrespective of their primary symptoms [15]. Antibiotics, easily available from hawkers and street-sellers in many places and from poorly regulated pharmacies, are the drugs of choice for many with symptoms of any illness at all. We have been slow to perceive the risk and react to it and are now faced with the almost impossible task across the world of reversing the assumptions and habits of decades, assumptions and habits to which health workers are as prone as the general population.

The decline in the risk of infectious diseases has resulted in complacency among those who never saw the ravages of mumps or polio or whooping cough (pertussis) and fail to understand the imperative of protecting society from their re-emergence and the great risks of not doing so. The success of primary health in Cuba has led to a great increase in life expectancy [16] and consequent increase in the prevalence of the illnesses and problems of old age; Japan and many other countries are seeing the same effects; solving one set of problems gives rise to new ones (See box, p. 27).

We should also remember the perverse response to good advice: dismissal or doing the opposite. Parents are all too familiar with this when they try to influences their children's behaviour or choices. There is a psychological phenomenon called *reactance* [17] which describes how people of any age may respond to anything that appears to reduce their freedom in some way, even in matters between marital partners [18]. Authoritarian or imperative demands or tone of voice are especially liable to prompt such responses. While groups may show deference and compliance with the instructions of trusted leaders, those leaders themselves may respond negatively to any kind of external intervention or control. Perception may not be focused exclusively on the intrinsic issue at hand (e.g. immunization or pandemic mask-wearing[7]), but on the extent to which autonomy or a cherished group identity or belief is being threatened or undermined. This problem has escalated in the era of bipartisan politics, tribalism and alternative facts. (See also *backfire effects*, p. 54.)

---

[7] There was a furious response by some groups of citizens in the US to regulations requiring the wearing of face-masks at a time when numbers of infections were escalating. See for example this CNN report from 29 June 2020: https://www.youtube.com/watch?v=cc4qgvXgLkc. Accessed 24 July 2020.

There is also the question of example. We can assume that, until all politicians, health professionals and officials are weight-controlled, moderate or abstemious-drinking non-smokers, perception of messages about obesity, alcohol and tobacco are going to be, at best, muddled, at worst cynical. Foreign-led initiatives (in all spheres) may be undermined by perception that the sponsors are disqualified because of their own unresolved social or other problems, as well as suspicion of subversive political or religious motives.

Reflection   Strict laws and enforcement may change behaviour and have the potential to change perception. Changing perception and behaviour without sanctions is a quite different and massive challenge. The law of unintended consequences[8] is a constant risk in social affairs. Sound advice may be resisted simply because it appears to threaten freedom, autonomy or individual or group identity.

15.4   How Does Risk Perception Differ in Developed and Developing Countries?

During the course of this chapter, some broad generalizations will be made about risk, risk perception and risk communication in the developing world. However, we shall find that many variables lie on a spectrum which encompasses most or all human beings, developed or developing, and that location on the spectrum is not determined by mere labels, economics or geography. One such variable is what so-called 'rational or scientific' thinking which has a profound effect on risk perception and assessment. It could easily be assumed that wealthy, urban, educated people might be clustered at one end of this spectrum, with poor, rural, uneducated people at the other. While there probably are partial clusters at each end, there is also very substantial scattering across the whole range. We know, for example, that there are many highly educated people who challenge the science of climate change or evolution or vaccination while there are many rural, uneducated people who grasp the reality of climate change only too well and understand and welcome, first hand, the immense benefits of immunization and disease-prevention programmes. (There is more discussion of the vexed question of the effects of education on risk perception and risky behaviour below (p. 37))

The assumption that the developing world is, in general, less rational than so-called advanced countries is also challenged by a host of other risk-taking behaviours which are more or less common everywhere: smoking, alcohol and narcotic

---

[8] '…the law of unintended consequences has come to be used as an adage or idiomatic warning that an intervention in a complex system tends to create unanticipated and often undesirable outcomes. Akin to Murphy's law, it is commonly used as a wry or humorous warning against the hubristic belief that humans can fully control the world around them.' Unintended consequences. Wikipedia. https://en.wikipedia.org/wiki/Unintended_consequences. Accessed 15 July 2020.

consumption are three prime issues; then there is driving motorbikes without a helmet; texting or talking on mobile phones while driving; unprotected sex; obesity and the abandonment of healthy eating habits; the fetishization of body-image. If superstition and irrational thinking drive perception and behaviour in some parts of some developing societies, we must also remember that they manifest themselves in Western society too: homeopathy, unproven dietary supplements and physical therapies, refusal of blood transfusions, as well as the larger issues mentioned earlier.[9] (We should not forget belief in alien abductions and landings and UFO sightings to which very large numbers of people in the West are attached.) Developed countries may have more exposure to scientific thinking, but it does not necessarily make their populations comprehensively more rational or scientific in their view of life. In recent times, the erosion of confidence in experts, evidence and the scientific method have accelerated the race towards irrationality. There is a plausible argument that the whole Enlightenment project—reason, liberty, progress and religious tolerance—is under radical threat [19]. Our work in science and medicine is being profoundly affected by such developments.

One of the most stunning examples of hostility to scientific thinking was during the time of Thebo Mbeki, President of South Africa from 1999 to 2008, and his Minister for Health, Manto Tshabalala-Msimang. They rejected the causal relationship between HIV and AIDS, denied antiretroviral treatment to South Africans for years, promoted the use of herbal remedies, lemon, beetroot and other daft substances and were responsible for the deaths of maybe 350,000 untreated AIDS patients [20]. This is a powerful example of the impact of national leadership on the risks a population faces and how risk is characterized in a country. President's Trump's suggestion that injecting bleach might save Americans from COVID-19 also highlighted the extent to which some world leaders promote dangerous nonsense [21]. More on this topic follows later (see pp. 30–31).

When we look at something as specific as rational use of medicines, which might be thought of as a taken-for-granted set of behaviours in the developed world, we find that the picture is inconsistent—and alarming—right across the continents. Irrational use of antimicrobials in humans, and their abuse in animal husbandry, infects every region of the world. Non-adherence is a major world problem across all frontiers (WHO suggests that at least 50% of patients are non-adherent in one way or another [22], and there is substantial evidence that the situation is worse in some places). Self-medication with unregulated substances from a range of illicit

---

[9] Joseph Mercola is a notorious but very popular proponent of 'natural' remedies in the US. He is rabidly anti-science and mocks and attacks the wisdom and practice of Western medicine. He makes a lot of money from the stuff he sells to a very large market. A typical headline in his engaging newsletter, arriving on the day I write this, is: 'Don't Believe Anything Your Conventional Doctor Says About Arthritis.' He does, from time to time, have arguments that are sensible and deserve attention, but they are lost in the turmoil of his relentless and unscientific war. The FDA insists that he places this caveat beneath all his claims: 'These statements have not been evaluated by the Food and Drug Administration. These products are not intended to diagnose, treat, cure, or prevent any disease.' But that does not divert his great multitude of camp-followers. Mercola. www.mercola.com. Accessed 15 July 2020.

sources (e.g. internet and street-sellers) and counterfeit and sub-standard drugs plague many countries. Multiple deaths and injuries from adverse reactions to medicines and negative interactions are widespread.[10] Polypharmacy is a common problem. Populations cling to out-dated beliefs about the benefits of supplements and other products and support huge, influential and very profitable industries at the same time (a recent example is the definitive debunking of the cardiovascular benefits of omega-3 oils, a multi-billion dollar industry [23, 24]).

These issues alert us to the fact that regions of the world do not necessarily fall into neat categories that adequately characterize the behaviour or priorities of the people. Every country, even districts within countries, have their unique characteristics (Oslo is probably the crystal meth user capital of Europe, for example [25]; at 44/100,000 annually, Guyana has the highest suicide rate in the world [26]; Swaziland at 27.4% has the highest HIV prevalence of any country [27]; lifetime prevalence of cannabis use in Fiji and Papua New Guinea is about 47% and 55%, respectively, the highest in the world [28]). There are some issues that do have greater prominence in consideration of the situation in the developing world, but these are not equally applicable to all developing countries, nor exclusive to them.

Risk *factors* do vary from country to country.[11] There are variations, for example, in the risk factors for suicide as between developed and developing countries [29]. There are, therefore, major implications for different kinds of preventive risk communication. The same applies to many other risk categories, including HIV and other STDs, for example [30, 31]. Social, economic and environmental risk factors have a significant impact on child development everywhere, but the situation in developing countries has particular and compelling features [32].

Without examining the world country by country, and each country by region, it is not possible to make large and plausible generalizations about 'the developing world'. Recognizing these complexities and divergences, this chapter will focus on the dimensions that influence risk and risk perception everywhere, identifying elements that may be particularly influential in the developing world, or parts of it.

---

[10] '...studies [on hospitalized patient populations] estimate that 6.7% of hospitalized patients have a serious adverse drug reaction with a fatality rate of 0.32%. If these estimates are correct, then there are more than 2,216,000 serious ADRs in hospitalized patients, causing over 106,000 deaths annually. If true, then ADRs are the 4th leading cause of death—ahead of pulmonary disease, diabetes, AIDS, pneumonia, accidents, and automobile deaths.' Preventable adverse drug reactions: a focus on drug interactions. U.S. Food and Drug Administration. https://www.fda.gov/drugs/developmentapprovalprocess/developmentresources/druginteractionslabeling/ucm110632.htm#ADRs:%20Prevalence%20and%20Incidence. Accessed 15 July 2020. These figures relate only to hospitalised patients and are, therefore, likely a considerable underestimate of injuries and deaths throughout the community. Studies in other countries have found comparable levels of harm from medicines.

[11] *Risk factors* are those aspects of individual psychology and social context that affect feeling, perception, behaviour and exposure to risk; examples are poverty, literacy, access to healthcare, support networks, gender roles, sanitation, safety on the streets and a multitude more.

This approach will also give us some clues as to how to identify the most effective methods of communicating risk in relation to particular circumstances.

Reflection The differences between some aspects of risk perception and behaviour in developed and developing countries may be less that they seem, though the socio-political and cultural contexts are dramatically different. Communications must be tailored to the exact profile of the target audience.

The nature of any chosen country can be assessed against all the issues discussed. This process will not result in a definitive picture or prescription, but it will allow intelligent priorities and plans for action to be proposed and explored. It must be remembered that human beings are infinitely varied; though we may be able to sketch some general characteristics of particular societies or regions, there will still be a great range of individual and group variation; the bell-curve may have long tails. Only on-the-ground research and engagement can discover these multiple variables.

What Is Risk?

In medicine, risk has come to mean the chance of something bad happening or of something good not happening to a patient or a population, immediately or over a period of time. As far as possible, risk in medicine is calculated on the basis of data from clinical trials or other large studies and is intended to indicate what percentage of individuals would, over a specified period of time, be likely to suffer the negative effects under discussion. (In pandemics, the safety data is generated through cumulative counting and through track and trace systems.) Risk is stratified in various ways such as 'common' and 'rare' and all their variants. ('Risk' has actually been confounded with 'harm' (and 'hazard,' or 'danger') when it is paired with 'benefit': 'risk' is the probability; 'harm' and 'benefit' describe the nature of the event that might or might not happen, though 'benefit' has taken on a measure of meaning as probability.)

Risk in commerce and finance is a slightly different animal, defined as much by instinct ('gut feeling') and conviction as by statistics: do I feel that this investment or innovation will be successful, that is to say, profitable [33]? Such instincts operate differentially depending on the ownership of liabilities and potential benefits (bankers take risks with other people's money, but not with their own bonuses). Facing and overcoming the risk of death or serious injury is the incentive, the adrenaline-rush, for lovers of extreme sports. Protecting themselves and their children from 'risk' (really, 'danger') is a common priority for parents and citizens in general. Health and safety legislation is designed to reduce the risk of citizens suffering injury or death in the course of their daily lives.

Paul Slovic [34] identified these four differing but overlapping definitions:

- Risk as a hazard: "Which risks should we rank?"
- Risk as probability: "What is the risk of getting AIDS from an infected needle?"
- Risk as consequence: "What is the risk of not paying your tax?"
- Risk as potential adversity or threat: "How great is the risk of riding a motorcycle?"

He also pointed out two crucial aspects of risk: risk as *feeling* and risk as *analysis*. All risks generate *affect*, the technical term for emotional response. 'Rational' thinking is also part affect, part analysis (cognition), and it is the integration of these two seemingly conflicting elements in coherent balance that leads to the most intelligent decisions and communications. In order to *think* about risk, we must first put aside our instant and spontaneous *feelings* about it. Communications about risk that do not address at least these two basic determinants of perception will fail. Communication in pharmacovigilance and medicine has often focused on cognition (data) to the exclusion of emotional affect. Statistics do not drive behaviour in the way that feelings do. The exercise of *empathy* is a critical skill.

In discussing risk perception, these various interpretations of 'risk'—and others—need to be borne in mind.

Social, Political, Religious, Intellectual and Cultural Influences on Risk and Risk Perception

1. Disposition towards risk

Willingness to tolerate risk and risk-aversion are powerful determinants of risk perception, as are the unavoidable endurance of risk and freedom from risk. The population of some countries, such as Sweden, exhibit risk-aversion as a strong national characteristic.[12] This seems to be a feature of many developed nations when they reach a certain level of sophistication in their national infrastructure and social affairs and the gross risks of daily life are well managed. The good management and reduction of serious risks can give rise to a preoccupation with minor risks and a culture of anxiety or fear which is disproportionate to the statistical risks of small hazards and to the harm they night cause. Risk-aversion is, in some senses, a luxury enjoyed by those whose lives are relatively stable and safe. It is the case, nevertheless, that some people who are risk-averse in matters subject to oversight by others, such as governments or regulators, may still take major voluntary risks in their own lives (extreme sports, reckless driving, abuse of drugs, unsafe sex, for example).

In recent times, we have seen millions of people from fractured, oppressed, unstable societies choose to take the ultimate risk of death for them and their families on perilous journeys in the pursuit of a better life. If there is a high risk of death where you live, and no hope of improvement, then the risk of death, already familiar, but in the search for security elsewhere is clearly a preferable, though still extreme, option. This illuminates an important aspect of human responses to risk: in extreme circumstances, people are willing to take great risks to manage them or escape them. This holds good also for extreme pain or terminal illness: patients will review benefits and harms and assess risks in ways quite different from their previous habits; to mitigate extreme pain or major illness, people may select alternative risks (e.g. of shortening their lives). The pursuit of quality of life may be an overriding consideration (a benefit) even if the risks are greater than those of the status quo or other available choices. Hindus will seek spiritual purification in the filthy waters of Mother Ganges, even when the risks to life and health are real.

---

[12] Though the welcoming of tens of thousands of refugees might raise some doubts about this assertion, risk-aversion is still probably a default cultural norm.

A significant percentage of the populations of many developing countries face daily problems of security and survival: disease; food; unpredictable water and power supplies (if they have either); fragile living conditions; deficient or dangerous infrastructure and transport; corrupt police and officials. Many live in degraded or polluted or overcrowded environments, are likely victims of drought or floods and have low incomes and few opportunities, little or no access to education or healthcare. (But let us not forget communities in the developed world who suffer some of the same problems, as, for example, the people of the poor community of Flint, Michigan, whose polluted public water supplies had unacknowledged and dangerously high levels of lead pollution during 2015 [35]; or the much lower life expectancy of Australian Aboriginal people [36]; or the homeless sleeping on the streets of great Western cities.)

Risk perception in these circumstances will focus almost entirely on the threats to survival: what risks must I take or manage today to ensure that I and my family are still alive and healthy when night falls? And within that agenda, what are the priorities that require most effort? (Siberian Kazakhs, for example, see cold in all its forms (weather, drinks, floors, seats) as the major life-risks to be managed, and tea as the principal remedy for most ills [37]; poor people everywhere will risk food-poisoning by eating cheap or discarded food.)

Other risks differ too:

A woman in sub-Saharan Africa has a 1 in 16 chance of dying in pregnancy or childbirth, compared to a 1 in 4,000 risk in a developing country—the largest difference between poor and rich countries of any health indicator [38].

While in an 'informal settlement' or favela the population will be struggling to survive, next door, or down the road, wealthy citizens will be obsessed with the risks to their property and physical safety posed by their disadvantaged and (sometimes justifiably) demonized neighbours. This powerful élite will share many of the social and financial preoccupations and risk perceptions of their fellows in advanced countries, radically different from those of the local, poor majority.

During COVID-19 pandemic lockdowns, the daily income of millions of people in the informal economies of developing countries disappeared; if they had options available to them at all, they had to choose between dying of hunger at home or risking infection by going out into the world, and the risk of sanction if they did.

Reflection Where the risks of daily life are high, the preoccupation will be with survival that may encourage habituation to risk and risky behaviour. Where there are fewer threats to survival, there may be a greater urge to manage and reduce some risks.

The ground-breaking work of Paul Slovic [39] enriched our understanding of the ways in which most people perceive risk and the multiple factors that influence the risk assessments they make in their own lives and environment. Here, I shall refer only briefly to the details of his important work and point readers to the fuller account referenced in this paragraph. The Box below includes a summary of Slovic's ten factors, with some additions from this author. In considering our own risk communications, we need to identify which factors might be influencing our audiences and their responses and to take measures to manage them.

Twelve Risk-Perception Factors Based on Slovic
This list has been elaborated from the original by this author.

Actual and perceived risk are often very different. Certain characteristics of risk prompt us to make snap-judgements that do not take account of true probabilities and possible harms. These reactions are mostly affective (emotional) and instinctive rather than rational and are often influenced by a range of biases, including the heuristic bias (patterns we're familiar with, 'rules of thumb') and the availability bias (what we've recently heard, seen or experienced, especially on social media).

1. *Dread*

   We tend to overestimate the risk and impact of events that we dread, even when they are actually rare. This exaggeration makes us assess the risk as being higher than it is and can prompt overreactive, short-term 'knee-jerk' measures. Anything that we believe has catastrophic potential will deeply influence our perception and response and what we might expect from official action. A sense of dread can be amplified by excessive or emotional attention in various media channels, including powerful and evocative anecdotes. Data has little impact in such circumstances.

2. *Control*

   When we feel we are in control of our lives and choices, we tend to underestimate the risks we take (e.g. driving, self-medication). Anxiety or anger may occur when we feel others are controlling the risks in our lives in ways we do not consent to. This negative response is exacerbated if those in control are not familiar or trusted, or if events are outside our common framework of accepted risks. (Tourists may be anxious about the safety of Jeepneys in the Philippines or buses in Bogota, while locals take it for granted, for example; communities may be alarmed by novel public health programmes that are taken-for-granted by officials and health workers (HPV vaccination is an example).) There is good reason to suppose that disillusionment with ruling élites and their disenfranchisement of populations (i.e. causing exposure to risk and the loss of control and agency) has had much to do with recent social and political turmoil and with the appeal of strong leaders.

3. *Nature* vs. *Man-Made*

   There may be a willingness to live with the risks of nature, or resignation to them, while man-made risks may prompt greater anxiety or hostility. Most people underestimate the risks of exposure to radiation from the sun, for example, while many are deeply (disproportionately) concerned about the risks from nuclear energy, electric power-lines and other relatively new technologies, where the risks are statistically much lower. Genetically modified crops and gene-therapy have provoked hostility because of their perceived novelty, unnaturalness and unknown risks.

4. *Choice*

This overlaps with the 'control' factor. If we have active choice, say, with one option, or between two equally risky issues, then we may well perceive that the risk is lower than it actually is, probably from the sense of control that having a choice gives us. We react badly to risks that are imposed on us, especially if they result in damage. We will commit ourselves more completely to living with risks that we choose, as in the process of informed consent to therapy. Limiting of choice or freedom may result in perverse outcomes (see reactance, p. 7)

5. *Children*

Risks that affect children prompt very strong protective emotions that may lead to overestimation of probabilities and excessive efforts to manage them; damage to children provokes outrage. We tend to react differentially to exposure of children and adults to the same risk. The overprotection of children is thought by some to lead to the weakening of their health and survival skills [40]. Communication challenges are particularly acute when there is any measure of outrage in public reaction; outraged audiences will hear nothing until their outrage has reduced or been acknowledged and managed.

6. *Novelty*

Risks that we have not encountered before cause uncertainty and anxiety and may lead us to overestimate their threat to us. This is true of early and continuing opinion about nuclear power, more recently about 5G communication networks. Even great risks that we have long lived with (such as road traffic deaths, skin cancer from excessive exposure to sunlight, the damage caused by alcohol) tend to be regarded with less concern. The unknown prompts anxiety; the familiar prompts complacency. The medical community has a long history of resistance to innovation and change [41], one symptom of innate conservatism that is common in all societies.

7. *Publicity and Awareness*

Major publicity or public concern over particular risks may lead us to become disproportionately worried about them and to overestimate their probability. This is true of some disease outbreaks (e.g. SARS) and for deaths from terrorist attacks in the developed world. Highly publicized events, even if extremely rare, tend to lodge in memory and influence perception of similar events subsequently. Vivid, single-case anecdotes can have a large and distorting effect on public perception of risk. Classic research by Renn et al. showed that 'perceptions and social responses are more strongly related to exposure to risk than to its magnitude' [42]. Data has little weight in the face of a powerful, emotional story.

8. *Propinquity*

If we are directly at risk (as a surgical patient, for example, or a pregnant mother) or those close to us are at risk (children, for example), we will tend to assess risk as higher than for those at some distance; we will certainly see it as an issue for more urgent resolution. Closeness in time is also an issue: risks in the far distant future (cancer from smoking; death from obesity) may seem much less persuasive than risks that are vivid and immediate, even if much smaller (vaccination, a disease outbreak). Risks that threaten our property, immediate environment, personal financial or employment opportunities prompt strong reactions. (The risks of COVID-19 were downplayed by many leaders and populations, while the disease was ravaging distant countries.)

9. *Uncertainty*

Most people are anxious in situations of uncertainty particularly if the unknown quantity relates to their health and safety. Although many people take risks with uncertain outcomes in their own lives, they are suspicious, even intolerant of official risk communications that lack certainty. The fantasy of zero-risk is pandered to by politicians and CEOs who declare, hubristically, after crises, that they will ensure that the event 'never happens again'. Communicating uncertainty, and the inevitability of risk, is one of the great higher-level challenges in the discipline of risk communication (see p. 67 and Kahnemann et al. [43]).

10. *Risk-Benefit Trade-off*

If there are opportunities as well as risks mixed up together and a choice could lead to benefits, this can make the actual risk being seen as less than it actually still is, or more acceptable even if properly understood. (A common manifestation of this is participation in national lotteries where the risk of losing cash is millions of times higher than the seductive chance of winning anything.) Some people make such calculations in choosing alternative medicines in the face of chronic illness. There is great individual variation in the assessment of trade-offs; it is an area of great psychological complexity [44] and is relevant at every stage of reaching informed consent. Thinking and emotion are both in play, with emotion often having the upper hand.

11. *Fairness*

Risks that are distributed through human agency in some way unfairly give rise to strong reactions from those adversely affected. The perceived innocence of victims—as individuals or groups—is a powerful influence.

12. *Trust*

Where the risk involves the actions or advice of others, how we assess the risk will be significantly affected by the extent to which we trust the other party or parties involved, including governments and industry. This has the most profound implications for risk communications. Perceived political or commercial or financial conflicts of interest or suspected hidden motivations will radically undermine communications. Communications are also likely to be ineffective if their originators are perceived to be arbitrary, distant or uncaring or have failed to engage in dialogue with the affected population. Recent years have seen a steep decline in the extent to which experts and ruling élites are trusted [45]. This is a major obstacle to scientific and medical risk communication and must be addressed in the formulation and delivery of messages of any kind at all. The handling by national leaders of the COVID-19 pandemic has led to enormous upheavals in levels of public trust, often profoundly negative.

Reflection When planning a risk communication, the influence of any of these 12 factors must be taken into account and specifically addressed. The challenge is to acknowledge, understand and engage with audiences and the realities of their thoughts and feelings (the exercise of empathy) on the journey to helping them manage the emotional response, so that they are receptive and the facts may become clearer and a more measured choice or decision can be made. Lack of trust in politicians and officials is a formidable obstacle to effective risk communication.

2. *Cause and Effect*

This chapter opened with commentary on the extent to which rational discourse and scientific thinking did or did not influence risk perception and public debate. Some years ago, we might have believed that there was some correlation between social status, educational level and the habit of rational thought, though it was by no means guaranteed. That assumption no longer holds good, with irrational, anti-scientific thinking now contaminating affairs at national and international levels (President Mbeki was a grim example; President Trump the most recent and terrifying). The converse is more certain: the lower a population's level of education, the less common will be rational, scientific thinking and, consequently, the greater will be the influence of myth, rumour and gossip (especially dispersed through social media) and of traditional or cultural modes of thought. The extent of association between education and risky behaviour is another matter, discussed further below (see p. 37).

There was a time in Ghana, for example, when excessive consumption of red oil or over-exposure to sunlight was thought to cause malaria [46]. Arabs may believe in possession by spirits on in the power of the evil-eye. Traditional Chinese people believe that most illnesses are caused by an imbalance of qi (vital force or energy) and yin and yang in the body [47]. The Filipino concept of health is based on the principle of balance—*timbang*: specific disorders are perceived to be caused by an excess intake of one type of food. Hot foods such as meat are thought to cause arthritis and hypertension; cold foods such as many fruits and vegetables may bring about cancer and anaemia [47]. The four most common treatment methods in South Korea are acupuncture, herbs, moxibustion (direct or indirect burning with a stick made of the mugwort plant) and cupping (applying heated glass cups directly to the skin, forming a vacuum) [47]. Central to the Hindu view of health is the concept of the three humours (doşa) and a confidence in mantras, yogas or divine or saintly intervention to cure ailments that 'far exceeds their clinically demonstrable results' [48]. While many of these will not seem 'rational' by Western standards, they embody ancient systems of thought which are credible ('reasonable' if not strictly 'rational') within the history of the culture and coherent within their own terms and their natural environment. There is familiarity in almost all cultures with the use or ingestion of substances for treatment of physical and spiritual ills of all kinds. This is an important element that Western and traditional cultures share. The corrupting forces of postmodernism (in which the existence of universal truths is denied and subjective experience is regarded as the touchstone of truth) have fuelled distrust of the scientific method and its assumption that nature is intelligible through observation and research [45].

In one way or another, based on the information and experience we have, all of us create mental models of the world, parts conscious, parts hidden from consciousness, through which we explain and make sense of our lives. It is these *heuristics* which underlie most of our actions and decisions. These include experiences and learning, values and preferences, biases and prejudices, theories and explanations, assumptions and habits, notions of cause and effect, and they have a profound impact on our perceptions and behaviour. These models are often deeply entrenched and are very difficult to reach, shift or influence (some of them are socio-structural and even more implacable). We tend to seek the company of those whose mental models of the world are similar to our own and avoid or become even actively hostile to those who differ. Social media 'filter-bubbles' and 'echo-chambers' demonstrate this kind of tribal, hostile partisan fragmentation. We resist or ignore communications or explanations that challenge our customary way of seeing the world; we are likely to change only when our settled habits of thought and feeling are uncomfortably out of line with some new insight or experience, sometimes as the result of a traumatic event; or when manipulating and moulding our perception of reality does not bring peace and we must struggle for a new accommodation. Evidence alone will not necessarily penetrate the defences of our fortress of habitual thinking; major events or disruptions that conflict with our common assumptions may, perversely, be perceived and explained within existing frameworks, rather than suggesting the need for new ways of seeing and understanding.

Cause and effect are two, inter-related concepts at the heart of scientific thinking: *mycobacterium tuberculosis* causes TB, HIV leads to AIDS, no contest. In traditional and superstitious cultures, disease, accidents and other misfortunes may be seen as the result of the interference of spiritual, ancestral or paranormal powers of one kind or another, which require pacification through ritual or other specific counter-measures. In such cultures, one of the primary risks to be managed will be that of offending gods or spirits or those humans who mediate their powers on earth. Refusing the guidance or treatment of traditional healers or fetish-priests, for example, may put one at risk of dark consequences. The enormous challenge of effective scientific communication against such a background is painfully obvious.

Reflection There are many ways of experiencing and interpreting the nature of human life. Effective communication must respect and engage with them as the basis for building trust in alternative views. Science knows important truths, but science is not the whole story of humankind, not by long way. Differences must be acknowledged, respected and negotiated for progress to be made. Access to the minds of those whose values and beliefs are different requires immense empathy and skill; the best solutions will contain elements that bridge divergent systems of thought and belief.

3. *Destiny and Avoidability*

For a variety of reasons, populations in different parts of the world may feel that little can be done to manage risk or avoid dangers and disasters. Fate or karma, or the will of the gods, may be seen as the determining factors in human affairs, leaving little or no space for human agency or intervention. Cause and effect are, by scientific standards, inaccurately attributed and individuals will submit to whatever may happen to them and to their future helplessness to influence the course of events. Such superior forces may be seen as benign or malignant or beyond prediction. Interference with the natural course of events may itself be seen as an offence. In Sierra Leone, for example, there are some who believe that the taking of medicines interferes with the will of God.

A colleague in Ghana reports the intriguing fact that in some parts of the country, local people perceive the land as belonging ineffably to them and their community, and that their confident sense of proprietorship leads to road accidents through inattention to hazardous vehicle incursions on their territory. Here, a settled belief is unaffected by the evident threat the behaviour it poses to personal safety.

Many women, in thrall to dominant, sometimes violent men, or subject to cultural practices that rob them of autonomy, endure a seemingly immutable fate imposed by human agency. For some, it represents the accepted nature of their community, to which they may be more or less socialized, and a negative analysis would be seen as ignorant and offensive. Such oppression may have the authority of religion or traditional practice or be the expression of secular male cultural values. Such women may have little control over their unique domestic risks or the common risks of womanhood and motherhood. One of the risks many of them face is the prohibition on accessing or simply communicating with outsiders, such as health workers; another, the dreadful reality of female genital mutilation.

Reflection Varying perceptions on the issue of human agency, the capacity to decide and act freely, affect risk perception and freedom to manage risk. Interventions cannot avoid negotiating within these parameters.

4. *Status and Deference*

Submission to fate may also be reflected in submission to the social status quo, especially the hierarchy of status and respect. Patients in Thailand and other southeast Asian countries, as well as many in Africa, are very unlikely to challenge or question their superiors, whether academics, officials or health professionals. They may secretly defy guidance or instruction but will not expose their disagreement or non-compliance in any form that might reach their ascribed superiors. This pattern is also evident in the behaviour of workers whose dissatisfactions may never be made explicit to managers and lead simply to their unannounced disappearance from employment.[13]

This pattern is related to the profound influence of the concept of maintaining face: to question a superior or to suggest that they might be wrong is to risk their losing face or to risk one's own face in the (humiliating) criticism that may follow. In such societies (Thailand is a good example), the expression of anger or strong emotions leads to loss of face, and there are multiple, complex mechanisms for avoiding such personal or social conflict. This, like many historic cultural patterns of thought, feeling and habit, is being diluted in the modern world but remains still deeply influential. Many Thai university students hunger for debate, interaction and challenge, but very few of their teachers are capable of breaking out of traditional patterns of lecturing to a passive and compliant audience.[14]

A specific manifestation of hierarchy is the disposition of paternalism which, though maybe benignly intended, disempowers its victims. In Nigeria and other countries, this is a persistent mode of relationship with patients. Japan's medical establishment has struggled towards greater openness and democracy in patient relationships from a history that is actually more autocratic than paternalistic [49]; informed consent and, therefore, mature risk communication, do not come easily in such cultures.

Throughout the world, there is good evidence that the most effective risk communication and the change it promotes arise out of dialogue between experts,

---

[13] This silent cultural submission in relation to employers is greatly exacerbated in all parts of the world by autocratic management cultures in government and commercial organisations. Risks perceived by staff at junior levels may never be exposed because of fear of reprisals; this is a fear amply justified by the fate of courageous whistle-blowers who can be punished and expelled. Even when junior staff raise issues, they may be ignored and this is one element in many major crises and disasters, such as the BP Gulf oil disaster and in the fate of the drugs Mediator and Vioxx (in these two latter cases it was doctors ignored by regulators).

[14] Thailand had one of the world's most successful, taboo-shattering safe-sex campaigns in the 1990s, run by national hero Meechai Viravaidya ('Mr. Condom'). It was part of a larger campaign to reduce child mortality and population growth. New HIV infections were reduced by about 90%. Its methods were stunningly radical and innovative and it remains one of the great models of effective public health communication. For an overview, see Mechai's TED talk at: Viravaidya M. How Mr. Condom made Thailand a better place for life and love. TEDxChange: TED Talks. 2010. https://www.ted.com/talks/mechai_viravaidya_how_mr_condom_made_thailand_a_better_place?language=en. Accessed 18 July 2020.

officials and the people; that change comes not through pronouncements, but through engagement; not through lectures and leaflets, but through conversations and activities in an ethos of trust and collaboration. We shall return to this theme again and again.

Reflection   While cultures of deference inhibit open discussion and debate, those in positions of influence have a duty to encourage open and frank conversations, especially on matters of health and in risk communication.

5. Sex

Men and women perceive risk differently and are subject to a very divergent catalogue of risks. I have written extensively on the topic of risk in medicine and women elsewhere [50] and will summarize just some of the issues here.

A recent report in the UK [51] powerfully exposed three of the serious dangers to which women have been (and, in some cases, still are) exposed in the West and elsewhere: valproate in pregnancy, the Primodos pregnancy test and pelvic mesh. The intrinsic risks of these products were shown to be seriously exacerbated by the recklessness of physicians, their failure to explain and manage the risks and their failure to take seriously women's reports of the harrowing consequences, particularly of pelvic mesh.

Women across the world are disadvantaged in life and healthcare in a number of profound ways. They are subject to violence and abuse in all parts of the world. Alcade's work [52] has illuminated the disturbing situation in Peru and Latin America, but the picture is bleak in Africa and many other places too.

In Sierra Leone, pregnant teenagers may seek the dangerous service of quack doctors for abortions, in order to avoid the shame and punishment following public disclosure. Millions of female foetuses or babies are at risk in many parts of the world, notably India and China [53]. Tens of millions of women have suffered from or are at risk of genital mutilation [54].

Inferior treatment and poor outcomes for heart disease [55], delay in brain-tumour diagnosis [56], and the neglect of menopause and pelvic pain as areas of research [57] are four further examples. Drug information, and risk communication in particular, has rarely taken into account the contextual risks of women's lives or been tailored to their specific needs and preferences.

Risk communication for women must take into account the multiple cultural, social, psychological and risk variables which impact their lives. These include their preferences for provider sex, sources of information and decision-making style; the degree of self-determination in their cultural setting and the level of subjection to male behaviour and expectations (including health professionals); their exposure to abuse and unwanted pregnancies; and their unique and diverse attitudes to motherhood, contraception, menopause, body-image and much more. Across cultures, these all vary enormously and no one model or profile can be adduced.

Young women face a particular series of risks in their lives that profoundly affect their health (e.g. alcohol, unprotected sex, eating disorders, body-image issues, depression and suicidality). Many of these are not disclosed to health professionals and therefore become a dimension of hidden risk that is not accounted for in diagnosis, risk communication and treatment. Risks and patterns of behaviour formerly exclusive to the developed world, such as eating disorders [58], are erupting in many parts of the developing world, threatening personal and public health in societies often ill-prepared to manage novel risks.

Specific challenges in risk communication for women, among many others, arise in the cases of ante-natal care, giving birth, HPV vaccination, HRT, epilepsy in pregnancy, a range of cancers and contraception.

Effective risk communication is a critical element in ethical therapeutic relationships that respect the autonomy and unique characteristics of individual patients. Risk communication for women is a major sub-set of the discipline in general, and one that requires radical reappraisal and reformed practice.

None of this is to say that men do not have their special, idiosyncratic risks and needs; they clearly do, but they are, on the whole, far less widely and deeply disadvantaged than women, when all other factors are equal. A negative aspect of men's dominant position is their difficulty in disclosing weakness or need which manifests itself, among other ways, in delayed presentation of symptoms of disease and a higher risk of suicide, but poor, rural women in the developing world have a more difficult time than do their men and much the same is true of affluent, urban women in developed countries. Most of the power is in the hands of men, and most of the systems, including healthcare, have been designed by men and are, still, largely, managed by men and run according to their habits and preferences. An indicator of this process is the extent to which several aspects of women's health and symptoms, including their experience of pain (especially pelvic pain), have been disparaged and undervalued by men.

A classic piece of risk perception research from 1994 [59] demonstrated that white males in the US 'on average, ... perceived risks as much smaller and much more acceptable than did other people'. Non-white males and females and white females all assessed risks as greater and less acceptable (see [Fig. 15.1]).

The differential for white males is striking and most likely explained by white males' dominant status in the culture and their innate sense of privilege and security. Similar research in Sweden in 2011 [60] found little difference between native males and females, but different results for immigrants. The authors concluded:

> The chief finding is that there is no WME [white male effect] in Sweden, which we concluded results from the relative equality between the sexes in the country. On the other hand, ethnicity serves as a marker of inequality and discrimination in Sweden. Consequently, ethnicity, in terms of foreign background, mediates inequality, resulting in high risk perception. Equality therefore seems to be a fruitful concept with which to examine differences in risk perception between groups in society, and we propose that the "societal inequality effect" is a more proper description than the 'WME'.[15]

---

[15]This became a headline issue in 2020, after the murder by police of George Floyd and in the excessive death-rate of black, Asian and minority ethnic people during the COVID-19 pandemic. Both of these thrust the 'social inequality effect' into dramatic and tragic relief.

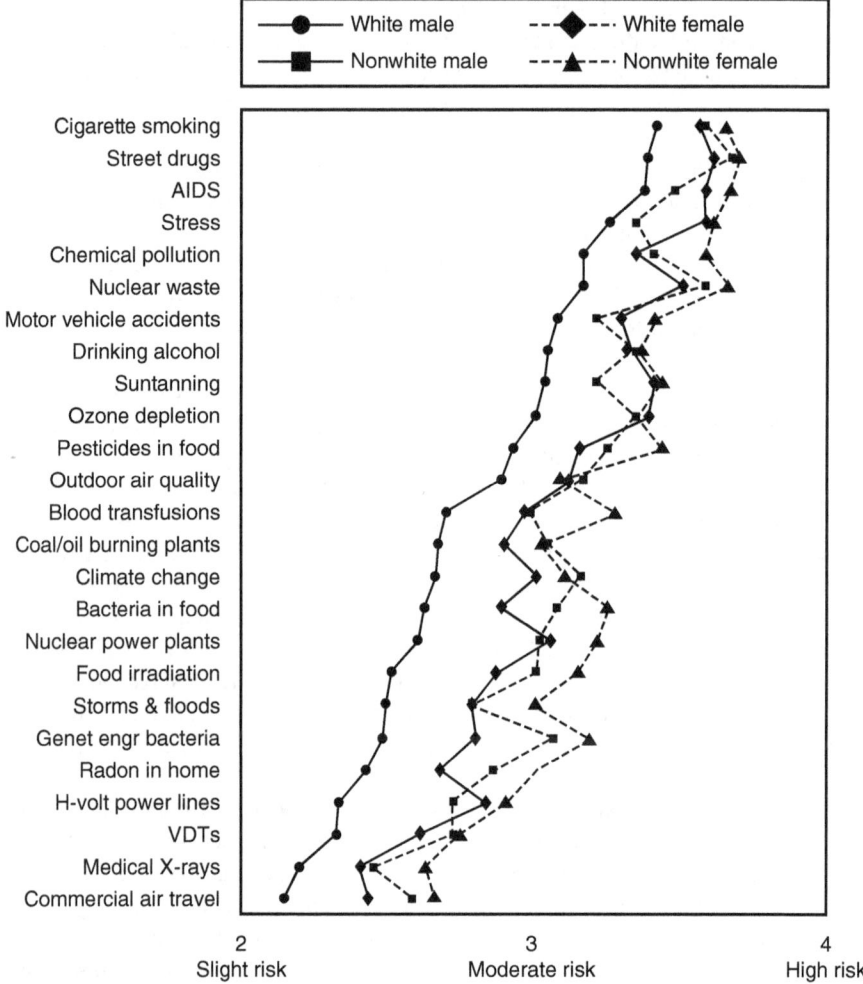

Fig. 15.1 Mean risk-perception ratings by race and gender. (Source: Flynn et al. [59])

If this finding holds good for societies across the world, then it has great implications for our understanding of risk perception and communication everywhere. It reinforces the evidence relating to the disadvantage of women as well as ethnic and other minorities. Those who enjoy secure, dominant status in society are more risk-tolerant than those who are disadvantaged, discriminated against and vulnerable. The 'societal inequality effect' requires us to tailor communications differentially to those with very different perceptions of risk, particularly noting those who may be more resistant to influence because they assess risks as lower (and, therefore, less of a threat) than others. This is simply one of the many variables to be factored into any interpretation of behaviour or communication about it.

Reflection   Doctors and patients have very different perceptions of risk, especially if they are opposite sex; male and female patients will have significantly different perceptions of risk and have differing needs and priorities in risk communication. Status in the social hierarchy and its associated sense of power or lack of it will influence perception of risk and communications about risk. Officials (especially male officials) will have radically different perceptions of risk than those in less dominant and privileged positions in the social hierarchy. Profound social-structural issues affect the risks people face and their perceptions of them.

6. Sexuality

Sexual identity and orientation are important and problematic issues in vulnerability to risk and in risk perception and risk communication. In many parts of the developing world, and many enclaves of the developed world, the LGBT+[16] population is deeply discriminated against, vulnerable even to injury and death for no reason beyond their sexual orientation. Even in relatively advanced countries, the stigma of heterodox sexuality is a significant threat to many. Russia and Uganda are two prime examples of such countries, while all Muslim countries and communities, as well as fundamentalist Christians and the Catholic Church, are hostile to same-sex or unconventional sexual liaisons. Progress is being made, but disparities are still enormous [61], especially in the developing world, where non-heterosexual sex is predominantly illegal.

For many members of this very large group of people, embracing all classes, all backgrounds and human types, risk perception will be occupied primarily with the threat of exposure and the potentially hideous consequences. Even where injury and death are not on the cards, there are children who are bullied at school or rejected by their parents, graduates who fail to get jobs, many who fear ridicule or humiliation at the hands of straight society or extreme politicians, many who remain silent and isolated, feeling that their chance of an open and happy life is negligible. Among this population, mental health problems, the consumption of excessive alcohol or illegal drugs, self-harm and suicide are all significantly higher than for the heterosexual population [62].

Reaching such an audience is immensely difficult, but crucial when the exceptional and everyday risks they face are urgent and compelling. The task is complicated also by the extent to which individuals may be secretive about the details of their lives and the risks they face. Some campaigns have reached and influenced these sexual minorities, notably those concerned with safe sex, but few examples of risk communication have addressed the wider issues of their lives and lifestyles.

Sex workers, both women and men, are a further minority (but large) population of importance to public health. The risks of their working lives are substantial

---

[16]Lesbian, gay, bisexual and transgender (people). This is the minimal acronym for the complex field of sexual orientation and gender variance; it does, many would (not unreasonably) claim, exclude several significant other groups; some would maintain that the acronym should be LGBTQIA+ (you'll find it on Google).

(infection, injury, especially) and their lives are also subject to other health and survival risks particularly in societies where they are stigmatized or criminalized. Energetic, creative and persistent HIV risk communication campaigns in some countries have reached and influenced sex workers and changed behaviour, but there are still many hard-to-reach populations, such as the housewives of Kolkata who become prostitutes to pay the bills [63], or the illegal and harassed sex workers of Ghana [64].

Reflection Sexual diversity is a fact of life; however, much of it may be hidden or demonized and has deep implications for all aspects of relationships and communication in healthcare. Hard-to-reach populations provide some of the greatest challenges to risk communication.

7. National Leadership and Political Culture

Those who live in countries where the authorities appear to understand, manage and care about the risks of daily life are likely to be less fearful and more resilient in the face of risk and uncertainty than those whose national authorities fail to deliver good policy and legislation and are unwilling or unable to regulate or enforce compliance to manage risk and enhance safety. This is true also of organizations, where a strong safety culture leads to safer practices, fewer accidents and a more confident and fulfilled workforce, whose perceptions and expectations are broadly positive. In both cases, the extent to which the population is informed, involved and engaged in risk management will influence the extent to which they feel more or less secure and engage in safe practices. Preparedness for natural disasters (including pandemics) is a sphere in which this particularly holds good.

On the other hand, largely stable, safe and well-regulated societies may be plunged into dangerous insecurity by the advent of shocking new risks such as epidemics, mass shootings, exceptional natural disasters or terrorism. In developing countries, where such risks and their consequences are more familiar, there is likely to be a much greater feeling of helplessness and resignation, even though the degree of human suffering is comparable. Communication must always take account of the prevailing political and social ethos, and the current preoccupations and perceptions of the population; it must meet and exceed low expectations if it is to make its mark. Sad to say, official communications often do not meet even low expectations.

The Case of Cuba

Cuba, a relatively poor country, has lower infant mortality than the USA and similar life-expectancy, at about one twentieth of the per capita cost. The major factor in this remarkable achievement is proactive preventive medicine: every family in the country is visited in their home annually by the local doctor and nurse for a complete health check-up; those who are at risk are monitored more frequently and advised or supported or treated as necessary. However, not all is well, as the BBC reports [65]:

> Ageing, an increase in obesity and problems with tobacco and alcohol mean Cuba's citizens are now dying of the same diseases claiming lives in higher income countries: heart disease, stroke and cancer.

The Government's response has been massive public health campaigns with front line risk and health communication being delivered directly into citizen's homes by local doctors and health staff.

That inspired method of work is a model for every aspect of effective engagement and communication with patients for the maximum possible effect. (See also HCP Uganda, p. 58, for a comparably radical approach.)

In Mbeki's South Africa, when the causal link between HIV and AIDS was denied, healthcare policy was driven by a fantasy, putting hundreds of thousands of people at risk. Sections of the population would have had their perception of the nature of HIV infection, its risks and treatment completely distorted. The same is true for populations whose leadership downplay the risks of infectious diseases and pandemics or demonize immunization, or other health interventions, or particular groups of people.

Nevertheless, well-intended campaigns that change behaviour can have negative, unintended consequences as well. In Ghana, for example, early, frightening messages about the risks of HIV infection did have an impact on behaviour, but they also left HIV+ patients stigmatized and alienated and contributed to myths about the transmission of the infection from toilets, shared utensils and non-sexual physical contact. This highlights the sometimes neglected truth that effective, relatively risk-free risk communication is a very complex and sophisticated aspiration.

In the West, the most powerful anti-science leadership is probably the US Republican party with its implacable resistance to climate-change science that has profoundly influenced the rise of science-sceptics in this and several other fields. Creationists and some so-called Greens have made their contribution too. The political Right, in many developed countries, especially in times of austerity, has stood in the way of healthcare and welfare provision and of educational opportunity for the poor in general and for sexual and ethnic minorities in particular. These movements have profound effects on the beliefs, perceptions and expectations, latent or provoked, of large numbers of people. They all have, to differing degrees, exposed populations to new risks, immediately and in the future. Social norms, which profoundly influence individual perception or risk, can very rapidly be driven in the direction of the prevailing political agenda.

Reflection Populations that feel their government is caring and capable will be more resilient in the face of risk, though they will be unforgiving in the event of preventable disasters; those living under corrupt or incompetent régimes will feel more vulnerable and exposed and, in some cases, angry. Powerful political agendas shift social norms and influence values and beliefs.

8. *Corruption*

There are many categories of risk in societies. One of these is the incipient risk of systems, bureaucratic, law-enforcement, political, regulatory and healthcare itself. In a society where corruption is endemic, perception of everyday risks, such as domestic security or disease, is mediated by perception of the risks associated with the behaviour and demands of the relevant systems and their agents. Two examples are the systems of law-enforcement and healthcare, both of which may be hazardous: police because of unethical agendas and the risks of not being able to afford bribes; healthcare because of under-resourced or over-stretched or compromised services or supplies.

Political corruption, particularly at elections with the risk of coercion, even violence, is a risk for many populations, perceived, understood and feared. Political corruption often means the diversion of funds from essential services and the neglect or even intensification of everyday social risks of all kinds (the neglect of all aspects of welfare and infrastructure are prime examples). Perception of these kinds of risks is more or less universal, with reactions that vary from country to country, from exasperated resignation or protest, to submission and acceptance. The developing world undoubtedly carries the greatest burden of gross, visible and petty corruption, but developed countries and systems also suffer persistently from all forms at all levels. The conducting of what might seem like ordinary, low level everyday business may be compromised by the real and perceived risk and reality of corruption, including access to medicines. Even without corruption, some systems are so impenetrable and complex that ordinary people may be utterly disempowered or excluded by them.

A subtler form of corruption comes in the form of improper influence in medical practice. Most common, in all parts of the world, is the influence of pharmaceutical companies on prescribing practice and procurement decisions, often resulting in higher costs and few benefits to patients [66]. Until recently, this was reported as a significant issue in Ethiopia, for example. In Georgia, pharmaceutical companies battled it out in public claiming that their rivals' drugs were unsafe.

Transparency International claims that in some countries up to two-thirds of hospital medicines supplies are lost to corruption and fraud [67].

Reflection In countries where corruption is endemic, people find workarounds or resign themselves to the way things are. Corrupt societies create and enhance risks of all kinds and inhibit the practical management of risk. Risk communication has a greater challenge to establish credibility in societies where officialdom is not trusted and where corruption is rife.

9. *Urban and Rural Living*

This categorization is, in some ways, distracting, because by no means the greatest disparities between communities exist simply in town or country: side-by-side with the wealthiest citizens in the greatest cities of the world live some of the poorest, most disadvantaged, unhealthiest and oppressed groups you can find anywhere.

It is true that remote rural populations in developing countries (and some developed countries) often suffer from multiple disadvantages and extreme survival risks: they may have little or no access to education or healthcare and be at enhanced risk of disease, maternal and child mortality, climate irregularities, water shortage, and so on; they may also be beyond the reach of modern communications.

Poor urban populations will perceive risk very differently from poor rural populations. For one thing, urban dwellers have, paraded daily for their oppression, the wealth and success of fellow citizens, whose privilege and affluence is accompanied by many fewer survival risks. Risk tolerance for these poor populations will be mediated by their differential beliefs in destiny or human agency and by the politics of opportunity.

Reflection The remoteness of rural populations is one of the extreme aspects of human deprivation that challenges traditional methods of service-delivery and communication. Urban living brings with it problems and risks that are different from rural living but requires equally ingenious approaches to reach and influence diverse communities.

10. *Politics and Religion*

The polio vaccination crises in northern Nigeria [68] and Pakistan [69] neatly and vividly illustrate the extent to which public perception and interpretation of science can be hi-jacked by political and religious priorities. Unlike its giant neighbour, India, Pakistan made only sluggish progress towards eradication of polio, even before the direct intervention of the Taliban and the killing of immunization health workers. The Taliban declared the vaccine 'poison' and part of a Western conspiracy to damage Muslim communities and make their women infertile.[17] (There are instances of such beliefs in other countries, for example, in parts of Sierra Leone.) There were also rumours that the vaccine contained substances derived from pigs. Similar allegations were made by Muslim clerics and community leaders in northern Nigeria, initially rejecting all argument and evidence to the contrary and refusing permission for vaccination to take place in their territory.

In Nigeria, the opposition to vaccination was eventually overcome by a huge collaborative effort to provide sufficient international opinion and evidence to demonstrate that the vaccine was safe; the programme was allowed to proceed. In Pakistan, in 2015, the authorities started arresting parents who refused to have their children vaccinated but the Taliban's position did not change. Perception of the real risk of

---

[17] In January 2016, 15 people were killed and many injured when a suicide-bomber detonated just outside the polio eradication centre in Quetta: Boone J. Bomb attack at polio vaccination centre kills 15 in Pakistani city of Quetta. Guardian. http://www.theguardian.com/world/2016/jan/13/bomb-attack-at-polio-vaccination-centre-kills-14-in-pakistani-city-of-quetta. Accessed 15 Jul 2020. Assassination of health workers occurred in January 2018: Aizenman N. Pakistan raises its guard after 2 polio vaccinators are gunned down. National Public Radio. 23 Jan 2018. https://www.npr.org/sections/goatsandsoda/2018/01/23/580002283/pakistan-raises-its-guard-after-two-polio-vaccinators-are-gunned-down?t=1532949664007. Accessed 15 July 2020.

polio (Pakistan accounts for the vast majority of polio cases globally [70]) is confounded by alternative versions of the disease's aetiology; by religious complexities, even reprisals (including brutal killings) and political allegations; and by forceful intervention by the State. Few 'simple' medical interventions can ever have been subject to such huge distortion and to such a wide range of collateral risks. Over the years, dozens of public health campaigns have been sponsored by the Government and NGOs, but even those who might have been convinced by the science (risk of polio, very high; risk of vaccination, extremely low) may have difficulty seeing things clearly and making a straightforward decision to have their children vaccinated.

For quite different reasons, but with similarly damaging effects on public health in Europe and the USA, the anti-MMR vaccine campaign flourished on the basis of criminally fraudulent work by Dr Andrew Wakefield. Unlike the clerics in Nigeria, many members of the American and UK public refused, over a decade, to be convinced by a massive amount of evidence that refuted the claims [71]; children became unnecessarily sick and some died; measles reasserted itself. There is little to choose between the minds and behaviour and the distorted perception of risk of those deaf to science, wherever they may live. Changing their views is massively complex and frequently subject to failure– and data will not do it.

People in many parts of the developing world are at risk of kidnapping, torture and death because of religious, ethnic, political and territorial conflicts. Safety and survival are the daily priorities in such situations, and many other needs (e.g. accessing healthcare or education) may be frustrated. People may perceive risks to their present and future chances in life but be helpless to take action beyond flight (a desperate solution so many are taking now).

Religion is an active influence, of course, in the whole moral and social sphere, shaping attitudes and perceptions to many issues, not least in medicine and public health. While religion has had some benign effects in many parts of the world, there is also a dark side when it comes to the health and welfare of populations. Catholicism inhibits family-planning and safe sex practices; outlaws abortion; contributes to the oppression of LGBT+ people and enhances their risks of medical and psychological problems (while colluding for decades with the abusers of children). Jehovah's Witnesses do not permit blood transfusions. Fundamentalist and some Evangelical Christians are anti-intellectual and anti-science, anti-gay and anti-abortion; they maintain the sanctity of marriage and abhor and punish extra-marital sex. Islam prohibits certain practices pertaining to food, drink, recreation and sex and among much else, proscribes extra-marital and same-sex relationships. Almost all religions disadvantage women to a greater or lesser extent. This, coupled with cultural norms of male-superiority in many developed and developing countries, puts women at great risk in many aspects of their health, safety and general welfare. Missionaries from all denominations have disrupted traditional cultures, often proselytizing with the promise of benefits in exchange, with little concern for the spiritual and anthropological risks, costs and losses.

While Hinduism and Buddhism are less prescriptive in terms of specific moral behaviours, various concepts of dharma, reincarnation and caste, deeply influence behaviour and perception, especially with regard to hierarchical submission and resignation to one's fate. Much misunderstood Haitian voodoo[18] (officially recognized as a religion since 2003 [72]) has the cause of healing at its centre, but there is also belief in the intervention of spirits and ancestors and a deep vein of fatalism.

On the banks of the Zambezi in Zambia, villagers have a profound and unshakable belief in witchcraft and its powers for good and evil. They attributed the killing of several of their number by aggressive hippopotamuses to demon-possession spells targeted at specific victims. In their view, the only remedy was an exorcism by the most powerful witchdoctor. This, incredible though it seemed to the investigating zoologist, appeared to bring the killings to an end [73]. In such a context, scientific discourse is all but impossible.

Haiti is of particular interest because the case prompts attention to an important element of all religious communities: that beneath the surface, there are all kinds of complexities and contradictions, especially in terms of behaviour. Haiti is often characterized as being, '70% Catholic, 30% Protestant, 100% Voodoo' [74]. Voodoo (or voodun) represents a range of very ancient beliefs and practices, probably originating in West Africa, later exported to the Americas during the era of the slave trade. Slaves were beaten and tortured to convert to Christianity, and though missionaries, one way or another, persuaded African populations to convert, ancient beliefs and practices persisted (and do persist) under the pretence of compliance.

This is one point at which religious and political realities intersect and compound: imperial adventures often had specific religious purposes, as well as economic and political ones, and many had the specific blessing of the Catholic Church, from persons as elevated as kings and popes themselves.

This dark and painful history has profound implications for modern-day perceptions of risk, of foreign materials or interventions and of whom to trust. If your ancestors were beaten into Christian submission, or annihilated in the pursuit of imperial ambitions, where do you turn for reassurance and physical and spiritual security? One choice is to stick with what you and your ancestors have always known and believed in and to remain highly sceptical about science and foreign interventions.

Behind the Nigerian polio crisis and the damaging de-worming eruption in Ghana [75], lay fears that the West was conspiring, once again to undermine the integrity and health of African communities. There have been a sufficient number of cases of disgraceful individual and commercial malpractice, African deaths and injuries, and ambiguous or poorly promoted interventions [76] for the suspicions and the rumours to have a plausible foundation.[19]

---

[18] For an excellent summary of the essence of Haitian Voodoo, see: Corbett B. Introduction to Voodoo in Haiti. 1988. http://faculty.webster.edu/corbetre/haiti/voodoo/overview.htm. Accessed 15 July 2020.

[19] The phoney immunization programme run by the CIA in Abbotabad in their pursuit of Osama Bin Laden did untold damage to the reputation of the West and the credibility of public health programmes. See: Shah S. CIA organised fake vaccination drive to get Osama bin Laden's family DNA. Guardian. 11 July 2011. http://www.theguardian.com/world/2011/jul/11/cia-fake-vaccinations-osama-bin-ladens-dna. Accessed 15 July 2020.

Breaking the Habit
Liver Flukes

In parts of north-eastern Thailand, the prevalence of liver cancer is more than five times the global average. It has been known for 40 years that the main cause of this was liver-fluke infestation from a popular dish made from fresh, uncooked fish [77]. In the last decade, community leaders have been involved in spreading information about the risk; there have been village meetings with music and songs; schools have included it in their teaching. Perceptions and habits have been changing, though there appears to be a minority who remain uninfluenced by the risk. Younger people, seeing many of their elders dying from liver cancer, have taken the message to heart.

Betelnuts

Across Asia and the Western Pacific, betelnut chewing, with or without added tobacco, has high prevalence [78, 79]. Along with alcohol, nicotine and caffeine, it is thought to be among the commonest mind-altering substances in daily use by millions of people, including children. In countries, like Taiwan, where the habit is common, rates of oral cancer are very high, the majority of cases attributable to the carcinogenic properties of the nut itself and the ingredients wrapped in the 'quid'. In many places, the nut is deeply ingrained in the culture, used in gifts, graveside offerings, and especially by working men to keep them alert and awake during long working periods, driving or fishing, for example. In spite of campaigning efforts in, for example, Taiwan, Thailand and India, the habit is still common. Like the cancers from liver flukes, those caused by betelnut chewing take decades to emerge; the activity perceived as harmless until it is too late. Such perceptions are very hard to shift.

Tobacco and Pregnancy

Studies in Latin America [80] and Africa [81] show that smoking, use of smokeless tobacco products and exposure to second-hand smoke (from domestic cooking fires too) are serious issues with regard to pregnant women and the health of their unborn babies. Not all populations have been exposed to the intensity of anti-smoking campaigning that has been seen in developed countries and some women appear not to know about the risks, while they remain vulnerable to advertising messages. While levels of tobacco use have fallen in developed countries, there is still a considerable number of women who are habitual users, before, during and after pregnancy [82].[20] This, as in the

---

[20] The characteristics of the women most at risk indicate the challenge of effectively influencing them to change their behavior: women with fewer resources living in Western or Eastern Europe are more likely not only to smoke before pregnancy but also to continue smoking during pregnancy. These high-risk women are characterized as living alone, having high school or less as highest education level, having low health literacy, being a housewife, having previous children, having unplanned pregnancy, and no use of folic acid.

examples above (and as for alcohol and obesity), reinforces the fact that being informed does not necessarily lead to change in behaviour, even for issues as critical as foetal health. Tools much more subtle than mere information are needed. Persistence, over many years, sometimes decades, is also a characteristic of campaigns that have had success in altering behaviour.

From the examination of this selective set of variables, we can see how complex is the question of risk perception: it is not just the risk of a substance or intervention that is relevant, but also the risk of the system through which it is offered, its history, its source and the motivation behind it. The more people affected—whole populations in immunization programmes—the more are such distorted or negative perceptions likely to take hold, especially in the era of social media.

No official communication—about risk or anything else—has any hope of success if it does not take into account and acknowledge some of these powerful, underlying issues.

11. *Public and Private*

There is one more twist in this important perspective in risk perception and communication: people may not always behave as their religion or politics, or public opinions might be assumed to predict they will, and people will very often not talk about the divergence between their public and private selves. Extra-marital sex, with all its potential risks, is a case in point: while Muslims and Hindus in developing countries report quite low levels of extra-marital sex, Christians and Jews appear to more liberal in their behaviour [83], but what is actually happening may not match what people claim. It is a matter for some surprise for a traveller in comprehensively Christian West Africa (e.g. Ghana), to find that, in spite of prayers before and after even the most serious scientific meetings, many of the local men, single and married, are drinking a lot and having affairs all over the place. More credible evidence about extra-marital sex in Nigeria, for married and cohabiting men aged 15–64, comes from Ovediran et al. [84], who brilliantly demonstrate the complexity of the picture across the country's regions and 389 ethnic groups, the multiple risk factors and the challenges for risk communication in this, as in any, field of concern:

> The results show that 16% engaged in extramarital sex in the 12 months preceding the survey and had an average of 1.82 partners. The results also show statistically significant association between extramarital sex and ethnicity, religion, age, age at sexual debut, education, occupation, and place of residence. Based on the study results, it could be concluded that significant proportions of Nigerians are exposed to HIV infection through extramarital sex…because of gender-based power imbalances within the family, a large number of the women are unable to negotiate consistent condom use by their partners.

People of all religions are notorious for drinking more alcohol than they admit, even in societies where it is prohibited. This has some similarities to the motor-cycle helmet issue discussed earlier: the perceived risk of these behaviours may be more that of discovery and social opprobrium or punishment than of harm from the activity itself. The risk of discovery is especially potent for LGBT+ people; the pressure for secrecy immense. A patient's loss of face, the protection of reputation and dignity, the preservation of liberty, even of life, are important elements of risk in communications with officials and health workers.

This has huge implications for risk communication. If, as we know, patients everywhere withhold, omit or fabricate information when talking to their doctors about their own risky behaviour which they regard with embarrassment or fear [85]; if they are in denial about any of the risks they take (smokers, philanderers, drinkers, users of illicit drugs), then the chances of reaching and influencing them are very slim indeed by anything but extraordinary means, and those means demand significant time and resources. Those who do not disclose their sexual habits, for example, are at risk of HIV and STDs and other diseases; those who do not admit to illicit drug-use or to taking alternative or OTC medicines expose themselves to all kinds of harm, such as new injuries or serious interactions.

Reflection   Religion or beliefs in supernatural powers may profoundly influence the risks people face and their perceptions of them. The influence of faith of all kinds may require special research and consideration in any category of communication. Religious or social pressures may encourage duplicity or dangerous secrecy among those at odds with prevailing rules and practices.

12. *Employment and Economics*

Unemployment and poverty are two of the great burdens suffered by too many of the world's population. They are among the overwhelming features of life that push almost all other risks very far down the list of preoccupations. These are by no means exclusive to developing countries, but the burden and the risk are that much greater when there is no safety net of social or welfare security. While welfare and healthcare budgets are being squeezed (even slashed) in many developed countries, there may be some official or voluntary resource to ensure that most citizens have food and shelter, though homelessness and hunger are becoming issues in many rich countries.

Around 30% of South Africa's population (maybe many more), among the highest figures in the world, are unemployed (July 2020) [86]. The situation is dire in many other countries too. The ability to feed oneself or one's family; maintaining rent and utility payments; being free to travel to seek work; managing and treating illness; supporting children at school; all these are threatened by poverty and unemployment and represent major life risks that oppress victims' lives. During the coronavirus pandemic, these risks escalated for many populations, at the same time as the threats to health and life from the disease were inflating.

Poverty is one of the powerful elements that forces people to take risks with their health: postpone treatment or ignore symptoms, share medicines, use traditional medicines even for serious disease, buy dubious medicines on the street, stop taking meds early to save tablets for future use, not return for refills for chronic diseases. If it is food or medicines, it is clear which choice will be likely to take precedence.

Reflection   Poor and unemployed people face increased risks of all kinds and may have limited resources or strength to manage them. Risk communications may bypass those for whom daily life is a struggle for survival.

13. *Education*

It is commonly assumed that those with higher levels of educational attainment will have a more sensitive and accurate perception of risk. There is evidence to support this, but it cannot be taken for granted. A 2007 study of HIV risk perception among 2213 military personnel in Nigeria [87], for example, concluded:

> ...among military personnel, educational attainment inversely correlates with HIV risk perception.

The authors speculate about the reasons for this surprising finding:

> ...despite higher educational attainment, this cohort may not be exposed to substantial and reliable information on risk factors for acquiring HIV infection. In this cohort of NMP [Nigerian military personnel], educational attainment may not necessarily translate to knowledge of HIV risk factors, which is necessary for increased risk perception, and higher education status may be associated with higher rank among NMP, which may precipitate denial syndrome.

There were other interesting findings, including an inverse correlation between HIV perception and age, that is to say older people were less aware of the risks of HIV than their juniors.

A study in rural Uganda in the early 1990s [88] supported the thesis that education was a predictor of risky behaviour and that specific interventions needed to be planned for that at-risk population. In the same district of Rakai, 20 years later, the trend seems to have been reversed, with rising school enrolment and socio-economic status among adolescents associated with declining risk for HIV and pregnancy [89]. (An interesting secondary contributory factor was the decline in numbers of single and double orphans because of improved survival rates for HIV+ parents.)

Some of the most recent work in Ethiopia [90] show clearly that the affluent and well-educated are at greater risk:

> HIV prevalence reached 10-21% in the central, eastern and western geographic clusters of Ethiopia. Multivariable analysis showed that individuals who were in the middle, richer and richest wealth quintiles had increased odds of having HIV over those in the poorest quintile. Adults who had primary, secondary and higher educational levels had higher odds of being HIV positive than non-educated individuals.

A similar pattern was found by Yang et al. [91] in a study of the HIV epidemic in one Chinese city Suizhou. Those men engaged in high-risk behaviour (unprotected anal sex) were young, educated and married but were, in some measure, amenable to targeted interventions to encourage condom-use.

On the other hand, a systematic review of studies of HIV infection risk according to educational level in 11 sub-Saharan countries [92] showed significant positive changes over time:

Studies on data collected prior to 1996 generally found either no association or the highest risk of HIV infection among the most educated. Studies conducted from 1996 onwards were more likely to find a lower risk of HIV infection among the most educated. Where data over time were available, HIV prevalence fell more consistently among highly educated groups than among less educated groups, in whom HIV prevalence sometimes rose while overall population prevalence was falling. In several populations, associations suggesting greater HIV risk in the more educated at earlier time points were replaced by weaker associations later.

This supports the common public health wisdom that those with higher educational attainment are more likely to be amenable to influence with regard to risk and more likely to change their behaviour. This is supported in many studies, for example, in Zambia [93] and Thailand [94], but it is not the whole story.

In *Thirty Years of the AIDS Epidemic in Argentina* [95], Lavadenz et al. demonstrate very clearly the complexity of the picture and the great variability within one country or region. For them, the measure is years in education and while they see some strong trend in positive association between number of years in education and lowered risk of HIV infection, it is far from universal: Argentina and Peru show a positive correlation over the years 2000–2010; Chile and Venezuela a negative one. In Argentina, the picture is mixed, with 'higher educational attainment…associated with higher HIV incidence at the provincial level…The City of Buenos Aires has the highest level of schooling and the highest incidence of HIV' (p. 108). (It must be noted that this is only an *association*: we do not know the prevalence of infection among educated and uneducated groups, nor their relative numbers.)

Here, we have seen the interplay of the variables of educational level, financial status and, to some extent, age and geographical location. We have not explored others, such as sex, marital status, electronic connectivity or religion. While HIV is, in some respects, a special case, it nevertheless highlights for us the enormous complexity of risk perception and communication and human behaviour in relation to all areas of life.

Literacy and numeracy are important variables in a population's capacity to make use of risk and other communications. Levels of both are much lower than might be expected even in highly developed countries [96]. Much medical and safety material is written at a level well beyond the reach of a large percentage of most populations.

Reflection Education is by no means a guaranteed gateway to rational, scientific thinking. Low levels of education, literacy and numeracy may raise substantial barriers to the understanding and acceptance of information and risk communication. Few assumptions can be made about exactly how to approach populations, educated and uneducated. Only extensive research and testing can generate useful materials.

15.5   Risk Perception and Healthcare and Medicines

1. Regulation and Enforcement

Most citizens in most parts of the world expect their governments to make some effort to manage risk, protect them from harm, and help them when things go wrong. While actual performance in those three vital aspects of social safety and wellbeing varies across the world from negligible to admirable, most citizens will hope that the authorities will not voluntarily or negligently subject them to harm through their medicines, healthcare systems or public health policy. In particular, they generally have an expectation that medicines will be safe and are shocked and upset when they learn that any medicine may cause harm; that no medicine is 100% safe for all people in all situations. Even among highly educated populations, this truth can be a disturbing revelation when it becomes known. This has huge implications for medicines use.

Perception of medicines and their safety can also be complicated by irrational beliefs, such as the notion, in Ghana, for example, that vomiting prompted by a medication indicates the presence of a powerful and effective substance. In 2020, some very weird notions circulated about the aetiology of COVID-19 in several countries and threatened management of the virus. The science may be clear, but that does not mean everyone will believe it or follow its wisdom.

15.5.1 Traditional Medicines

Regulation and testing of traditional medicines (TM) and complementary and alternative medicines (CAM) in most parts of the world are at elementary stages compared with the systems for regulation of pharmaceuticals (see Chap. 13). Traditional medicines in all their forms are widely used in many developed countries but are the primary source of therapy for many hundreds of millions in developing countries, for more than half the population in China and Sierra Leone, for example. In many places, the traditional healer is often the first port of call even for serious illnesses; failures may lead to patients arriving at formal health facilities only when they are in a critical state. On the other hand, anecdotes abound of those who felt failed by modern medicine but found effective treatment by traditional methods. A 2011 study in rural Ghana [97] pinpoints why TM maintains such a powerful hold in many places:

> The role of TM is significant particularly in rural Ghana in the treatment of life-threatening and dreadful ailments. TM is affordable, readily available, hence, easily accessible and therefore utilized as such. There are other complex psycho-social and cultural factors associated with TM use. It is seen to be embedded in the personal values, religious and health philosophies of people.

That TM is embedded in complex aspects of everyday life and perception gives it a credibility and inevitability which is largely absent from perceptions of Western medicine in such countries. It means that people are familiar with the benefits and the harms and that they are comfortable with the risks and probabilities and know how to manage and accept them.

The growth in popularity of complementary and alternative medicines (CAM) and therapies in developed countries, a market worth tens of billions of dollars, is one of the remarkable phenomena of recent years. The naïve perception that CAM is natural and therefore safe is common in societies where there is no embedded history of its use. There is resistance to scientific evidence (e.g. with regard to homeopathy) and a proliferation of anecdotes that appear to show very positive, even miraculous, effects. Beyond our knowledge about substances and therapies that have no possible scientific basis for effectiveness, and the few that do, good evidence for the benefits and risks of CAM is hard to find. Users are engaged more in an act of faith than in a rational choice based on evidence. One brand marketing message in the UK conflates the issues: 'Powered by nature; proven by science,' leaving a sceptic wondering just what the science behind such products might be.

15.5.2   Regulation and Safety of Pharmaceuticals

The situation in relation to the safety of medicines in sub-Saharan Africa and beyond is vividly described in a report from the Strengthening Pharmaceutical Systems (SPS) Programme [98]:

> Several studies documented how ADRs[21] contribute to patient morbidity and hospitalization in Africa—4.5–8.4 percent of all hospital admissions were related to ADRs, 1.5–6.3 percent of patients were admitted as a direct result of ADRs; and 6.3–49.5 percent of all hospitalized patients developed ADRs. Moreover, ADRs accounted for the most frequent reason (45.5 percent) for treatment modification and interruptions in patients on ART...
>
> Counterfeit medicine is a growing threat across the world, accounting for up to USD 75 billion in sales in 2010. WHO estimates that more than 30 percent of the medicines for sale in some areas in Africa can be counterfeit. In Kenya alone, about USD 65 to 130 millions' worth of counterfeit medicines are being sold each year. The use of substandard and counterfeit medicines can lead to therapeutic failure, drug resistance, or even death. In Nigeria in 2008, more than 80 children died and many others were hospitalized after being given My Pikin Baby Teething Mixture®, a syrup containing a high level of the poisonous solvent diethylene glycol (DEG). In 2005, more than 60,000 people in Niger were inoculated with a counterfeit meningitis vaccine resulting in about 3,000 deaths. The extent of morbidity and mortality caused by counterfeit medicines is unknown, since most events are not detected and reported because of weak regulatory systems, lack of enforcement and the presence of unregulated markets.
>
> ...
>
> The US Institute of Medicine in 2006 estimated that more than 1.5 million Americans are injured every year by medication errors. The analysis of a database in Morocco shows that 14 percent of all suspected ADRs were associated with preventable medication errors.
>
> Insufficient and inadequate resources to monitor safety of medicines; the unreliable supply of quality, safe and effective medicines; the lack of trained health workers, and the weak state of the health systems in Africa are likely to contribute to significant medicines-related harm.[22]

---

[21] Adverse drug reactions.

[22] A recent scandal in Shandong Province, PR China (July 2018), involved the administration of tens of thousands of doses of sub-standard vaccines; the problems are not limited to Africa. See: Kuo L. 'They are devils': China's parents demand answers over vaccine scandal. Guardian. 25 July 2018. https://www.theguardian.com/world/2018/jul/25/china-vaccine-scandal-parents-demand-answers-rabies. Accessed 15 July 2020.

For multiple references for the content of this extract, please consult the original document.

In the 2010 report, Assessment of medicines regulatory systems in sub-Saharan African countries [99], the WHO team concluded:

> Structures for medicines regulation existed in the countries assessed, and the main regulatory functions were addressed, although in practice the measures were often inadequate and did not form a coherent regulatory system. Common weaknesses included a fragmented legal basis in need of consolidation, weak management structures and processes, and a severe lack of staff and resources. On the whole, countries did not have the capacity to control the quality, safety and efficacy of the medicines circulating on their markets or passing through their territories.

This echoes the conclusions of the George Institute report [100], published in the same year:

> Over 40 African MRAs were considered insufficiently functional and needing significant capacity building to perform fundamental regulatory tasks.

In an Institute of Medicine review of regulatory functioning in 12 countries [101], the authors found that:

> …regulators abroad face problems with: adhering to international standards, controlling supply chains, infrastructure, their laws, their workforce, institutional fragmentation, surveillance, communication, and political will.

The public profile and perceived integrity and effectiveness of a regulatory authority will have a profound effect on the public's confidence and risk perception. A weak, vacillating authority with a low profile will preclude confidence and leave question or doubts about the safety of medicines unanswered. In such a situation, people will turn to other sources of information such as traditional printed or broadcast media or social media, family and friends and where there is access, the Internet. They will also become critical or alienated and maybe resistant to guidance, as happened in the Ebola crisis in West Africa and in the USA and Spain (things were calmer and more controlled in the UK and Germany) [102]. On the other hand, the effective management of safety issues, such as the crisis arising from kidney failure from children's cough syrup containing diethylene glycol and contaminated tooth powder in Nigeria [103], do much to establish the credentials of an authority, even though some people will still believe that the danger should have been anticipated and prevented.

   The COVID-19 global pandemic presented the most extreme challenges in risk assessment, communication and management in modern times. Some governments met the challenge with effective performance in most aspects (South Korea, Singapore, New Zealand, Germany, Denmark among them), while others displayed denial, delay, incompetence and mixed messaging. In all cases, public perception of the pandemic and its risks were largely determined by communication from politicians and healthcare leaders; where these were strong and clear, positive perception led to positive behaviour. The USA, the UK and Brazil were among the worst performing countries, with tens of thousands of deaths attributable to the virus and huge numbers of excess deaths resulting from failures of systems under pressure.

Risk assessments were faulty or distorted by political interests; communications were driven by political priorities and were ambiguous or contradictory; risk management was beset by prior underfunding and inadequate procurement, prevarication and delay and fundamental failures of leadership. Trust has been fatally damaged in many places. In the greatest threat to public health in recent generations, many governments utterly failed their people and killed multitudes.

15.5.3 Perceptions of Medicines, Disease and Health Issues in Developing Countries

This section contains some examples of the varying perceptions of health-related risks in different parts of the developing world. Its purpose is to highlight the range and complexity of risk perception and behaviour and to alert us again to the fact that risk communication can hope to be effective only with an intimate prior knowledge of the target community.

An intelligent interest in the quality of drugs they are taking is an important element in the safety and health of patients. There is much evidence that many patients are buying drugs of doubtful quality without any real understanding of the risks. A study of drug-sellers and their patients in Lao PDR [104] highlighted some of the—alarming—issues in this area of interest:

> There was inadequate scientific drug knowledge among drug sellers. Only a few customers were aware of the existence of low quality drugs. Only one drug seller knew what constitutes a good quality drug according to the given criteria, and only two drug sellers knew the correct temperature for drug storage. Forty-four per cent had correct knowledge on drug labelling and 73% could read the expiry date. Fifty-eight per cent stated that they bought some drugs from unauthorized sources. Both drug sellers and consumers also elaborated on a local definition of drug quality. They determined drug quality by its perceived efficacy in the sense that a drug is good if it takes the disease away. They also trusted the responsible authorities not to provide them with low quality drugs. A majority of the consumers (73%) did not worry about the quality of the drugs, their greatest problem being financial constraints. People living in urban districts had significantly more knowledge on aspects of drug quality than those living in rural and remote areas.

Given the preoccupation with ability to pay among this sample of customers, it is odd that poor people were not concerned about value for their precious cash, that is, having good quality medicine. The cause and effect issue about taking medicines and recovering from illness is also one that leaves many questions unanswered. (The report of this research is greatly enriched by verbatim quotations from participants, some of which leave one deeply anxious about Laotian patients: for example, 'We don't care if it is with or without a label as long as it is a drug we take it. We don't know anything—if it is a poison it will not be sold to us'. The level of risk-blindness and uncritical trust in dubious sources is notable.)

In South Africa, there are problems in the perceptions of patients and health workers with regard to generic drugs: a lack of confidence in their quality [105].

Here, an important aspect of public health policy and communication has clearly been inadequate to influence the minds of many of the population.

A survey in Afghanistan [106] showed a public preoccupation with the regulatory issues of quality and price.

Pharmacy students in Malaysia [107] had a mature and integrational view of complementary and alternative medicine (CAM):

> This study reveals a high percentage of pharmacy students who were using or had previously used at least one type of CAM. Students of higher professional years tend to agree that CAMs include ideas and methods from which conventional medicine could benefit.

15.5.3.1 Perceptions of Epilepsy and Diabetes

A fascinating piece of work by Akhtar and Aziz [108] demonstrates the extraordinary range of perceptions of the aetiology (and therefore the risks) of epilepsy in a number of Muslim countries. It forces us to face the huge challenge of unscientific assumptions and thinking and their implications for every aspect of risk perception and communication with populations anywhere in the world:

> The perception of epilepsy varies in Muslim countries, according to the local cultural beliefs. In Nigeria, epilepsy is commonly thought to be contagious, even among medical students; hence persons with epilepsy are avoided. In Burkina Faso, Africa, epilepsy is considered to be contagious (by 44%) and hereditary (by 40%); while only 15% link it to a problem in the head and 7.8% think it being due to worms in the head. In Senegal, Africa, epilepsy is most frequently considered as a religious or magic mental affliction. In Afghanistan most rural people think it is caused by djinn. A study in a largely rural Muslim population in Kelantan, Malaysia showed 20% objected to their children associating with a person who sometimes had seizures, 48% objected to their children marrying someone who sometimes had seizures, and 58% thought that people with epilepsy should not be employed in jobs like other people. In another study among school teachers in Indonesia, where Muslims form the majority of population, 57% thought that epilepsy was a mental illness, and 20% thought that epilepsy was contagious.

References for all the cited studies can be found in the original article which is listed in the references at the end of this chapter.

The most commonly ascribed cause of Type 2 diabetes among a group of 523 Metropolitan Libyans was the will of Allah. More than one-third of them reported low adherence to their medication, with employed males showing the worst results.

15.5.4 Sanitation

A public health issue as apparently simple as promoting the use of latrines to reduce disease turns out to be much more complex than might be imagined. Thys et al. [109] showed how taboos and traditional practices shape perception and can stand in the way of change.

The study objective was to assess the communities' perceptions, practices and knowledge regarding latrines in a *T. solium* endemic rural area in Eastern Zambia inhabited by the Nsenga ethno-linguistic group, and to identify possible barriers to their construction and use.

Their findings took them into the very heart of the culture and values of the community:

Men expressed reluctance to abandon the open-air defecation practice mainly because of toilet-associated taboos with in-laws and grown-up children of the opposite gender. When reviewing conceptual frameworks of people's approach to sanitation, we found that seeking privacy and taboos hindering latrine use and construction were mainly explained in our study area by the fact that the Nsenga observe a traditionally matrilineal descent.

Their suggestions for communication were clear:

...in this local context latrine promotion messages should not only focus on health benefits in general. Since only men were responsible for building latrines and mostly men preferred open defecation, sanitation programmes should also be directed to men and address related sanitary taboos in order to be effective... In order to contribute to breaking the vicious cycle between poverty and poor health among livestock owners in developing countries, disease control strategies should always consider the socio-cultural context.

In India, almost half the population has no access to toilets; for them, defecation in the open is the norm. It is, of course, an enormous public health issue. A state council in the Gujarati city of Ahmedabad is trying to address the issue by paying children one rupee every time they use a public toilet [110]. Some adults perceive public toilets as the abode of witches or kidnappers and will not use them; some refuse on the grounds that the toilets are not clean (there could be some truth in this). The official message is 'Behave well and you'll be rewarded', in the hope that where children lead the way and change their behaviour, adults will follow. This campaign has not attempted prior communication of the complex and serious health risks of open defecation by appeal to cognitive faculties, but only to change behaviour, which may open the way to later understanding. (It is notable that women have a strong perception of the risk to their personal safety of going out to relieve themselves in the dark; nothing but a social revolution and domestic toilets will reduce that risk.)

This chapter is about the multiple, complex variables that shape risk perception and influence behaviour. The case of latrines illuminates profound issues among them, not least those who may perceive a risk but feel they are helpless to do anything to manage it.

15.6 Risk, Risk Perception and Change

Risk perception is not necessarily constant over time. New information, new experiences, changes in group or community opinion, stories on social media, pronouncements by national leaders or change in the socio-economic environment may modify or intensify perceptions of risk. Hayter et al. [111] found that rural village development had very mixed effects on the feelings and perceptions of people in rural India; while they perceived some benefits, participants

> ...believed their communities were currently less healthy, more polluted, less physically active, and had poorer access to nutritious food and shorter life expectancies than previously. There were contradictory perceptions of the effects of urbanization on health within and between individuals; several of the participants felt their quality of life had been reduced.

How far this perception of new risks was matched by the reality of new risks cannot be judged from the research, but the perception of new risks will almost certainly have been influenced by the eroding of traditional community values and security. Estimation of new risks is always likely to be more fearful than that for familiar risks.

The migration of rural people to urban environments exposes newcomers to some new specific risks, such as those associated with greater opportunity for sexual adventure and hence greater risk of HIV and other infections (see Ovediran above, ref. 84). There are also the more generalized risks of losing the security and familiarity of village relationships, values, customs and behaviour. This applies to internal migration (e.g. in Indonesia) [112] as well as external migration [113].

Men in Tonga are the most obese in the world and the women are close behind [114]; up to 40% of the population is thought to have Type2 diabetes [115]. Perception of the risk is complicated by the fact that physical size has traditionally been associated with success, wealth and attractiveness (this echoes the kudos of the full female physique in regions of Africa). Obesity became a national epidemic in the last half of the twentieth century as imports of fatty meat (especially cheap breast of lamb from New Zealand) and sugary drinks displaced the traditional basic diet of locally caught fish, vegetables and water as the principal beverage. While sumptuous feasting is also a characteristic of the nation's pleasures, it alone does not account for the massive surge in the population's weight.

Older people appear to understand the dramatic nature of the change and perceive the risks more clearly than the young. In an inspired act of leadership by example, King Taufa'ahau Tupou IV reduced his weight from a spectacular 209 kg in 1976 to 130 kg in 1997 [116], but the effort was not influential. Government action appears to have been ineffective in altering risk perception of obesity and changing behaviour, a failure of risk communication. (Multiple examples demonstrate that being informed does not necessarily lead to changing behaviour.)

The findings of the Lancet study show that developing countries are now carrying the greatest burden of obesity, while there has been slowing down in developed countries:

> Worldwide, the proportion of adults with a body-mass index (BMI) of 25 kg/m2 or greater increased between 1980 and 2013 from 28·8%...to 36·9%...in men, and from 29·8%...to 38·0%...in women. Prevalence has increased substantially in children and adolescents in developed countries; 23·8%...of boys and 22·6%...of girls were overweight or obese in 2013. The prevalence of overweight and obesity has also increased in children and adolescents in developing countries, from 8·1%...to 12·9%...in 2013 for boys and from 8·4%...to 13·4%...in girls. In adults, estimated prevalence of obesity exceeded 50% in men in Tonga

and in women in Kuwait, Kiribati, Federated States of Micronesia, Libya, Qatar, Tonga, and Samoa. Since 2006, the increase in adult obesity in developed countries has slowed down [114].

Strong, comprehensive public health initiatives over many years in Finland have shown remarkable results in improving health and longevity and in reducing many risks, such as death from smoking-related cancer and cardiovascular disease [117].

15.6.1   Access to Healthcare

Kenyans perceive many obstacles to accessing emergency care, although there appears to be an understanding of the time-critical nature of medical emergencies [118]. The risks of postponing early symptoms of illness seem not so well understood, though this may be influenced by the difficulties in accessing services and associated costs. This is one of the quite rare situations where there is no gap between the perception of risk and the risk itself: lack of emergency care is seen to be risky and undesirable and, of course, it is.

Once again, we are alerted to the multiple issues:

Socioeconomic and cultural factors play a major role both in seeking and reaching emergency care. Community members in Kenya experience a wide range of medical emergencies, and seem to understand their time-critical nature. They rely on one another for assistance in the face of substantial barriers to care—a lack of: system structure, resources, transportation, trained healthcare providers and initial care at the scene.

Access to healthcare is one of the elements in the worldwide problem of stillbirths. Studies published in The Lancet [119] estimate that there are around 2.6 million stillbirths a year,[23] 98% of which occur in low and middle income countries, more than 90% of which are preventable with high quality ante-natal care; 78% are in sub-Saharan Africa and south Asia. In sub-Saharan Africa, two thirds of stillbirths occur in rural areas; worldwide, about 40- million women give birth unattended each year. The highest rates are in Pakistan, Nigeria and Chad, while Rwanda has made progress in significantly reducing the numbers. The issues and risks here relate to access and to quality of care, both of which deeply affect perceptions of maternal risk and actual life-chances for many communities. While perception may be that these tragedies are more or less inevitable, the truth is that they are not. Improvements can come only through positive risk management, when governments provide the resources and individuals understand that they can take a measure of control.

It is worth pausing briefly to consider the case of Rwanda where great progress has been made in reducing maternal and child mortality [120]. There was been strong,

---

[23] We should note that a comparable number of children, maybe more, die from malnutrition every year. See: Maternal and child nutrition. Lancet. 6 June 2013. http://www.thelancet.com/series/maternal-and-child-nutrition#sthash.C9OeY0ui.dpuf. Accessed 15 July 2020.

visionary leadership from the Ministry of Health, especially from Minister Agnes Binagwaha. Forty-five thousand community health workers were elected, officially appointed and trained as front-line representatives of healthcare. They deal with vaccination programmes, screening for malaria and all simple maladies and are also able to recognize conditions that need professional help, especially the most urgent and critical. Management Sciences for Health (MSH) helped the Government introduce a simple text-messaging system (RapidSMS) that puts easy contact with other levels of the health service into the hands of community health workers, many of whom had never seen a mobile phone prior to the scheme being introduced.

A Save the Children UK report [121] points out:

> They have [also] improved female empowerment, education, nutrition, water and sanitation... [which] also affect children's chance of survival.

The same report points out the hazards of averaged national statistics about issues like this: some countries have improved their statistics but have achieved this by tackling the 'low-hanging fruits' and actually increasing the disparity between the privileged and the disadvantaged.

15.6.2 Quality of Health Professionals

Medicine is fundamentally an altruistic profession, that is, it is focused on the welfare of others, even though there may be less admirable elements such as profit, reputation, status and so on that drive some practitioners.

While the global impact of medicine in the last century has been staggeringly positive and benign, its practice, nevertheless, gives rise to many risks beyond the intrinsic risks of medical science itself. Those risks are associated with the nature of the individuals and the systems in which they work.

Here are a few of the risk factors that affect the safety and welfare of patients in many developing countries[24]:

- Inadequate staff resources for growing demand: This puts immense pressure on time and on the length of patient consultations and has inevitable consequences in risks of misdiagnosis, inappropriate prescribing, patient dissatisfaction, rational use and compliance [122].
- Inadequate training for pharmacists: patient encounters with dispensing pharmacists are often seconds rather than minutes (e.g. 52 second in Nepal [123]), involving little in the way of checking prescriptions or providing benefit-risk information.

---

[24] In this section, I have referenced some examples from Nepal, drawing on the literature review, Irrational Use of Drugs in Nepal, carried out by Pramesh Koju, at the School of Global Studies, Thammasart University, under the supervision of Dr Stephane.P. Rousseau. Similar findings would come from many other countries.

- Unqualified pharmacy staff and illegal sales: Many pharmacies in the developing world are not staffed by qualified pharmacists and sale of prescription-only medicines is common [124].
- Poor regulation and enforcement leave the market open to informal, unqualified sellers hawking poor quality or counterfeit drugs on the streets.
- In authoritarian, hierarchical or paternalistic social or professional cultures, the voice of patients may not be heard and critical information about the patient's disease, risks, concerns, priorities and life in general may never be discovered.
- Corrupt or poorly managed supply-chain management may introduce dangers even into the official healthcare system. (A stunning recent example was the fake heart drugs scandal in Pakistan) [125, 126].
- Improper pressure from the pharmaceutical industry may negatively affect drug choices and prescribing practices [127].
- The costs of service and medicines may inhibit patients from seeking treatment at all or prompt them to risky behaviours such as medicine-sharing, stopping taking medicines to accumulate them for future use, or seeking unreliable and potentially dangerous, cheaper alternatives [128].

15.7   Risk Communication

There is an enormous literature on risk perception and risk communication. Important work was done in the last century and much of it still stands strong, particularly the founding work of people like Slovic, Kasperson and Fischoff. Many of the older generation are still writing and working. Gigerenzer, Sandman, Spiegelhalter and Löfstedt have been influential recently. An excellent, very short introduction can be found in Public Risk Perception and Environmental Policy, from the University of the West of England [129], and a comprehensive review of all aspects including methods and practice in the fifth edition of *Risk Communication: A Handbook for Communicating Environmental, Safety and Health Risks* [130]. Making Health Communication Programmes Work (known as 'The Pink Book') from the US National Cancer Institute is an intelligent, helpful, clear account of most of the essential issues, downloadable and free [131]. This chapter can do no more than touch on some of the multiple issues and challenges.

15.7.1   Why Do We Communicate Risk?

The purpose of risk communication is to help individuals and communities make good decisions. Most often, there is a persuasive, argumentative element promoting a particular choice or behaviour that would reduce harm or loss of benefit for individuals or society at large. Immunization, smoking-cessation, rational use of antibiotics, vector control against mosquitoes, hand-washing, prescription adherence, safe-sex, seeking ante-natal care, and increased exercise are prominent medical and public health examples. At other times, communication is aimed at informing an audience about choices and their differing consequences when neither benefit nor harm is conclusive. Alternatives for treatment of cancers and other diseases, the benefits and harms of HRT or statins or screening for breast or prostatic cancer fall into this group. The former intends to change behaviour in a particular direction for individual and common good; the latter to facilitate decisions that meet individual wishes and priorities, which include their level of risk-tolerance.

We must note here, again, that information itself is not sufficient to bring about change or to help patients make good decisions. The enterprise of risk communication is much more complex than that.

There are two primary domains in risk communication: individual, as with a single patient, and public, as in public health and other communal concerns such as disaster-preparedness or pandemic response. We shall pay less attention to the second category in this chapter.[25]

Many of the principles of good risk communication are common to both, so we shall look at the overall picture before focusing principally on individuals.

Reflection In pharmacovigilance, one of the principal communications objectives is to provide simple, clear information about the benefits and harms of medicines, vaccines and devices and their use. The core information must be tailored to multiple channels and audiences, directly or via intermediaries, such as regulators or health professionals. Health professionals must have the skills to help patients make sense of it and make their decisions. Information itself may not be sufficient to help people manage risk and make good decisions.

15.7.2 Trust

Of all the variables in the pursuit of effective risk communication, trust in the communicator and confidence in their judgement are probably the most essential. Kasperson identified four critical elements in the establishment of trust:

- Commitment
- Competence
- Care or empathy
- Honesty

It is very difficult to establish such qualities at all, let alone overnight or in the short-term. Authorities, organizations and health professionals need to have a

---

[25] But see the author's Expecting the Worst for a thorough review of risk and crisis communication in all sectors of healthcare (available in English, Chinese, Japanese and Spanish). Uppsala Monitoring Centre, Sweden (English edition, 2010). Downloadable pdf in English at: Uppsala Monitoring Centre. www.who-umc.org. Accessed 15 July 2020.

long-term track record of credibility if they are to have the best chance of reaching and influencing audiences and if, collectively, they are to be trusted. If there is public memory of less than satisfactory performance in the past, then that is an additional and substantial obstacle to new communication projects. Regulators and institutions need to have a constant programme of communications so that they are regularly in the public ear and eye, even when there are no urgent issues to address (see also Media below, p. 70). Communicators need to be trusted, and therefore, they need to be familiar to their audiences as features of the common landscape and as entities who have earned their trust. Among the qualities essential for trust is the perception that the audience's feelings and priorities are understood and cared about and that's where empathy starts to play its part. This is as true of organizations and communities as it is of health workers and individual patients. Some of the serious problems, and some of the deaths, associated with the Ebola outbreak in 2014–2015 were attributable to poor (often late) communications from authorities who were not trusted [102]. Nothing destroys trust more completely than the revelation that risk information has been withheld from the public or that officials have lied or prevaricated; evident mismanagement (as in the COVID-19 pandemic) is a fatal threat to trust and, of course, to compliance and risk reduction.

15.7.3   Empathy: Dialogue, Understanding and Engagement

No communication between free adults (e.g. as opposed to those between autocrat and subject) can work if there is not a high level of mutual understanding, trust, respect and empathy. Empathy is the ability to see and feel the world through the eyes of another and to sense exactly what it is like to be another person. Not all problems and conflicts could be solved through empathetic engagement, though many can, but it is certain that most attempts to reach and influence others cannot succeed without the exercise of genuine empathy, followed by action that accords with the insights gained. Helping others reach their own, voluntary decisions that are satisfactory for them (e.g. about therapy or lifestyle issues) can rarely be achieved by the one-way transmission of edicts, information, advice or guidance, unless they are perfectly tailored to the audience's feelings and values and arrive at a time of readiness. Guidance on diet and alcohol consumption has failed to have much effect on behaviour, for example, because the population does not perceive or understand the risks or wish to change their habits.[26] Even when provisions have legal force, they may have little or no effect if they do not match the preferences of the population and there is no effective enforcement.

---

[26] It is also the case that scientific guidance on diet has been through so many versions and revisions, some involving complete U-turns (the whole saturated fat and cholesterol question being one such reversal), that the public may not know what to think, who to trust or what to take seriously.

Communities may resist decisions that are imposed on them without prior discussion and negotiation even when there could have been a plausible chance of influencing them in the early planning stages. This is almost certainly true of the polio crisis in northern Nigeria, where the mindset of local leaders and communities was never explored prior to implementation.

Reflection Communications delivered by those who are perceived as thinking they know best are likely to prompt resistance and cynicism. Communication will work only when there is a deep, empathetic grasp of the reality of the lives of the target audience that is perceived and felt by them.

15.7.4 Risk Communication Principles

- Prior to any intervention, explore and research the values, perceptions, preferences, demography and culture of the target population. (The first part of this chapter provides a rich basis for thinking about the research agenda in this area.)
- Ensure that plans for any intervention are shaped by the knowledge gained from prior research and engagement in the community *and by the wishes and capacity of the target population and by the extent of its willingness to co-operate.*
- Ensure that the audience genuinely feels that they have been listened to and taken seriously and that there is evidence of their contribution in the final plans.
- With patients, ensure a comprehensive, empathetic grasp of the patient's experience, priorities, perceptions and wishes before presenting options or making (joint) decisions about therapy.
- Ensure that the patient feels that the reality and complexity of their lives, in principle or in detail, are understood and respected and are driving the communication
- Present risk information in a way that meets to patient's abilities, preferences and priorities

15.7.5 Beware! Bureaucracy and Safety

There are aspects of bureaucracy and some bureaucrats that are inimical to effective, open communication: sluggishness, secretiveness, cautiousness, distance, arrogance, use of jargon among others. Many bureaucrats are remote from the populations they serve, either geographically, socially or psychologically; they exist behind high walls in centralized institutions with loyalties divided between political or commercial masters, establishment traditions, rules and priorities, the public and their own self-serving career priorities. The odds are weighed against empathy, engagement, influence and impact. There are benign and effective bureaucracies, but the risk of failure and corruption is always present. (For a detailed discussion of these issues, see this author's work in Drug Safety [132].) There is also a great risk to coherence and continuity in the developing world from the constant moving of staff from post to post, often just at the point they are beginning to achieve some competence and mastery of their responsibilities.

Anyone working within a bureaucracy must understand the risks of institutional distance from people and issues, and blindness to needs and preoccupations in the outside world, to false priorities that are driven by hidden institutional biases and pressure. They must understand that the public often view bureaucracies with great cynicism and that to reach and influence people requires almost revolutionary vision and effort.

Bureaucracies are enthusiasts for statistics and data (and forms) and often perceive the world through a lens of numbers. Most people see the world through the lens of their feelings; even when statistics were widely trusted, they were not necessarily influential in determining behaviour, and in the third decade of the twenty-first century, their credibility has declined further. People may not only ignore statistics or number-based arguments (e.g. the low number of children harmed by vaccination) but may have their negativity intensified by what is known as the *backfire effect*: cascading information and data, far from persuading or converting, simply increases a sense of being under attack and results in a consolidation of a previous position. If predominant emotional realities are not understood and engaged with, facts (in whatever form) are irrelevant and useless.

Pharmacovigilance has been built on a bureaucratic model: the filling in of forms and their processing by remote, centralized officials [133]. Officials need data; they create forms and consequential paperwork and manual processes and make entirely unreasonable demands on over-stretched professionals. Over-stretched professionals ignore these demands about which they were never consulted resulting, in this case, in the well-known phenomenon of under-reporting of ADRs—to a huge and tragic extent [134].

While electronic and mobile reporting have become familiar in Europe and the USA, developing countries have been slow to catch up. Kenya was the first African country to ditch the ineffective, old-fashioned paper-based approach to this vital, urgent contemporary issue [135]. In 2013, the Pharmacy and Poisons Board launched digital reporting, using mobile technology alongside their existing web reporting tool. Uganda is researching the potential [136]. In India, there is an Android reporting app [137, 138]. Things are moving, and the dead hand of paper is weakening.

Two important issues arise from these observations and developments: first, if the ultimate purpose of pharmacovigilance and risk communication, that is, the greater safety of patients, is to be achieved, there must be effective communications throughout the network of officials, health professionals, patients and the public. Promoting ADR reporting throughout healthcare, and among patients, is, in itself, a great communications challenge. It requires not only research, engagement and dialogue, but also the right methods and tools, as well as evaluation and follow-up. It requires a decentralized, user-centred focus, which many officials and official systems find very hard to embrace. It also requires creativity and the willingness to take risks. The Uppsala Monitoring Centre's Take&Tell campaign is a good example of a lively and engaging approach to the serious issue of encouraging patients to report adverse events to their physicians [139] in a surprising and novel way, but regulators and PV personnel often do not have the imagination, courage or the skills to strike out in new ways.

Mobile Health (m-Health) in all its forms—Telemedicine, also known as Telehealth and Telecare—in India [140], Africa [141], Australia [142] and, emerging in Europe [143], and Remote Patient Monitoring (RPM) are transforming access to medical care and delivery with affordable, effective, popular services for everyone, though the impact is particularly dramatic for dispersed rural populations and housebound patients, poor or not. The vision of these schemes is radical; the embrace of technology is uncompromising; the communications are fluid, vivid and direct.

SMART Health India [144] is one such programme:

> ...a unique low-cost, high-quality healthcare delivery system that enables both community health workers and doctors to provide state-of-the-art healthcare for common chronic diseases for a fraction of the price it would otherwise cost. It utilizes advanced mobile health technologies that provide the healthcare worker with personalized clinical decision support to guide the Systematic Medical Appraisal Referral and Treatment (SMART) of individual members of the community.

At the heart of this, and several other of the innovative Indian schemes, are Accredited Social Health Activists (ASHAs), who are mature members of village communities, usually women (there are 650,000 villages in India). Across the globe, the term Community Health Worker (CHW) has been adopted to identify a wide range of participants in comparable schemes [145]. The radical impact of these initiatives relates to *decentralization*: a substantial fraction of diagnostic and treatment services are removed from institutions (primarily urban) and from centralized professional monopoly, dispersed, placed firmly in the middle of everyday, neighbourly life. Regulators and PV centres have not begun to react to these imperatives of dispersal and decentralization (indeed many are going in the opposite direction), especially, to the genius of local people on the ground as agents of change.

Reaching the People: Imaginative and Radical Solutions

The world's first hospital train, the Lifeline or Jeevan Rekha Express [146], was launched in India in 1991. In China, there is the 'Eye Train' Lifeline express [147]; in South Africa, the two Phelophepa Trains of Hope [148]. These have reached and treated millions of poor rural people who would otherwise have had no access to health facilities. Different environments require different solutions: to reach isolated communities in the shifting riverine and delta landscape of Bangladesh, hospital ships cruise the inland waterways [149]; the Orbis flying eye hospital [150] reaches communities far from health resources in south-east Asia. These are all icons of compassionate and effective outreach, challenging traditional notions of centralized, institutional service and communication. They change people's perception of healthcare and of risk beyond recognition.

Sundar Subramanian et al. make the point vividly in a recent article in the Harvard Business Review [151]:

In a few years, the idea of receiving medical treatment exclusively at a doctor's office or hospital will seem quaint. Wearable technologies, implanted devices, and smartphone apps allow continuous monitoring and create a ubiquitous, 24/7, digitized picture of your health that can be accessed and analysed in real-time, anywhere. Data gathering isn't the only force moving treatment out of the doctor's office; telemedicine, home diagnostics, and retail clinics increasingly treat patients where they live and work. In the next decade, these trends will create a veritable gold rush in patient data and consumer options.

These developments do not just relate to diagnosis and treatment, but to the availability of data, safety data in particular, on a scale that is as yet unimagined. Apps and devices in the hands of patients—and health professionals—offer enormous new opportunities.

Reflection Paternalism and bureaucratic processes stand in the way of open, trusted communications. Increasingly, audiences everywhere are demanding more transparent, collaborative, effective relationships and methods.

15.7.6   The Printed Word Is Not Sufficient

Reliance on the transmission of important information through the passive printed word is still the method favoured by many bureaucracies (one-size-fits-all package inserts are the prime example in our field). In the past, when there were few alternatives, there was some justification, but in the middle of the third decade of the twenty-first century, with so many vibrant alternatives, there is no excuse. Although patient information leaflets have, in some places, been produced in the minority languages of the country, even in Braille—gestures towards diversity—rarely is there a range of leaflets targeting the different populations using the same language, providing, for example, for those with the lowest levels of literacy and numeracy,[27] or for women.

Many of the old ways must be phased out in favour of the rich new possibilities. Nevertheless, there is one traditional method—woefully neglected—that needs reviving and invigorating: conversation between prescriber or dispenser and patient—the most powerful, influential approach to managing the risks that patients face with their medications. If physicians cannot find the time, then pharmacists must. They are the final safety net for patients, and they meet almost every patient in the world both in health facilities and in retail outlets. They are central to the future of risk communication and patient safety and possibly for the vigorous growth of ADR reporting too.

---

[27] I owe this insight to Prof David Spiegelhalter; see: Cambridge University. Professor David Spiegelhalter: Communicating risk and uncertainty. YouTube. 17 Aug 2011. https://www.youtube.com/watch?v=JhfMkmzaNdU. Accessed 15 July 2020.

If face-to-face is not possible, then alternatives, with access to people's homes and lives through the human voice, are phone and radio. In Uganda, radio is heard by a large majority of the population; carefully tailored health information (and distance learning materials for village health teams, see above) have had a significant impact. The Uganda national health hotline [152] has also had an immense appeal and response, especially in reaching men. Text messaging is a rich and important channel (Tanzania's healthy pregnancy text messaging service is a good example [153]).

15.7.7   Routine Public Health Campaigns Are Not Enough

Research into the effects of the UK's Change4Life (C4L) campaign to reduce childhood obesity showed that awareness of the campaign was increased, but that there was almost no change in attitudes or behaviour among the target population of parents and children [154]. The notorious case of the FDA's lengthy campaign to reduce the contra-indicated use of cisapride showed how intractable were the habits of prescribing physicians and how little they paid attention to official guidance [155]. Researchers concluded:

> The FDA's 1998 regulatory action regarding cisapride use had no material effect on contra-indicated cisapride use. More effective ways to communicate new information about drug safety are needed.

On the other hand, successful campaigns show a degree of innovation, creativity, and, especially outreach and engagement, through mobile staff, TV, radio and the active use of whatever broadcast or electronic media as are available [156]. Such campaigns include:

- Zambia: Helping each other act responsibly together (Heart) to reduce HIV
- Bangladesh: Oral rehydration therapy for diarrhoea
- World Vision India HIV awareness campaign for people with a disability
- Tanzania: Wazazi Nipendeni (Love me, parents)
- The Americas: Vaccination Weeks
- Thailand: Safe sex and HIV prevention (see footnote 14, p. 22)

The Health Communication Partnership Uganda was a particularly successful example of an ambitious, nationwide, broad-front public health campaign, with rich and varied resources addressing different populations about a wide range of issues (HIV prevention and treatment, domestic violence and the position of women, safe male circumcision, TB and malaria prevention, contraception and much more). The Final Report (2012) [157] is a record of remarkable achievements and of the multifarious techniques and strategies employed throughout the campaign. It serves as an emblem of best practice, of use to audiences anywhere in the developing (and developed) world.

The key learning points from the whole project were these (p. 12):

15.7.8   Key HCP Project Learnings

- Communities and individuals are the creators of health; health communication needs to provide balanced information that allows people to make informed choices.
- A collaborative and participatory approach to health communication design and implementation strengthens partnerships and ownership of project outcomes and leads to lasting changes in health communication and service delivery.
- Effective communication strategies draw on evidence-based practices, a thorough analysis of health issues, input from audience representatives, and utilization of relevant behavioural theories.
- Strengthening capacity for health communication at all levels from individuals at household level to service providers, community leaders, the media, and national leaders improves the reach and effects of communication efforts.
- Health communication that addresses barriers to change at more than one level of society is more likely to result in adoption of health practices.
- Communication is a two-way process. Monitoring and evaluation are necessary in order to get feedback and adjust messages and approaches so the messages reach the right people, are understandable and relevant.
- National communication efforts need a minimum of 2 years to allow for proper design and at least a year of implementation.
- Project documentation should begin from the first day of the project.

Two years for planning; at least 1 year for implementation: yes, it takes time. Fifty-odd years to reach a point where smoking is, in the West, socially unattractive and on the decline.

Reflection Successful communications projects in the twenty-first century almost always ditch the sluggish old centralized modes of thinking and action and show qualities of creativity, adventurousness, agility, outreach and empathy.

15.7.9   Experts and Amateurs

While we should not set the barriers too high, we must understand that communication is a sophisticated speciality, with, not least, a vast body of research and experience already behind it. The task cannot reasonably just be handed to any member of the team or tagged onto a project as some kind of after-thought. It requires embedding in planning and specialist knowledge and skills.

Fischoff, in an excellent, if somewhat technical chapter called Risk Perception and Communication, in a first class book on the subject [158], sets out the range of expertise needed to reach and influence those making decisions (e.g. communities, or patients):

In order to communicate effectively, organizations require four kinds of expertise:

(a) Subject matter specialists, who can identify the processes creating and control-
    ling risks (and benefits)
(b) Risk and decision analysts, who can estimate the risks (and benefits) most per-
    tinent to decision makers (based on subject matter specialists' knowledge)
(c) Behavioural scientists, who can assess decision makers' beliefs and goals,
    guide the formulation of communications, and evaluate their success
(d) Communication practitioners, who can manage communication products and
    channels, getting messages to audiences and feedback from them

In simpler language, this means you need specialists in

- The topic (e.g. pharmaceuticals, cancer therapy, tropical disease)
- Assessing and characterizing risks and what implications they have for action
- Understanding the complex reality of audiences, how they can be reached and
  listened to and how communications might be evaluated
- Doing the communications job and interacting with audiences.

We should add anthropology as a further discipline of relevance and importance.

If there is only one person responsible for risk communication, they must
embrace all these elements of knowledge and skill or have access to other expert
resources for consultation. But there are other, deep problems, as we shall see in the
next section. And essential are the talents of professional graphic designers and
social and general media whizz-kids.

In the HCP Uganda campaigns, the personnel involved and committed ranged
from the Minister of Health, though healthcare professionals, radio and TV person-
alities and producers, designers, teachers, community leaders, volunteers, and
many, many more—and, of course, large numbers of Ugandans from all regions and
walks of life: a coalition of multiple partners.

15.7.10   The Realities of Target Audiences

There is an elegant and comprehensive review of all the technical and statistical
ways in which risk can be expressed (relative risk, odds ratio, number needed to
treat, and so on) by Mahmoud Elbarbary [159] and similar coverage in many other
articles and texts. Risk communication personnel need to understand all the technical stuff and be able to assess and deconstruct trial results and research outcomes.

It is very clear that relatively few people, including doctors, fully understand
health statistics and risk data. In the introduction to one of the most brilliant reviews
of the whole topic anywhere, Gigerenzer et al. [160] observe:

Many doctors, patients, journalists, and politicians alike do not understand what health
statistics mean or draw wrong conclusions without noticing. Collective statistical illiteracy
refers to the widespread inability to understand the meaning of numbers. For instance,
many citizens are unaware that higher survival rates with cancer screening do not imply
longer life, or that the statement that mammography screening reduces the risk of dying
from breast cancer by 25% in fact means that 1 less woman out of 1,000 will die of the

disease. We provide evidence that statistical illiteracy (a) is common to patients, journalists, and physicians; (b) is created by nontransparent framing of information that is sometimes an unintentional result of lack of understanding but can also be a result of intentional efforts to manipulate or persuade people; and (c) can have serious consequences for health.

This is a serious, disconcerting issue. Along with low levels of literacy and numeracy and the substantial category of low health-literacy/numeracy across all populations (widespread, maybe 50%, in even well-educated communities [161]), the enterprise of risk communication begins to look deeply challenging.

Different populations will require different kinds and levels of risk information expressed in quite different ways. A campaign for HPV vaccination has multiple and complicated risk communication demands that are quite different from, for example, those of a woman with ductile carcinoma in situ (DCIS).

For public acceptance of HPV vaccination, the prevalence of the virus and the causal link between it and cervical and related cancers must be believed; the effectiveness and safety of the vaccine and the integrity of its origins and of those running the programme must be trusted; the advisability (and moral sensitivity) of vaccinating young, even pre-pubertal girls, must be understood. These issues alone touch on many of the multiple aspects of risk perception raised in this chapter: scientific discourse, cause and effect, belief in evidence, credibility of officials and programme managers, source and quality of vaccines, religion and traditional beliefs (particularly relating to the sexual component of HPV transmission), the influence of sceptics, the evidence for benefits and harms; and the whole sphere of ethics and the realms of perception and emotion about the welfare of children. There is no doubt that low- and middle-income countries carry the greatest burden of cervical cancer, with 'mortality rates in some parts of Africa being 15 times higher than in North America' [162], and the scale and the urgency of the problem has to be grasped if people are going to be willing to consider taking action.

Though more than 200 million girls have been vaccinated worldwide, public responses to the programmes have been very varied: uptake in Australia has been exceptional, in the UK excellent, in the USA relatively low. Concerns about side effects led to the abandonment of the programme in Romania [163] (a country with the highest burden of cervical cancer in Europe) and to the cessation of active promotion of vaccination in Japan. Question about complex regional pain syndrome (CRPS) and postural orthostatic tachycardia syndrome (POTS) and other conditions following HPV vaccination have resulted in considerable negative publicity and genuine doubt among some scientists, though the WHO's Global Advisory Committee on Vaccine Safety (GACVS) continues to assert that the evidence for harms is weak and inconclusive [164]. With plans to introduce HPV vaccination to developing countries, the need for active surveillance is pressing. GACVS remarks:

> The greatest health benefit globally is anticipated in countries without routine cervical cancer screening, where the vaccine is yet to be introduced. Enhanced spontaneous reporting of adverse events following immunization should be put in place to ensure that those who could benefit the most from the intervention are vaccinated with adequate safety monitoring.

The challenges for risk communication are considerable: first, to characterize adequately the risks of cervical and associated cancers and the benefits of vaccination; second, to counter the negative narratives promoted by vaccine sceptics and hostile media, especially vivid anecdotes of alleged harm[28]; third, respond to the genuine concerns of some scientists; fourth, to overcome the resistance of parents to their perception of the moral and behavioural resonance of putting their young daughters forward for vaccination against a sexually transmitted virus.

Though there is little evidence for long-term harm, even the best evidence list of known harms [165] might alarm a sensitive parent, and anecdotes of alleged adverse effects are alarming and persuasive. The undoubted population benefit is unlikely to be sufficiently persuasive for an anxious parent; the real issue is: what is the risk of my child suffering harm from the vaccination weighed against the risk of life-threatening cancer in the future? Different people will assess those risks differently. However, successful programmes, such as those in Australia and the UK, do strongly suggest that the quality and range of communications have a radical effect on public perception and uptake.

In the past, for women diagnosed with DCIS, surgery or radiation would almost certainly have been proposed as a matter of urgency. However, new evidence reported by the National Cancer Institute (NCI) [166] suggests that women with DCIS:

...generally have a low risk of dying from breast cancer. In addition, treating these lesions may help prevent a recurrence in the breast but does not appear to decrease the already-low risk of dying from the disease, even after 20 years of follow-up... The overall death rate from breast cancer at 20 years after diagnosis was 3.3 percent, a rate similar to that of the general population.

Specific groups had differential death rates:

Some women with DCIS may be at an increased risk of dying from breast cancer, including those diagnosed at a younger age and African Americans, the study showed. Death rates were higher for women diagnosed before age 35 than for older women (7.8 percent versus 3.2 percent), and higher for African Americans than for Caucasians (7 percent versus 3 percent).

The implications of all this for risk perception and communications are profound. While the new evidence is provisional and awaits more studies for corroboration, it needs to be part of the material provided for a woman with a new diagnosis. In addition there are all the complex issues of benefit and harm, and uncertainty, associated with breast cancer screening and treatment.

The authors of the NCI report note

...a potential parallel with prostate cancer and the development of careful follow-up, rather than initial surgery, to manage screen-detected early stage cancers.

---

[28] This issue is comprehensively discussed in an excellent MedScape report by Zosia Chustecka: Chustecka Z. Case reports of 'syndrome' appearing after HPV vaccination. 18 Sept 2015. http://www.medscape.com/viewarticle/851186. Accessed 15 July 2020.

Decisions about both DCIS and prostate cancer involve complex issues of evidence and personal preferences based on a host of individual characteristics. For the active and literate, there are rich resources available; for those less capable—the great majority in the world—there is no substitute for thoughtful, empathetic, individual counselling.

Reflection Risk and risk statistics are poorly understood even among professionals; that and limited public understanding, along with confounding issues of anxiety and perceived harm, raise the communications stakes very high.

15.7.11 Expressing Risk

Good decisions must be made about what forms of risk expression to use. Gigerenzer advises us:

> A major precondition for statistical literacy is transparent risk communication. We recommend using frequency statements instead of single-event probabilities, absolute risks instead of relative risks, mortality rates instead of survival rates, and natural frequencies instead of conditional probabilities.

These are important observations:

- Explain probability by how often events occur (3 in 1000, etc.) and over what period of time
- Use absolute numbers for expressing increase or decrease in risk (increase from 3 in 1000 to 6 in 1000, for example, not 'a doubling of risk'; in addition, use the same denominators for comparing risks)
- Use all-cause mortality data (e.g. for screened and unscreened groups); survival rates are almost meaningless because of lead-time bias and other problems

We have to be sure that the population that the statistics refer to is relevant to the patient in front of us in terms of age, sex, lifestyle, disease history, ethnic characteristics and so on. In developing countries, we must check that the population originally tested shares the same ethnic and genetic profile as the patient (the anti-malarial Lapdap was a signal example of this problem [167]); medicines approved in Western countries for Western populations may have quite different effects elsewhere. We must also remember that epidemiology, and clinical trials in particular, give us information about populations, not about individuals; the reality of *this* patient in *this* situation may not be reflected in the results of big studies.

We need to be aware of issues like *framing*: we influence others by the order in which we present information and by our own implicit preferences that may influence how we present information or ask questions. If you talk about the figures for those who benefit from a particular option, the numbers who do not benefit may not be so vivid; the reverse is true too: promote the number who experience no effect or are harmed, and the benefits may be shadowed. One method for managing this dilemma is the use of pages of patient icons or pictographs (e.g. 100, or 1000) where the entire sample is visible, with both benefits and harms equally presented. John Paling has done particularly useful work in this field [168]. (There are excellent examples on Pinterest [169].)

A Good Result?

The simplest of language may give rise to misunderstandings.

Is a 'positive' result to a test for disease a good or bad result? Not everyone will understand the special meaning of the word in this context, nor that a 'negative' result is a very good thing. It may be best to avoid the taken-for-granted jargon altogether.

Clarity and simplicity of language in all matters is essential. An audience's level of comprehension must be rigorously tested before any materials are produced.

CDC has excellent reference materials [170] and a clear communication widget [171] for all aspects of communication in English. The principles apply to all languages and audiences: for example, use only language that is part of the everyday vocabulary of the target audience [172]; ensure the main message is the first thing to catch the reader's eye [173]. Many of the first principles seem obvious, but they are frequently neglected.

Every patient will have different abilities and preferences with regards to the form in which risk information is presented. Some will manage with the best figures, as characterized by Gigerenzer; some will need charts or graphics to make sense of the figures; some will need help with the whole notion of probability and the unsettling fact of uncertainty (see p. 67 for more on this). Some will want verbal explanations, supported by paper or web-based information; some may prefer informative videos or animations; some may want to use their phones. Some will value text message reminders about their medications, their appointments or other matters.

Decision aids and option grids are two important tools in risk communication, and there is good evidence that they have a positive impact, as a Cochrane review [174] reported:

> Trials of decision aids indicate that they are superior to usual care interventions in improving knowledge and realistic expectations of the benefits and harms of options; reducing passivity in decision making; and lowering decisional conflict stemming from feeling uninformed.

The most sophisticated decision aids will help patients calculate their risk based on their unique profile and on the best evidence available. An excellent example of such a tool is the Mayo Clinic Statin Choice Decision Aid [175]. Smokers and ex-smokers can calculate their lung cancer risk and the wisdom of screening with tools from shouldiscreen.com. In the field of breast cancer treatment, there is a 'a web-based tool that provides automated risk assessment and personalized decision support designed for collaborative use between patients and clinicians' [176]. NHS

England has a range of tools for shared decision making, covering several types: 'including one-page sheets outlining choices (e.g. option grids), more detailed leaflets (e.g., brief decision aids and shared decision making sheets), computer programmes to DVDs, mobile apps and interactive web-sites (e.g. patient decision aids)' [177].

No single method for any issue or medication can ever reach even a fraction of the total interested population. Package inserts, or some highly developed, creative version of them, apps, web-based or on paper, may provide the foundation information for any medication, for access by health professionals or patients. While such tools are invaluable starting points for investigation, few of them can ever match the existential reality and needs of any individual patient. That can happen only through empathetic interaction with another human being and through tools and resources chosen for and perfectly matched to that patient.

The concept of community health workers, outlined above, holds the primary key to patient safety in communities of all kinds in all kinds of environments. It also holds the key to safety surveillance and the rapid reporting of problems of any kind with medicines. Where patients can access regular health facilities, the burden of responsibility for risk communication must be on the shoulders of prescribing physicians; when they fail (and they commonly do in this respect), it is static or mobile pharmacists or health workers who must take up the task and provide what we may regard as the beginning of true community healthcare.

Few physicians or pharmacists consistently follow up their patients and learn the outcomes of therapy. Few patients report back about their experience of medicines unless they have some disturbing problem, and not all of those return to their provider or say anything. We know too little about all aspects of medicines use and safety, especially in the community (almost all research on ADR prevalence, for example, takes place in hospitals).

15.7.12   What To Do

Some decisions that patients and communities need to make are preference-sensitive, that is, they involve a choice as between several different courses of action with differing risks and the need to choose between different benefit-harm trade-offs, determined partly by quality-of-life preferences; this is true of treatment choices for a range of cancers, for example. Some decisions are binary (e.g. treatment/no treatment; vaccination/no vaccination). In a helpful review of aspects of best practice, Fagerlin et al. [178] make these recommendations for risk communication for cancer patients, though they have applicability to a much wider range of circumstances:

1. Use plain language to make written and verbal materials more understandable.
2. Present data using absolute risks.

3. Present information in pictographs if you are going to include graphs.
4. Present data using frequencies.
5. Use an incremental risk format to highlight how treatment changes risks from pre-existing baseline levels.
6. Be aware that the order in which risks and benefits are presented can affect risk perceptions.
7. Consider using summary tables that include all of the risks and benefits for each treatment option.
8. Recognize that comparative risk information (e.g. what the average person's risk is) is persuasive and not just informative.
9. Consider presenting only the information that is most critical to the patients' decision making, even at the expense of completeness.
10. Repeatedly draw patients' attention to the time interval over which a risk occurs.

While this advice is entirely sound, it focuses on the cognitive aspects of risk communication. We have already referred to the very large spontaneous, emotional element in risk perception; consideration of the impact of this must be a constant aspect of risk communication. A patient receiving a disturbing diagnosis will be fully occupied with the emotional impact of the news, maybe shocked, angry, distressed, overwhelmed. Initially they will be in no state at all to apply their brains to the cognitive aspects of the diagnosis, treatment options, prognosis and so on. The first duty of risk communication in such a situation is to reduce the extent of emotional arousal by providing empathetic attention and support. It may be hours or days before a patient is in any kind of state to talk coolly about treatment, risk-benefit and all those important issues. This is a single instance of one of the major themes of this chapter: for individuals or communities, we must know their entire state of mind and emotions at the point we communicate with them. Our behaviour must be perfectly calibrated to their situation, and they must be in a state of readiness to engage with us.

15.7.13 Communicating Uncertainty

Mary Politi is one of the leading lights in the field of communicating uncertainty. In an overview of the field [179], she records patients' desire for certainty and providers' urge to comply, in spite of the risks of later problems. The risks of expressing uncertainty badly include less patient satisfaction with decisions, lower perceived credibility of the provider, lower adherence by the patient. However, patient-centred care and shared decision-making principles require that:

> ...to better support patients' decisions, clinicians should, at the very least, acknowledge uncertainty, clarify its sources, and communicate to patients as partners to help them through the emotionally laden process of grappling with unknowns.

Failure to admit uncertainty can lead not only to loss of credibility, but even to disaster.[29] Patients will not be pleased if they have a negative outcome the possibility of which they were not alerted to (in litigious nations, patients are also likely to sue). Assertion of unwarranted confidence can also be perilous, as the US CDC found when it declared that management of Ebola cases on home-soil was under control and it turned out to be far from the case [180]. Few medical interventions come with any precise degree of certainty of positive or negative outcomes; though probabilities may be well defined at population level, what will happen to *this* patient in *this* situation is much more uncertain. The use of web-based risk-calculators for individuals is a very positive start to discussions. (One example is the Mayo Clinic's Heart Disease Risk Calculator for patients' own use [181].)

Uncertainty—that is the range of probabilities—can be expressed in many ways: numerically ('from 4 in 100 to 7 in 100,' or 'between 4% and 7%') with or without graphical representation of the range; as a fan chart, showing the risk range over time; as icon arrays in blocks or scattered pattern; as coloured icons that fade or blur through the range of uncertainty; as bar charts, pie charts or graphs. The choices are many for both acute and chronic risks. Every communicator needs to be familiar with such different methods and to use those that are matched with the preferences and abilities of the audience (see box, p. 69).

Reforming the Presentation of Medical Information: Examples
This is just a tiny selection from a host of good work that has been done in recent years. What they all illustrate is that with a fresh, creative mind and the patient or a community firmly at the centre of concern, complex information can be made accessible and attractive.

1. Animated risk information
   Cochrane reviews provide the highest quality evidence for a wide range of conditions and treatments. One such is *Surgery or radiotherapy for early cervical cancer of the adenocarcinoma type* [182]. The summary of results is a complex page of data. This has been translated into an elegant and helpful animation by understanduncertainty.com [183]. It is a perfect tool to use as the basis for discussion between a patient and physician about risks and benefits on the road to making decisions about treatment.

---

[29] A non-medical example demonstrates the risks vividly: 'The levées of the Red River in Grand Forks, North Dakota, are built to withstand 51-ft water levels. In 1997, the National Weather Service predicted a flood, but despite a 35% margin of error for previous estimates, it emphasized that the river would crest at 49 ft at most. When the waters rose to 54 ft, wreaking havoc on the area, local inhabitants were shocked and angry'. See: Rosenbaum [180].

2. The Drug Facts Box

   Schwartz et al. developed and tested a Drug Facts Box for Tamoxifen, a simple, tabular presentation of benefit-risk information. After more than a decade, it remains one of the best examples of accessible, elegant presentation of complex drug information for an audience with basic literacy and numeracy skills [184].

3. The Blood Test gets a Makeover

   In this brilliant piece of re-imagining of the presentation of test results with sophisticated graphic design, pages of data largely incomprehensible to patients are made meaningful and helpful (examples here are basic workup, prostate and heart disease tests). These examples were published in Wired [185], under the influence of the talented Thomas Goetz (see his TED talk on YouTube [186], watched four and a half million times).

4. Mobile health apps for Africa

   (a) 'Smart Health' app: 'The free application called "Smart Health" is the first Android "Made for Africa" mobile health and wellness platform that encourages behavioural changing practices to help reduce the transmission and infection rates of AIDS, Malaria, and Tuberculosis...Future releases will include information on nutrition and Prenatal / Postnatal mother and newborn care'. [187]

   (b) Drugs of abuse: 'The Drug Free World app (created by Lightworx Ltd.) provides mobile access to information on the most commonly abused drugs, youth can instantly view at the time they need it most–when they are being exposed to drugs...The app is tailored to appeal to youth, and incorporates the edgy graphics, award-winning videos and virtual booklets shown on this site. It provides the history of each individual drug, its effects on the body and mind.' [188]

   (c) AFRICA: Mobile phones for health [189]: for a summary of projects in Kenya, Ghana, Nigeria, Ethiopia, South Africa and Uganda see the web page.

5. Carefully targeted websites, such as kidshealth.org

6. The WEB-RADR mobile reporting app (the 'White app'), originally developed for the UK, the Netherlands and Croatia, now live in Zambia and Burkina Faso with potential for the whole continent (https://web-radr.eu/)

Part of risk communication is accustoming patients to the degree of uncertainty in any intervention. While using the best evidence will always be the touchstone of good practice, even the best evidence will provide only probabilities.

15.7.14   Assessing Impact

We have discussed the importance of intense research and planning and the pre-testing all kinds of communications with representatives of the real intended audience. None of this, nor indeed any other communications activity, has credibility if impact is not assessed: did attitudes, beliefs or behaviour change and to what extent? If so, why? If not, why not? We can assess the extent of change only if we have some measure of the situation before the intervention which requires research prior to any aspect of planning or implementation to provide a baseline for comparison.

Qualitative assessment of communications can be made without baseline data. When a physician has completed a risk communication session with a patient, that patient's level of satisfaction with the encounter can be reviewed along with the elements that they liked or disliked and those that they found influential or problematic. (We should note that self-reported data or observations can be very unreliable.) This is a large—and vital—field of enterprise that we cannot deal with here with more than a token mention. There is a very substantial literature on assessing health and risk communication effectiveness, three examples of which appear in these references [190–192].

15.7.15   The Media

Radio, TV, newspapers, Internet and social media all play major roles in the fields of medicine and patient safety. They shape risk perception; they are constantly generating fast, creative, influential communication that can reach the remotest communities and cross national boundaries; they may misrepresent science or fan the flames of controversy or crisis, but they are also critical partners in the pursuit of improved public health and patient safety, and we underestimate or ignore them at our peril.

Building partnerships with journalists and bloggers does not guarantee that our messages will be transmitted uncritically, but ignoring or villifying them will mean we have no influence whatsoever and are likely to be criticized more often than supported. Journalists, bloggers and vloggers (video bloggers), influencers must be among the audiences we frequently engage with in an active and mutual collaboration: we need their reach and influence; they need our information and materials to fill their pages and air-time.

The most progressive and successful organizations establish and nurture relationships with the primary journalists and bloggers in their region and work as colleagues. There is a constant flow of communication and information between them, ensuring that the best information is rapidly made public and, in crises, that quick and accurate responses reduce anxiety and uncertainty. In many countries, there are regular health information columns and radio or TV programmes (e.g. Bhutan, Ghana) that are produced in collaboration between officials and media outlets.

There is a predominant view among officials that journalists are dangerous and unreliable and should be avoided. This often arises because of bad experiences in the past, when the degree of distance or alienation between officials and media meant that there was no consultation and no possibility of a balanced view being presented. Collaboration does not put us beyond criticism, especially if there have been bad decisions or failures of some kind, but it hugely increases the chances of the official view being put forward and reaching the public.

There should always be a serious media relations policy, including designated spokespersons, regular dialogue with all relevant professionals in the media and a conscientious programme of active dissemination of information. PV centres and regulatory authorities need skilled press officers who are the channel through which important information is disseminated and feedback collected. Some of the problems of media reporting (e.g. neglect of denominators in safety issue stories) result from journalists being provided with information that they have trouble interpreting (clinical trial results, for example), material that has not been tailored for them *as a specific and influential audience*. Many health stories are written by non-specialists with little or no knowledge of science and medicine. Where there are specialists or health journalist associations (e.g. Uganda), or where collaborative training is offered (as in Ethiopia), health reporting is usually more balanced and responsible. Such specialists and specialist groups should be embraced and supported.

15.7.16   Social Media

Smartphones and social media hold an even greater potential for reach and influence and are already playing a significant part in healthcare and patient safety. Text messaging with the cheapest and most basic mobile phones is reaching remote audiences. These are now essential channels for healthcare support and risk communication.

In the USA, The Mayo Clinic is a leader in digital communications of all kinds [193], offering examples and methods for organizations everywhere. The potential in the developing world is even greater [194] and no regulatory authority, public health programme or clinic can afford to remain on the sidelines of this escalating phenomenon, as some of the examples in this chapter have shown. X (Twitter), Facebook, WhatsApp, YouTube, podcasts, and many others have a major role; use of these platforms is essential to engagement with modern populations and it requires expert, agile, energetic management.

Smartphones can also play a part in checking the quality and safety of medicines with new forms of medicine packaging, smartphone-enabled for recognition of authenticity.

15.7.17   Intermediaries

Risk communication in medicine inevitably depends on intermediaries in order to reach its audience. Customarily, such intermediaries are health professionals and media personnel of all kinds. However, there are many others, who may play a unique and effective part in the process of reaching audiences. Some of the examples already quoted illustrate the importance of religious and civic leaders; then there are teachers and village elders; community health workers in all their varieties; and representative members of target communities or groups—pregnant women, sex workers, HIV+ citizens, TB patients, and so on. We have talked about choosing the appropriate technical channels for communication (radio, print, text message, etc.) but need always to think of the possibility of human channels with their immense potential for influence. There are many situations in which the obvious methods won't reach their targets. The preferences of pregnant women in rural Tibet for sources of peri-natal information are a vivid example of this issue [195]. The study authors concluded:

> Despite recent efforts in Tibet to use group teaching, television/radio programmes, and health professionals visiting patients' homes as health communication modalities, participants preferred to learn pregnancy-related health messages from their close family, especially their mothers. Future health communication interventions in rural Tibet and similar communities should consider targeting close family members as well as pregnant women to maximize acceptability of advice on healthy pregnancy and delivery

This is a useful object lesson on which to end this chapter: our best attempts to reach our audiences will fail if we do not pay sensitive and realistic attention to their habits, wishes and preferences.

15.8   Conclusions

We have seen that risk perception is a complex phenomenon. It is influenced by a host of elements that must be understood and factored into any kind of risk communication at population or individual levels. Risk perception will influence feeling and behaviour in the management of everyday life and in response to medical and public health issues. Risk perception is acutely specific to individuals and communities and to particular hazards, threats or probabilities; feeling and behaviour with regard to one category of risk will not necessarily predict feeling and behaviour in relation to another.

While the conditions of life vary enormously for people across the world, the mechanisms of risk perception and the feelings and behaviour associated with them appear to be common to all humanity, infinitely variable though they may be. Equally, it seems that, for all humanity, the principal agents for change are empathy, trust, engagement and collaboration; the major obstacles to change are imposition, alienation, distrust.

Risk communication at individual and population levels is a complex and demanding discipline. At one end of its spectrum, it is a creative, imaginative socio-cultural pursuit; at the other, the routine transmission of technical and scientific data and information. Activities at those extremes, and at the multiple points in between, must be tailored exactly to the wishes, needs, values, preferences and abilities of the target population. The mature purpose of risk communication is to facilitate the making of voluntary decisions and choices by individuals and communities that will please them and bring the benefits they want or are persuaded they should want for themselves and their neighbours.

Key Points

- The purpose of risk communication in clinical practice and public health is to inform and protect; to support wise, balanced and rational decisions that match patients' and citizens' wishes and needs and keep them safe.
- In this chapter, we use the term 'pharmacovigilance' in its widest, modern sense: a concern with the safety of patients and citizens in relation to the use of vaccines, allopathic and traditional medicines, devices and other interventions, and in particular, with identifying and communicating any kind of adverse effects or associated problems and preveting harm.
- At the individual patient level, risk communication is about helping patients and physicians come to the best possible joint decision about the options available, especially the trade-offs in possible benefits and harms.
- There is immense variance in the perceptions, thoughts and feelings about risk across all individuals and populations.
- While risk is officially associated with data, for most people the primary association is emotional.
- Risk perception has deep sources embedded in personal, social, economic, cultural and a host of other factors.
- Behaviour change is a hugely ambitious project.
- Communication will not succeed if it is not tailored precisely to the reality of the audience and is not developed and delivered in ways that are perceived to be respectful, empathetic, engaged, collaborative and relevant,
- Communication will succeed only when it is seen to come from sources that are trusted
- Poorly designed communication risks causing perverse effects and damaging unintended consequences.
- Risk communication may have to negotiate with influential forces that are neither rational nor scientific.
- Risk communication must reach groups (e.g. women, sex workers and homosexuals) who, oppressed, in some locations, have low levels of self-determination and freedom of movement or expression and live with other influential, often hidden, risks
- Remote bureaucracies are particularly ill-equipped to communicate effectively with diverse audiences.
- Effective risk communication requires specialist skills and resourceful, creative, innovative methods and relationships.
- Literacy, health literacy and numeracy are issues that require special attention in risk communication, as does a generally poor level of risk literacy among professionals and lay people.
- Uncertainty is one of the great challenges of risk communication: the urge for comforting certainty is strong and must be managed skilfully.

Acknowledgements A number of friends and colleagues have contributed their wisdom and experience during the preparation of this chapter; I am grateful for their kindness and commitment: Jigme Tenzin (Bhutan), Assegid Mengistu (Ethiopia), Shota Jibuti (Georgia), Yvonne Yirenkyiwaa Esseku (Ghana), Yathendra Madineni (India), Dinesh Thapa (Nepal); Ambrose Isah (Nigeria), Wiltshire Johnson and Onome Thomas Abiri (Sierra Leone), Helen Ndagije (Uganda).

Katrina Fray capably and cheerfully helped me through the wilderness of referencing the chapter, bringing a sublime degree of meticulous attention to the task.

References

1. Boholm Å. Anthropology and risk. London: Routledge; 2015.
2. Rappaport RA. Risk and the human environment. Ann Am Acad Pol Soc Sci. 1996;545:64–74. https://doi.org/10.1177/0002716296545001007.
3. Sharot T. The optimism bias. Curr Biol. 2011;21:941–5. https://doi.org/10.1016/j.cub.2011.10.030.
4. Roy MM, Liersch MJ. I am a better driver than you think: examining self-enhancement for driving ability. J Appl Soc Psychol. 2013(43):1648–59. https://doi.org/10.1111/jasp.12117. *Summary at:* When it comes to driving, most people think their skills are above average. Association for Psychological Science. 28 Aug 2014. http://www.psychologicalscience.org/index.php/news/motr/when-it-comes-to-driving-most-people-think-their-skills-are-above-average.html. Accessed 12 July 2020.
5. Kruger J, Dunning D. Unskilled and unaware of it: how difficulties in recognizing one's own incompetence lead to inflated self-assessments. J Pers Soc Psychol. 1999;77:1121–34. https://doi.org/10.1037/0022-3514.77.6.1121.
6. Bench SW, Lench HC, Liew J, Miner K, Flores SA. Gender gaps in overestimation of math performance. Sex Roles. 2015;72:536–46. https://doi.org/10.1007/s11199-015-0486-9.
7. Dunlap RE, Gallup GH Jr, Gallup AM. Of global concern: results of the health of the planet survey. Environ: Sci Policy Sustain Dev. 1993;35:7–39. https://doi.org/10.1080/0013915 7.1993.9929122.
8. Chang EC, Asakawa K. Cultural variations on optimistic and pessimistic bias for self versus a sibling: is there evidence for self-enhancement in the West and for self-criticism in the East when the referent group is specified? J Pers Soc Psychol. 2003;84:569–81. https://doi.org/10.1037/0022-3514.84.3.569.
9. Atkinson S. The optimism divide. Ipsos Global Trends; 2017. https://www.ipsosglobaltrends.com/2017/04/the-optimism-divide/. Accessed 17 July 2020.
10. Bray A. Young men 'much more reckless' than women. Irish Independent. 2 Jan 2013. http://www.independent.ie/irish-news/young-men-much-more-reckless-than-women-28953329.html. Accessed 11 July 2020.
11. In the region of 1.35 million road traffic deaths per year throughout the world (2020). Road traffic injuries. WHO. 7 Feb 2020. https://www.who.int/news-room/fact-sheets/detail/road-traffic-injuries. Accessed 17 July 2020.
12. What evidence is there that cycle helmets save lives? Bicycle helmet research foundation. http://www.cyclehelmets.org/1012.html. Accessed 11 July 2020.
13. Study of bicycle helmets reveals how dangerous they are. Freestyle cyclists. 1 Jan 2014. https://www.freestylecyclists.org/study-of-bicycle-helmets-reveals-how-dangerous-they-are/. Accessed 11 July 2020.
14. Nikolov P. Does AIDS treatment stimulate negative behavioral response? A field experiment in South Africa. Harvard University. 19 Feb 2011. http://www.iaen.org/library/30_nikolov.pdf. Accessed 17 July 2020.
15. Yee TH. Antibiotic abuse killing thousands in Thailand. Straits Times. 12 Nov 2016. https://www.straitstimes.com/asia/se-asia/antibiotic-abuse-killing-thousands-in-thailand. Accessed 11 July 2020.

16. Cuba life expectancy at birth. IndexMundi. https://www.indexmundi.com/cuba/life_expectancy_at_birth.html. Accessed 11 July 2020.
17. Reynolds-Tylus T. Psychological reactance and persuasive health communication: a review of the literature. Front Commun. 2019. https://doi.org/10.3389/fcomm.2019.00056.
18. Chartrand TL, Dalton AN, Fitzsimons GJ. Nonconscious relationship reactance: when significant others prime opposing goals. J Exp Soc Psychol. 2007;43:719–26. https://doi.org/10.1016/j.jesp.2006.08.003.
19. Kakutani M. The death of truth. Glasgow: William Collins; 2018. This is one among a slew of significant contemporary writings on the topic.
20. Chigwedere P, Seage GR, Gruskin S, Lee T-H, Essex M. Estimating the lost benefits of antiretroviral drug use in South Africa. J Acquir Immune Defic Syndr. 2008;49:410–5. https://doi.org/10.1097/qai.0b013e31818a6cd5.
21. Coronavirus: outcry after Trump suggests injecting disinfectant as treatment. BBC News. 24 Apr 2020. https://www.bbc.co.uk/news/world-us-canada-52407177. Accessed 12 July 2020.
22. Sabaté E. Adherence to long-term therapies: evidence for action. Geneva: WHO; 2003.
23. New Cochrane health evidence challenges belief that omega 3 supplements reduce risk of heart disease, stroke or death. Cochrane. 18 July 2018. https://www.cochrane.org/news/new-cochrane-health-evidence-challenges-belief-omega-3-supplements-reduce-risk-heart-disease. Accessed 12 July 2020.
24. Greenberg P. Fool's gold: what fish oil is doing to our health and the planet. Guardian. 25 July 2018. https://www.theguardian.com/lifeandstyle/2018/jul/25/fish-oil-hype-health-planet-supplements-study-no-benefit. Accessed 12 July 2020.
25. Oslo is the crystal meth capital of Europe. Local. 5 June 2015. http://www.thelocal.no/20150605/oslo-methamphetamine-capital-of-europe. Accessed 12 July 2020.
26. H P. 25 countries with the highest suicide rates in the world. 21 Feb 2015. http://list25.com/25-countries-with-the-highest-suicide-rates-in-the-world/5/. Accessed 12 July 2020.
27. HIV and AIDS in East and Southern Africa regional overview. Avert http://www.avert.org/professionals/hiv-around-world/sub-saharan-africa/overview. Accessed 12 July 2020.
28. Smith D. Drug capitals of the world. Economy Watch. 5 May 2011. http://www.economywatch.com/economy-business-and-finance-news/drug-capitals-of-the-world.06-05.html. Accessed 12 July 2020.
29. Vijayakumar L, John S, Pirkis J, Whiteford H. Suicide in developing countries (2): risk factors. Crisis. 2005;26:112–9. https://doi.org/10.1027/0227-5910.26.3.112.
30. Smith Fawzi MC, Lambert W, Boehm F, Finkelstein JL, Singler JM, Léandre F, et al. Economic risk factors for HIV infection among women in rural Haiti: implications for HIV prevention policies and programs in resource-poor settings. J Women's Health. 2010;19:885–92. https://doi.org/10.1089/jwh.2008.1334.
31. Amirkhanian YA, Tiunov DV, Kelly JA. Risk factors for HIV and other sexually transmitted diseases among adolescents in St. Petersburg, Russia. Fam Plann Perspect. 2001. https://doi.org/10.1363/3310601.
32. Walker SP, Wachs TD, Gardner JM, Lozoff B, Wasserman GA, Pollitt E, et al. Child development: risk factors for adverse outcomes in developing countries. Lancet. 2007;369:145–57. https://doi.org/10.1016/S0140-6736(07)60076-2.
33. Loewenstein GF, Weber EU, Hsee CK, Welch N. Risk as feelings. Psychol Bull. 2001;127:267–86. https://doi.org/10.1037/0033-2909.127.2.267.
34. Slovic P, Weber EU. Perception of risk posed by extreme events. Columbia University; 2002. http://www.rff.org/files/sharepoint/Documents/Events/Workshops%20and%20Conferences/Climate%20Change%20and%20Extreme%20Events/slovic%20extreme%20events%20final%20geneva.pdf. Accessed 12 July 2020.
35. Laughland O, Felton R. 'It's all just poison now': Flint reels as families struggle through water crisis. Guardian. 24 Jan 2016. http://www.theguardian.com/us-news/2016/jan/24/flint-michigan-water-crisis-lead-poisoning-families-children. Accessed 12 July 2020.
36. AIHW. Deaths in Australia. Australian Institute of Health and Welfare. 2019. https://www.aihw.gov.au/reports/life-expectancy-death/deaths/contents/life-expectancy. Accessed 17 July 2020.

37. Wolkowicz J. When modern medicine and traditional culture collide. Helix Magazine. 27 Jun 2011. https://helix.northwestern.edu/blog/2011/06/when-modern-medicine-and-traditional-culture-collide. Accessed 12 July 2020.
38. Goal: improve maternal health. UNICEF. http://www.unicef.org/mdg/maternal.html. Accessed 12 July 2020.
39. Slovic P. Perception of risk. Science. 1987;236:280–5. https://doi.org/10.1126/science.3563507.
40. Rosin H. The overprotected kid. Atlantic. 2014. http://www.theatlantic.com/magazine/archive/2014/04/hey-parents-leave-those-kids-alone/358631/. Accessed 12 July 2020.
41. Flitter MA, Riesenmy KR, van Stralen D. Current medical staff governance and physician sensemaking: a formula for resistance to high reliability. Adv Health Care Manag. 2012;13:3–28. https://doi.org/10.1108/s1474-8231(2012)0000013006.
42. Renn O, Burns WJ, Kasperson JX, Kasperson RE, Slovic P. The social amplification of risk: theoretical foundations and empirical applications. J Soc Issues. 1992;48:137–60. https://doi.org/10.1111/j.1540-4560.1992.tb01949.x.
43. Kahneman D, Slovic P, Tversky A. Judgement under uncertainty: heuristics and biases. Cambridge: Cambridge University Press; 1982.
44. Ubel PA. Beyond costs and benefits: understanding how patients make health care decisions. Oncologist. 2010;15(Suppl 1):5–10. https://doi.org/10.1634/theoncologist.2010-S1-5.
45. Nichols T. The death of expertise: the campaign against established knowledge and why it matters. New York: Oxford University Press; 2017.
46. Tanka Bawa J. Malaria: from myths to management. Malaria Vaccine Initiative. 30 Apr 2012. https://www.malariavaccine.org/news-events/news/malaria-myths-management. Accessed 12 July 2020.
47. Dixon B. Cultural traditions and healthcare beliefs of some older adults. Red River College. 2009. http://www.virtualhospice.ca/Assets/cultural%20traditions%20and%20healthcare%20beliefs%20of%20older%20adults_20090429151038.pdf. Accessed 12 July 2020.
48. Sharma A. The Hindu tradition: religious beliefs and healthcare decisions. Park Ridge Centre. 2002. https://www.advocatehealth.com/assets/documents/faith/hindufinal.pdf. Accessed 12 July 2020.
49. Leflar RB. The cautious acceptance of informed consent in Japan. Med Law. 1997;16:705–20.
50. Hugman B. Chapter 18: Perspectives on risk communication and gender issues. Chapter 19: Risk communication and specific medicines for women. In: Harrison-Woolrych M, editor. Medicines for women. ADIS; 2015. p. 531–83, 585–627.
51. First do no harm – the report of the IMMDS Review. Independent Medicines and Medical Devices Safety Review. 8 July 2020. https://www.immdsreview.org.uk/downloads/IMMDSReview_Web.pdf. Accessed 18 July 2020.
52. Alcalde MC. The woman in the violence: gender, poverty, and resistance in Peru. Nashville: Vanderbilt University Press; 2010.
53. Anand G, Woo J. Asia struggles for a solution to its 'missing women' problem. Wall St J. 26 Nov 2015. http://www.wsj.com/articles/asia-struggles-for-a-solution-to-its-missing-women-problem-1448545813. Accessed 12 July 2020.
54. Female genital mutilation (FGM). WHO. http://www.who.int/reproductivehealth/topics/fgm/prevalence/en/. Accessed 12 July 2020.
55. New study: women more likely to die after a heart attack due to unequal treatment. World Heart Federation. 10 Jan 2018. https://www.world-heart-federation.org/news/new-study-women-likely-die-heart-attack-due-unequal-treatment/. Accessed 17 July 2020.
56. Finding myself in your hands: the reality of brain tumour treatment and care. Brain Tumour Charity. https://www.thebraintumourcharity.org/about-us/our-publications/finding-myself/. Accessed 12 July 2020.
57. George R. Menopause: a condition that affects half the population is woefully neglected. Scroll.in. 30 Jan 2016. http://scroll.in/article/776077/menopause-a-condition-that-affects-half-the-population-is-woefully-neglected. Accessed 12 July 2020.

58. Makino M, Tsuboi K, Dennerstein L. Prevalence of eating disorders: a comparison of Western and non-Western countries. MedGenMed. 2004;6:49.
59. Flynn J, Slovic P, Mertz CK. Gender, race, and perception of environmental health risks. Risk Anal. 1994;14:1101–8. https://doi.org/10.1111/j.1539-6924.1994.tb00082.x.
60. Olofsson A, Rashid S. The white (male) effect and risk perception: can equality make a difference? Risk Anal. 2011;31:1016–32. https://doi.org/10.1111/j.1539-6924.2010.01566.x.
61. Meeting the unique health-care needs of LGBTQ people. Lancet. 2016;387:95. https://doi.org/10.1016/S0140-6736(16)00013-1.
62. Friedman M. The psychological impact of LGBT discrimination. Psychology Today. 11 Feb 2014. https://www.psychologytoday.com/blog/brick-brick/201402/the-psychological-impact-lgbt-discrimination. Accessed 13 July 2020.
63. Kotiswaran P. Dangerous sex, invisible labor: sex work and the law in India. Princeton: Princeton University Press; 2011.
64. Spectator. Sex worker leaks secrets. Modern Ghana. 4 Oct 2008. https://www.modernghana.com/lifestyle/483/16/sex-worker-leaks-secrets.html. Accessed 13 July 2020.
65. Hill F. Prevention better than cure in Cuban healthcare system. BBC News. 13 Dec 2015. http://www.bbc.com/news/health-35073966. Accessed 13 July 2020.
66. Lyn TE. Drug companies influence prescribing, study finds. Reuters. 19 Oct 2010. http://www.reuters.com/article/us-doctors-influence-idUSTRE69I6DK20101019. Accessed 13 July 2020.
67. Good governance for medicines: curbing corruption in medicines regulation and supply. WHO. 2007. http://www.who.int/medicines/areas/policy/goodgovernance/GGM.pdf. Accessed 13 July 2020.
68. Kano shuns Nigeria polio campaign. BBC News. 12 Dec 2003. http://news.bbc.co.uk/2/hi/africa/3313419.stm. Accessed 13 July 2020.
69. Jawaid A. Pakistan's polio workers targeted for killing. Al Jazeera. 17 Dec 2013. http://www.aljazeera.com/indepth/features/2013/12/pakistan-polio-workers-targeted-killing-201312118364851379.html. Accessed 13 July 2020.
70. Pakistan arrests parents for refusing polio vaccine. BBC News. 2 Mar 2015. http://www.bbc.com/news/world-asia-31703835. Accessed 13 July 2020.
71. Moftah L. Vaccination controversy: no autism, MMR vaccine link, new study finds. International Business Times. 21 Apr 2015. http://www.ibtimes.com/vaccination-controversy-no-autism-mmr-vaccine-link-new-study-finds-1891420. Accessed 13 July 2020.
72. Voodoo recognized as an official national religion of Haiti. World History Project. 4 Apr 2003. https://worldhistoryproject.org/2003/4/4/voodoo-recognized-as-an-official-national-religion-of-haiti. Accessed 13 July 2020.
73. Salmoni D. World's deadliest towns. Animal Planet. Bristol: Icon Films; 21 Feb 2011. *See short synopsis here:* World's deadliest towns. Icon Films. https://iconfilms.co.uk/wp-content/uploads/2018/05/imported-Worlds%20Deadliest%20Towns%20Publicity%20Notes.pdf. Accessed 17 July 2020.
74. Guynup S. Haiti: possessed by voodoo. National Geographic. 7 July 2004. https://www.nationalgeographic.com/news/2004/7/haiti-ancient-traditions-voodoo/#:~:text=In%20Haiti%20these%20rituals%20are,voodoo%20for%20over%20a%20decade. Accessed 13 July 2020.
75. Dodoo A, Adjei S, Couper M, Hugman B, Edwards R. When rumours derail a mass deworming exercise. Lancet. 2007;370:465–6. https://doi.org/10.1016/S0140-6736(07)61211-2.
76. Drakard M. Why some Africans fear Western medicine. MercatorNet. 10 Aug 2007. http://www.mercatornet.com/articles/view/why_some_africans_fear_western_medicine/2398. Accessed 13 July 2020.
77. Head J. Deadly dish: the dinner that can give you cancer. BBC News. 13 June 2015. http://www.bbc.com/news/health-33095945. Accessed 13 July 2020.
78. Sui C, Lacey A. Asia's deadly secret: the scourge of the betel nut. BBC News. 22 Mar 2015. http://www.bbc.com/news/health-31921207. Accessed 13 July 2020.

79. New report reveals high prevalence of betel, tobacco chewing in Western Pacific. WHO. 23 Mar 2012. https://www.who.int/westernpacific/news/detail/23-03-2012-new-report-reveals-high-prevalence-of-betel-tobacco-chewing-in-western-pacific. Accessed 13 July 2020.

80. Bloch M, Althabe F, Onyamboko M, Kaseba-Sata C, Castilla EE, Freire S, et al. Tobacco use and secondhand smoke exposure during pregnancy: an investigative survey of women in 9 developing nations. Am J Public Health. 2008;98:1833–40. https://doi.org/10.2105/AJPH.2007.117887.

81. Chomba E, Tshefu A, Onyamboko M, Kaseba-Sata C, Moore J, McClure EM, et al. Tobacco use and secondhand smoke exposure during pregnancy in two African countries: Zambia and the Democratic Republic of the Congo. Acta Obstet Gynecol Scand. 2010;89:531–9. https://doi.org/10.3109/00016341003605693.

82. Smedberg J, Lupattelli A, Mårdby A-C, Nordeng H. Characteristics of women who continue smoking during pregnancy: a cross-sectional study of pregnant women and new mothers in 15 European countries. BMC Pregnancy Childbirth. 2014;14:213. https://doi.org/10.1186/1471-2393-14-213.

83. Hsu C. Muslims least likely to engage in premarital and extramarital sex, study suggests. Medical Daily. 19 Oct 2012. http://www.medicaldaily.com/muslims-least-likely-engage-premarital-and-extramarital-sex-study-suggests-243190. Accessed 13 July 2020.

84. Oyediran K, Isiugo-Abanihe UC, Feyisetan BJ, Ishola GP. Prevalence of and factors associated with extramarital sex among Nigerian men. Am J Mens Health. 2010;4:124–34. https://doi.org/10.1177/1557988308330772.

85. Irwin K. Patient deception of doctors. Software Advice. 22 Sept 2014. http://www.softwareadvice.com/medical/industryview/patient-deception-report-2014/. Accessed 13 July 2020.

86. South Africa unemployment rate. Trading Economics. 2020. https://tradingeconomics.com/south-africa/unemployment-rate#:~:text=Looking%20forward%2C%20we%20estimate%20Unemployment,according%20to%20our%20econometric%20models. Accessed 18 July 2020.

87. Essien EJ, Ogungbade GO, Ward D, Ekong E, Ross MW, Meshack A, et al. Influence of educational status and other variables on human immunodeficiency virus risk perception among military personnel: a large cohort finding. Mil Med. 2007;172:1177–81. https://doi.org/10.7205/milmed.172.11.1177.

88. Smith J, Nalagoda F, Wawer MJ, Serwadda D, Sewankambo N, Konde-Lule J, et al. Education attainment as a predictor of HIV risk in rural Uganda: results from a population-based study. Int J STD AIDS. 1999;10:452–9. https://doi.org/10.1258/0956462991914456.

89. Santelli JS, Mathur S, Song X, Huang TJ, Wei Y, Lutalo T, et al. Rising school enrollment and declining HIV and pregnancy risk among adolescents in Rakai District, Uganda, 1994–2013. Glob Soc Welf. 2015;2:87–103. https://doi.org/10.1007/s40609-015-0029-x.

90. Lakew Y, Benedict S, Haile D. Social determinants of HIV infection, hotspot areas and sub-population groups in Ethiopia: evidence from the National Demographic and Health Survey in 2011. BMJ Open. 2015;5:e008669. https://doi.org/10.1136/bmjopen-2015-008669.

91. Yang F, Shi X, He W, Wu S, Wang J, Zhao K, et al. Factors of the HIV transmission in men who have sex with men in Suizhou City from 2009 to 2013. Sex Med. 2015;3:24–31. https://doi.org/10.1002/sm2.55.

92. Hargreaves JR, Bonell CP, Boler T, Boccia D, Birdthistle I, Fletcher A, et al. Systematic review exploring time trends in the association between educational attainment and risk of HIV infection in sub-Saharan Africa. AIDS. 2008;22:403–14. https://doi.org/10.1097/QAD.0b013e3282f2aac3.

93. Michelo C, Sandøy IF, Fylkesnes K. Marked HIV prevalence declines in higher educated young people: evidence from population-based surveys (1995–2003) in Zambia. AIDS. 2006;20:1031–8. https://doi.org/10.1097/01.aids.0000222076.91114.95.

94. Hargreaves JR, Glynn JR. Educational attainment and HIV-1 infection in developing countries: a systematic review. Trop Med Int Health. 2002;7:489–98. https://doi.org/10.1046/j.1365-3156.2002.00889.x.

95. Lavadenz F, Pantanali C, Zeballos E. Thirty years of the HIV/AIDS epidemic in Argentina: an assessment of the national health response. Washington, DC: World Bank; 2015.
96. Health literacy. National Library of Medicine. https://www.nlm.nih.gov/medlineplus/health-literacy.html. Accessed 13 July 2020.
97. Gyasi RM, Mensah CM, Osei-Wusu Adjei P, Agyemang S. Public perceptions of the role of traditional medicine in the health care delivery system in Ghana. Glob J Health Sci. 2011;3:40–9. https://doi.org/10.5539/gjhs.v3n2p40.
98. Strengthening Pharmaceutical Systems (SPS) Program. Safety of medicines in Sub-Saharan Africa: assessment of pharmacovigilance systems and their performance. Submitted to the US Agency for International Development by the Strengthening Pharmaceutical Systems (SPS) Program. Arlington: Management Sciences for Health; 2011. https://www.msh.org/sites/msh.org/files/Safety-of-Medicines-in-SSA.pdf. Accessed 25 July 2020.
99. Assessment of medicines regulatory systems in sub-Saharan African countries: an overview of findings from 26 assessment reports. Geneva: WHO; 2010.
100. Moran M, Guzman J, McDonald A, Wu L, Omune B. Registering new drugs: the African context: new tools for new times. Sydney: George Institute of International Health; 2010.
101. Buckley GJ, Riviere JE. Ensuring safe foods and medical products through stronger regulatory systems abroad. National Academies Press; 2012.
102. Böl GF. Risk communication in times of crisis: pitfalls and challenges in ensuring preparedness instead of hysterics. EMBO Rep. 2016;17:1–9. https://doi.org/10.15252/embr.201541678.
103. Sandle T. Justice at last? The Nigerian baby mixture scandal. Digit J. 31 May 2013. http://www.digitaljournal.com/article/351252. Accessed 13 July 2020.
104. Syhakhang L, Freudenthal S, Tomson G, Wahlström R. Knowledge and perceptions of drug quality among drug sellers and consumers in Lao PDR. Health Policy Plan. 2004;19:391–401. https://doi.org/10.1093/heapol/czh054.
105. Patel A, Gauld R, Norris P, Rades T. Quality of generic medicines in South Africa: perceptions versus reality – a qualitative study. BMC Health Serv Res. 2012;12:297. https://doi.org/10.1186/1472-6963-12-297.
106. Bashaar M, Hassali MA, Saleem F, Shafie AA. Evaluation of public perception towards medicine quality and prices in six zones of Afghanistan. Int J Innov Healthc Res. 2015;3:4–11.
107. Hasan SS, Yong CS, Babar MG, Naing CM, Hameed A, Baig MR, et al. Understanding, perceptions and self-use of complementary and alternative medicine (CAM) among Malaysian pharmacy students. BMC Complement Altern Med. 2011;11:95. https://doi.org/10.1186/1472-6882-11-95.
108. Akhtar SW, Aziz H. Perception of epilepsy in Muslim history; with current scenario. Neurol Asia. 2004;9(Suppl 1):59–60.
109. Thys S, Mwape KE, Lefèvre P, Dorny P, Marcotty T, Phiri AM, et al. Why latrines are not used: communities' perceptions and practices regarding latrines in a Taenia solium endemic rural area in Eastern Zambia. PLoS Negl Trop Dis. 2015. https://doi.org/10.1371/journal.pntd.0003570.
110. Tewari S. Paid to poo: combating open defecation in India. BBC News. 30 Aug 2015. http://www.bbc.com/news/health-33980904. Accessed 13 July 2020.
111. Hayter AKM, Jeffery R, Sharma C, Prost A, Kinra S. Community perceptions of health and chronic disease in South Indian rural transitional communities: a qualitative study. Glob Health Action. 2015;8:25946. https://doi.org/10.3402/gha.v8.25946.
112. Lu Y. Mental health and risk behaviors of rural-urban migrants: longitudinal evidence from Indonesia. Popul Stud. 2010;64:147–63. https://doi.org/10.1080/00324721003734100.
113. Bhugra D, Becker MA. Migration, cultural bereavement and cultural identity. World Psychiatry. 2005;4:18–24.
114. Ng M, Fleming T, Robinson M, Thomson B, Graetz N, Margono C, et al. Global, regional, and national prevalence of overweight and obesity in children and adults during 1980–2013: a systematic analysis for the Global Burden of Disease Study 2013. Lancet. 2014;384:766–81. https://doi.org/10.1016/S0140-6736(14)60460-8.

115. How to tackle Tonga's obesity crisis? BBC News. 19 Jan 2016. http://www.bbc.com/news/world-asia-35349544. Accessed 14 July 2020.

116. Gates S. Trouble in paradise. Guardian. 3 Aug 2006. http://www.theguardian.com/lifeand-style/2006/aug/03/healthandwellbeing.health. Accessed 14 July 2020.

117. *See, for example:* Willingham E. Finland's bold push to change the heart health of a nation. Knowable Magazine. 3 July 2018. https://www.knowablemagazine.org/article/health-disease/2018/finlands-bold-push-change-heart-health-nation. Accessed 14 July 2020.

118. Broccoli MC, Calvello EJB, Skog AP, Wachira B, Wallis LA. Perceptions of emergency care in Kenyan communities lacking access to formalised emergency medical systems: a qualitative study. BMJ Open. 2015;5:e009208. https://doi.org/10.1136/bmjopen-2015-009208.

119. Blencowe H, Cousens S, Jassir FB, Say L, Chou D, Mathers C, et al. National, regional, and worldwide estimates of stillbirth rates in 2015, with trends from 2000: a systematic analysis. Lancet. 2016;4:e98–e108. https://doi.org/10.1016/S2214-109X(15)00275-2.

120. How has Rwanda saved the lives of 590,000 children? BBC News. 29 Apr 2015. http://www.bbc.com/news/world-africa-32438104. Accessed 14 July 2020.

121. Roche JM, Wise L, Gugushvili D, Hanna L. The lottery of birth: giving all children an equal chance to survive. London: Save the Children; 2015. http://www.savethechildren.org.uk/resources/online-library/lottery-birth. Accessed 14 July 2020.

122. Dahal P, Bhattarai B, Adhikari D, Shrestha R, Baral SR, Shrestha N. Drug use pattern in primary health care facilities of Kaski District, western Nepal. Sunsari Tech Coll J. 2012;1:1–8.

123. Ghimire S, Nepal S, Bhandari S, Nepal P, Palaian S. A prospective surveillance of drug prescribing and dispensing in a teaching hospital in western Nepal. J Pak Med Assoc. 2009;59:726–31.

124. Wachter DA, Joshi MP, Rimal B. Antibiotic dispensing by drug retailers in Kathmandu, Nepal. Trop Med Int Health. 1999;4:782–8. https://doi.org/10.1046/j.1365-3156.1999.00476.x.

125. Hughes S. Contaminated cardiac drugs kill more than 100 in Pakistan. Medscape. 27 Jan 2012. http://www.medscape.com/viewarticle/757657. Accessed 14 July 2020.

126. Shah SA, Khawaja HA. Unethical marketing practices of pharmaceutical companies in Pakistan: a case study of Sukkur Division. In: Proceedings book of ICEFMO. Handbook on the economic, finance and management outlooks. PAK Publishing Group; 2013. p. 627–35. http://www.conscientiabeam.com/ebooks/ICEFMO-297-627-635.pdf. Accessed 18 July 2020.

127. Alam K, Shah AK, Ojha P, Palaian S, Shankar PR. Evaluation of drug promotional materials in a hospital setting in Nepal. South Med Rev. 2009;2:2–6.

128. Panth N, Paudel KR, Chaudhary B, Thapa KK. A study on the price variability among the oral antibiotics available in a Western Region Hospital – a context of Nepal. World J Pharm Pharm Sci. 2014;3:1529–35.

129. European Commission DG Environment, University of the West of England, Science Communication Unit. Public risk perception and environmental policy. 2014. https://ec.europa.eu/environment/integration/research/newsalert/pdf/public_risk_perception_environmental_policy_FB8_en.pdf. Accessed 18 July 2020.

130. Lundgren RE, McMakin AH. Risk communication: a handbook for communicating environmental, safety and health risks. 5th ed. Hoboken: John Wiley & Sons, Inc.; 2013.

131. National Cancer Institute (U.S.), Office of Cancer Communications. Making health communication programs work: a planner's guide. United States Department of Health and Human Services. http://www.cancer.gov/publications/health-communication/pink-book.pdf. Accessed 14 July 2020.

132. Hugman B. Protecting the people?: risk communication and the chequered history and performance of bureaucracy. Drug Saf. 2012;1:1005–25. https://doi.org/10.2165/11635210-000000000-00000.

133. Hugman B. The fatal love of forms. Drug Saf. 2011;1:705–7. https://doi.org/10.2165/11595130-000000000-00000.

134. Hazell L, Shakir SAW. Under-reporting of adverse drug reactions: a systematic review. Drug Saf. 2006;29:385–96. https://doi.org/10.2165/00002018-200629050-00003.
135. Otieno Y. Pharmacovigilance reporting goes digital in Kenya. Management Sciences for Health. 29 Apr 2013. https://www.msh.org/news-events/stories/pharmacovigilance-reporting-goes-digital-in-kenya. Accessed 14 July 2020.
136. Adedeji AA, Babirye J, Nsooli O, Kamowa D, Tikare OA, Okoruwa AG, et al. Use of mobile phones for monitoring adverse drug reaction in pharmacy and drug stores in Ishaka, Uganda – a pilot assessment of willingness to report. Br J Pharm Res. 2014;4:2245–60. https://doi.org/10.9734/BJPR/2014/8065.
137. Shirodkar SN. IPC launches android mobile application for ADR reporting facilities. Pharmabiz.com. 19 June 2015. http://www.pharmabiz.com/NewsDetails.aspx?aid=89002&sid=1. Accessed 14 July 2020.
138. Prakesh J, Joshi K, Malik D, Mishra O, Sachan A, Jumar B, et al. "ADR PvPI" Android mobile app: report adverse drug reaction at any time anywhere in India. Indian J Pharmacol. 2009;51:236–42. https://doi.org/10.4103/ijp.IJP_595_18.
139. Take & Tell. Uppsala Monitoring Centre. http://www.takeandtell.org/. Accessed 14 July 2020.
140. Srinivasan S. Coronavirus has become the booster shot that telemedicine was waiting for in India. Quartz India. 6 Apr 2020. https://qz.com/india/1833374/coronavirus-to-boost-telemedicine-apps-mfine-and-practo-in-india/. Accessed 18 July 2020.
141. Wamala DS, Augustine K. A meta-analysis of telemedicine success in Africa. J Pathol Inform. 2013;4:6. https://doi.org/10.4103/2153-3539.112686.
142. Telehealth: specialist video consultations under Medicare. MBS Online. http://www.mbsonline.gov.au/telehealth. Accessed 14 July 2020.
143. Vinegar D. Telehealth: small scale initiatives can reduce costs and help patients. Guardian. 16 Dec 2013. http://www.theguardian.com/healthcare-network/2013/dec/16/telehealth-reduce-costs-help-patients. Accessed 14 July 2020.
144. SMART Health India. George Institute for Global Health, India. http://www.georgeinstitute.org/sites/default/files/smart-health-india-brochure.pdf. Accessed 14 July 2020.
145. Lehmann U, Sanders D. Community health workers: what do we know about them? Geneva: WHO; 2007. https://www.who.int/hrh/documents/community_health_workers.pdf. Accessed 14 July 2020.
146. Projects. Impact India Foundation. http://www.impactindia.org/lifeline-express.php#content-start. Accessed 14 July 2020.
147. Lifeline Express. https://lxenglish.com/about/. Accessed 14 July 2020.
148. The train of hope: South Africa's Phelophepa. Future Rail. https://rail.nridigital.com/future_rail_dec18/the_train_of_hope_south_africas_phelophepa. Accessed 17 July 2020.
149. Crouch L. Doctors on the move: getting healthcare to far-flung places. BBC News. 24 Jan 2016. http://www.bbc.com/news/health-35372495. Accessed 14 July 2020.
150. Orbis. http://www.orbis.org/feh. Accessed 14 July 2020.
151. Subramanian S, Dumont C, Dankert C, Wong A. Personalized technology will upend the doctor-patient relationship. Harvard Business Review. 19 June 2015. https://hbr.org/2015/06/personalized-technology-will-upend-the-doctor-patient-relationship. Accessed 14 July 2020.
152. Namaganda AK. Make a free call to get health solutions. Daily Monitor. 7 Sept 2012. https://www.monitor.co.ug/artsculture/Reviews/Make-a-free-call-to-get-health-solutions/691232-1498370-hhtv9z/index.html. Accessed 18 July 2020.
153. Tanzania's healthy pregnancy text message service reaches 100,000 subscribers in 15 weeks. OAfrica. 3 Apr 2013. http://www.oafrica.com/mobile/tanzanias-healthy-pregnancy-text-message-service-reaches-100000-subscribers-in-15-weeks/. Accessed 14 July 2020.
154. Croker H, Lucas R, Wardle J. Cluster-randomised trial to evaluate the 'Change for Life' mass media/ social marketing campaign in the UK. BMC Public Health. 2012;6:404. https://doi.org/10.1186/1471-2458-12-404.

155. Smalley W, Shatin D, Wysowski DK, Gurwitz J, Andrade SE, Goodman M, et al. Contraindicated use of Cisapride: impact of food and drug administration regulatory action. JAMA. 2000;284:3036–9. https://doi.org/10.1001/jama.284.23.3036.
156. Leach A. Five memorable movements in public health. Guardian. 6 June 2014. http://www.theguardian.com/global-development-professionals-network/2014/jun/06/five-memorable-movements-in-public-health. Accessed 14 July 2020.
157. Health Communication Partnership Uganda: final report May 2012. Johns Hopkins Bloomberg School of Public Health. http://ccp.jhu.edu/documents/HCP%20Uganda%20 2007-2012%20Final%20Project%20Report.pdf. Accessed 14 July 2020.
158. Fischoff B. Chapter 1: risk perception and communication. In: Fischoff B, editor. Risk analysis and human behavior. Abingdon: Earthscan; 2012. p. 3–32.
159. Elbarbary M. Understanding and expressing 'Risk'. J Saudi Heart Assoc. 2010;22:159–64. https://doi.org/10.1016/j.jsha.2010.04.002.
160. Gigerenzer G, Gaissmaier G, Kurz-Milcke E, Schwartz LM, Woloshin S. Helping doctors and patients make sense of health statistics. Psychol Sci Public Interest. 2007;8:53–96. https://doi.org/10.1111/j.1539-6053.2008.00033.x.
161. Kickbusch I, Apfel F, Pelikan JM, Tsouros AD. Health literacy: the solid facts. Geneva: WHO; 2013.
162. Part 4: increasing global HPV vaccination. President's cancer panel annual report 2012–2013. http://deainfo.nci.nih.gov/advisory/pcp/annualReports/HPV/Part4.htm#sthash.imuZW8XQ.dpbs. Accessed 14 July 2020.
163. Balanescu V. Prevention is better than cure, say Romanian doctors. Bull World Health Organ. 2011;89:248–9. https://doi.org/10.2471/BLT.11.030411.
164. Global Advisory Committee on Vaccine Safety. Weekly epidemiological report [22 Jan 2016]. WHO. 2016;91:21–32.
165. HPV vaccine side effects. NHS http://www.nhs.uk/conditions/vaccinations/pages/hpv-vaccine-cervarix-gardasil-side-effects.aspx. Accessed 14 July 2020.
166. NCI Staff. Risk of breast cancer death is low after a diagnosis of ductal carcinoma in situ. National Cancer Institute. 26 Aug 2015. http://www.cancer.gov/news-events/cancer-currents-blog/2015/dcis-low-risk. Accessed 14 July 2020.
167. Luzzatto L. The rise and fall of the antimalarial Lapdap: a lesson in pharmacogenetics. Lancet. 2010;376:739–41. https://doi.org/10.1016/S0140-6736(10)60396-0.
168. Paling Palettes in Pads. Risk Communication Institute. https://www.riskcomm.com/products_palettes.php?p=2. Accessed 14 July 2020.
169. Healthcare communications [search result]. Pinterest. https://www.pinterest.co.uk/search/pins/?rs=ac&len=2&q=healthcare%20communications&eq=healthcare%20communications&etslf=24044&term_meta[]=healthcare%7Cautocomplete%7C0&term_meta[]=communications%7Cautocomplete%7C0. Accessed 17 July 2020.
170. Trainings, tools, & templates. Centers for Disease Control and Prevention. https://www.cdc.gov/healthcommunication/toolstemplates.html. Accessed 17 July 2020.
171. The CDC Clear Communication Index. Centers for Disease Control and Prevention. http://www.cdc.gov/ccindex/index.html. Accessed 14 July 2020.
172. Everyday words for public health communication. Centers for Disease Control and Prevention. 2016. https://www.cdc.gov/other/pdf/EverydayWordsForPublicHealthCommunication.pdf. Accessed 14 July 2020.
173. Is the main message emphasized with visual cues? Centers for Disease Control and Prevention. http://www.cdc.gov/ccindex/tool/page-3.html. Accessed 14 July 2020.
174. Stacey D, Légaré F, Lewis K, Barry MJ, Bennett CL, Eden KB, et al. Decision aids for people facing health treatment or screening decisions. Cochrane Database Syst Rev. 2017;12:CD001431. https://doi.org/10.1002/14651858.CD001431.pub5.
175. Statin Choice decision aid. Mayo Clinic. https://statindecisionaid.mayoclinic.org/index.php/statin/index. Accessed 14 July 2020.
176. Ozanne EM, Howe R, Omer Z, Esserman LJ. Development of a personalized decision aid for breast cancer risk reduction and management. BMC Med Inform Decis Mak. 2014;14:4. https://doi.org/10.1186/1472-6947-14-4.

177. National Institute for Health and Care Excellence. https://www.evidence.nhs.uk/search?o
m=%5b%7b%22ety%22:%5b%22Patient%20Decision%20Aids%22%5d%7d,%7b%22s
rn%22:%5b%22National%20Institute%20for%20Health%20and%20Care%20Excellence%
20-%20NICE%22%5d%7d%5d. Accessed 18 July 2020.

178. Fagerlin A, Zikmund-Fisher BJ, Ubel PA. Helping patients decide: ten steps to better risk communication. J Natl Cancer Inst. 2011;103:1436–43. https://doi.org/10.1093/jnci/djr318.

179. Politi MC. Helping patients and clinicians manage uncertainty during clinical care. Institute for Public Health. 16 July 2015. https://publichealth.wustl.edu/helping-patients-and-clinicians-manage-uncertainty-during-clinical-care/. Accessed 14 July 2020.

180. Rosenbaum L. Communicating uncertainty – Ebola, public health, and the scientific process. N Engl J Med. 2015;372:7–9. https://doi.org/10.1056/NEJMp1413816.

181. Heart disease risk calculator. Mayo Clinic. https://www.mayoclinichealthsystem.org/locations/cannon-falls/services-and-treatments/cardiology/heart-disease-risk-calculator. Accessed 17 July 2020.

182. Baalbergen A, Veenstra Y, Stalpers L. Surgery or radiotherapy for early cervical cancer of the adenocarcinoma type. Cochrane Syst Rev. 2013. https://doi.org/10.1002/14651858. CD006248.pub3.

183. Visualisation of Cochrane summary of findings table. Understanding uncertainty. http://understandinguncertainty.org/files/animations/CochraneAnimation/CochraneSlides.html. Accessed 15 July 2020.

184. Schwartz LM, Woloshin S, Welch HG. The drug facts box: providing consumers with simple tabular data on drug benefit and harms. Med Decis Making. 2007;27:655–62. https://doi.org/10.1177/0272989X07306786.

185. Leckart S. The blood test gets a makeover. Wired. 29 Nov 2010. http://www.wired.com/2010/11/ff_bloodwork/. Accessed 15 July 2020.

186. TED. Thomas Goetz: it's time to redesign medical data. YouTube. 27 Jan 2011. https://www.youtube.com/watch?v=bCGlWQnzDVE. Accessed 15 July 2020.

187. Pennic J. New mobile health app to fight AIDS, malaria in 7 African countries. HIT Consultant. 24 Mar 2014. http://hitconsultant.net/2014/03/24/new-mobile-health-app-to-fight-aids-malaria-in-7-african-countries/. Accessed 15 July 2020.

188. Drug-free world brings information on drugs to apple iPhone. Foundation for a drug-free world. http://www.drugfreeworld.org/news/iphone-ipod-app.html. Accessed 15 July 2020.

189. Mobile phones for health. New Humanitarian. 3 Dec 2010. http://www.irinnews.org/report/91287/africa-mobile-phones-for-health. Accessed 15 July 2020.

190. Impact of communication in healthcare. Institute for Healthcare Communication. 2011. http://healthcarecomm.org/about-us/impact-of-communication-in-healthcare/. Accessed 15 July 2020.

191. Infanti JJ, Sixsmith J, Barry MM, Núñez-Córdoba JM, Oroviogoicoechea-Ortega C, Guillén-Grima F. A literature review on effective risk communication for the prevention and control of communicable diseases in Europe: insights into health communication. Stockholm: ECDC; 2013.

192. Dusetzina SB, Higashi AS, Dorsey ER, Conti R, Huskamp HA, Zhu S, et al. Impact of FDA drug risk communications on health care utilization and health behaviors: a systematic review. Med Care. 2012;50:466–78. https://doi.org/10.1097/MLR.0b013e318245a160.

193. Pennic J. 5 reasons why Mayo Clinic dominates social media in healthcare. HIT Consultant. 17 Feb 2014. http://hitconsultant.net/2014/02/17/5-reasons-mayo-clinic-dominates-social-media-in-healthcare/. Accessed 15 July 2020.

194. McNab C. What social media offers to health professionals and citizens. Bull World Health Organ. 2009;87:565–644. https://doi.org/10.2471/BLT.09.066712.

195. Le PV, Jones-Le E, Bell C, Miller S. Preferences for perinatal health communication of women in rural Tibet. J Obstet Gynecol Neonatal Nurs. 2009;38:108–17. https://doi.org/10.1111/j.1552-6909.2008.00312.x.

Chapter 16
Training and Capacity Building Opportunities in Pharmacovigilance

Karine Palin, Stéphane Liège, Christa Naboulet, and Francesco Salvo

16.1 Pharmacovigilance Needs in Low- and Middle-Income Countries

Medicines and vaccines are disseminating among unprecedented numbers of people in low- and middle-income countries (LMICs). These products have huge potential to save lives and reduce suffering. However, many of the countries in which these products are used need to have the capacity to effectively monitor post-marketing drug safety. International initiatives have been developed to address this need but have not attracted significant public or private support, nor political agreement and resources from governments of LMICs [1].

Pharmacovigilance programmes (PV) in most LMICs are recent, poorly funded and are only minimally supervised by legal or regulatory documents. On the one hand, rigorous regulations are needed so that the local pharmaceutical industry and healthcare professionals are more involved. On the other hand, PV regulations must be applied and monitored through good governance practices. In particular, LMICs should be able to collect sufficient and relevant drug safety information to accurately and rapidly inform the medicines-stakeholders involved. Finally, LMICs must develop the data analysis skills necessary to be able to independently assess the benefits and risks of medication use [1].

It is essential to deliver PV training at undergraduate and graduate levels in higher education institutions for all healthcare professionals at the worldwide level. Public health actors must urgently initiate PV programmes. In particular, academic institutions should provide PV training at undergraduate and graduate levels, so that

K. Palin (✉) · S. Liège · C. Naboulet · F. Salvo
Université de Bordeaux, Eu2P Central Office, Department of Pharmacology – Case 36, Bordeaux Cedex, France
e-mail: karine.palin@u-bordeaux.fr

© Springer Nature Singapore Pte Ltd. 2025
S. R. Ahmad (ed.), *Special Issues in Pharmacovigilance in Resource-Limited Countries*, https://doi.org/10.1007/978-981-96-6154-1_16

the roles of new healthcare professionals in documenting, collecting, reporting and learning about medication risk experience, including medication errors, are well known, understood and anticipated [1].

16.2 Training Opportunities in Pharmacovigilance for Low- and Middle-Income Countries

PV systems have been introduced for several years in some LMICs where health-related staff had basic PV knowledge. Nowadays, these professionals wish to develop in-depth skills related to the medicines' benefits and risks beyond these basics.

These advanced and relevant postgraduate training programmes are not accessible yet in LMICs as they have limited resources. Only a few higher education institutions in high-income countries offer targeted and relevant PV programmes [2]. It must be emphasized that the development of national programmes in LMICs mainly depends on the few locally trained individuals and their ability to be willing and able and to have time to train their fellow volunteers. This has nevertheless been the case in Accra since 2009 and in Rabat since 2011 [1]. Finally, although appointed members of the PV committees associated with the WHO and members of the executive committee of the International Society of Pharmacovigilance (ISoP) or its Education and Training Project Group (ETP) regularly describe and update relevant topics in PV, few universities offer specific courses in PV [3]. This is again particularly true for countries with limited financial resources.

In 2008, in the framework of the Innovative Medicines Initiative Joint Undertaking, the European Commission has launched a call in order to build and deliver a full online training programme in pharmacovigilance and pharmacoepidemiology [4–7]. This challenge was driven by seven European Universities, the European and French Medicines Agencies and fifteen Pharmaceutical Companies who have put their strengths together in order to build the European programme in Pharmacovigilance and Pharmacoepidemiology (Eu2P) [8].

Since 2011, Eu2P is the only one consortium in the world to deliver and jointly award full online academic courses in Pharmacovigilance and Pharmacoepidemiology, which are accessible anytime, any pace, anywhere. Eu2P targets worldwide specialists such as pharmacists, physicians, scientists and experienced professionals but also non-specialists such as media representatives, laypersons and patients. The Eu2P training programme particularly emphasizes hands-on training to maximize post-training employment opportunities.

Eu2P courses have been developed and are delivered using a unique and innovative modular approach integrating face-to-face lectures, e-teaching (live videoconferences) and e-learning formats (quiz, wiki, forums) through the Eu2P e-learning platform available in the English language. Besides, Eu2P has developed e-learning methods to provide opportunities to train all stakeholders when no local training is available in drug safety. The platform course activities are optimized for slow Internet connectivity (including files weight) and different world time-zones are taken into account with a large majority of asynchronous activities (24/7 access, forum discussion, and recording of all scheduled live meetings). Exams are also organized on a distant basis, using web-based facilities as well as research project oral defences thanks to the use of online conferencing. This enables trainees from everywhere to easily complete their curriculum.

Eu2P users are offered custom-built training programmes that lead to academic certificates, full Master's or PhD diplomas depending on the options chosen. The trainees can choose among specialties in benefit assessment, regulatory aspects, risk identification and quantification, benefit-risk assessment, public health and risk communication in order to be awarded accredited postgraduate diplomas.

Eu2P offers a certain number of grants to Master and PhD selected applicants to partially cover Master and PhD tuition fees. The Eu2P grants are proposed by the Eu2P consortium and private members on the appraisal of the applicant's status depending on their academic performance, professional ambition and environment, personal situation and also any special and financial circumstances that may affect their training performance. The application procedure and the selection process are the same for all applicants regardless of whether the trainees come from Eu2P partners or not, from European or other countries.

Therefore, Eu2P appears to be an efficient tool to train medicines-related stakeholders living in LMICs in real-world evidence of drug safety management.

16.3 The Place of Trainees from Low- and Middle-Income Countries in Eu2P Training Programme

As part of its commitment to provide a worldwide flexible learning, Eu2P has to comply with an increasing geographical variety of its trainees who register to its online Certificates, Master and PhD curricula (cf. Fig. 16.1). Out of 1059 registrations between September 2011 and October 2022, the European origin (53.6%) registrants were the most common, but Eu2P has geographically widened and registered trainees also come from North America (12.7%), South America (7.1%), Africa (15.9%), Asia (10.3%) and Oceania (0.4%).

16.3.1 Breakdown of the Number of Eu2P Registered Trainees from Resource-Limited Countries

Between September 2011 and October 2022, the 1059 registrants were classified depending on trainees' country of residence according to the last World Bank economical classification from July 2022. Then two groups of the Eu2P registrants

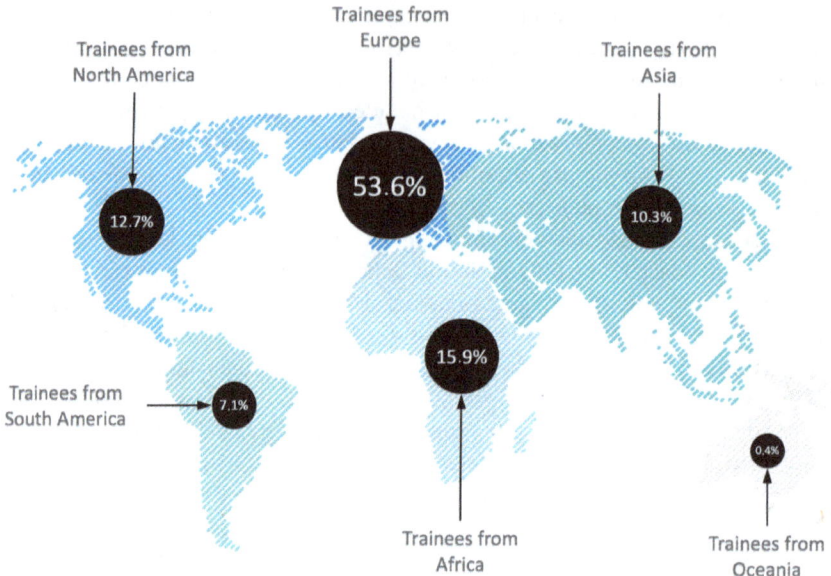

Fig. 16.1 Geolocalization of the Eu2P registrations to Certificates, Master and PhD programs (2011–2022)

were compared: the "low- and middle-income countries" (LMICs) group and the "high and upper middle income countries" (HUMICs). It is important to note that between 2011 and 2022, 17% of the Eu2P registrants ($n = 180$) originated from LMICs and 83% ($n = 879$) from HUMIC (cf. Fig. 16.2). These absolute figures, measured between September 2011 and October 2022, have been used to make the following calculations of Eu2P registrants' description.

Among the Eu2P registrants originating from LMICs, 19 different countries were represented: thirteen countries from Africa, six from Asia, one from Europe and one from North America. Among them, Egypt ($n = 30$), Nigeria ($n = 25$), Kenya ($n = 21$), India ($n = 13$) and Cameroon ($n = 11$) were the most represented countries among the LMICs registrants (cf. Fig. 16.3).

16.3.2 Breakdown of the Eu2P Course Diplomas' Interest in Resource-Limited Countries

The proportions of Eu2P course registrants have been compared between LMICs and HUMICs groups depending on the type of the diploma: Certificate versus Masters versus PhD (cf. Fig. 16.4). Trainees from LMICs were mostly registered in Masters and PhD curriculum, while trainees from HUMIC were mostly registered in Certificate curriculum. This would tend to show that LMICs trainees mostly need a broad and complete postgraduate training in PV rather than more specific topic

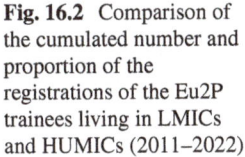

Fig. 16.2 Comparison of the cumulated number and proportion of the registrations of the Eu2P trainees living in LMICs and HUMICs (2011–2022)

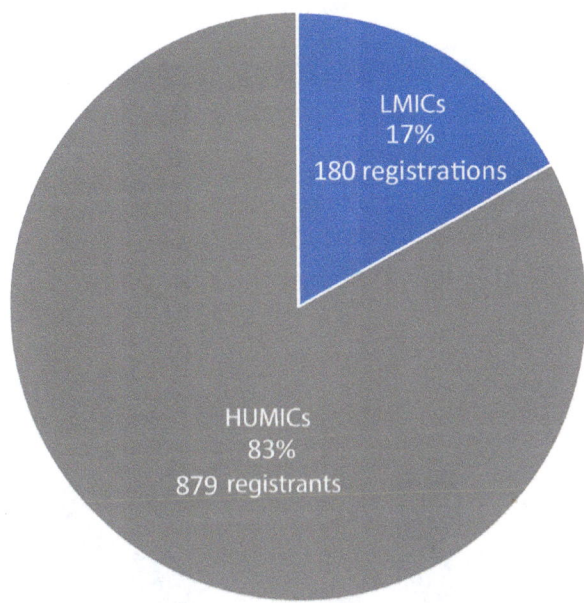

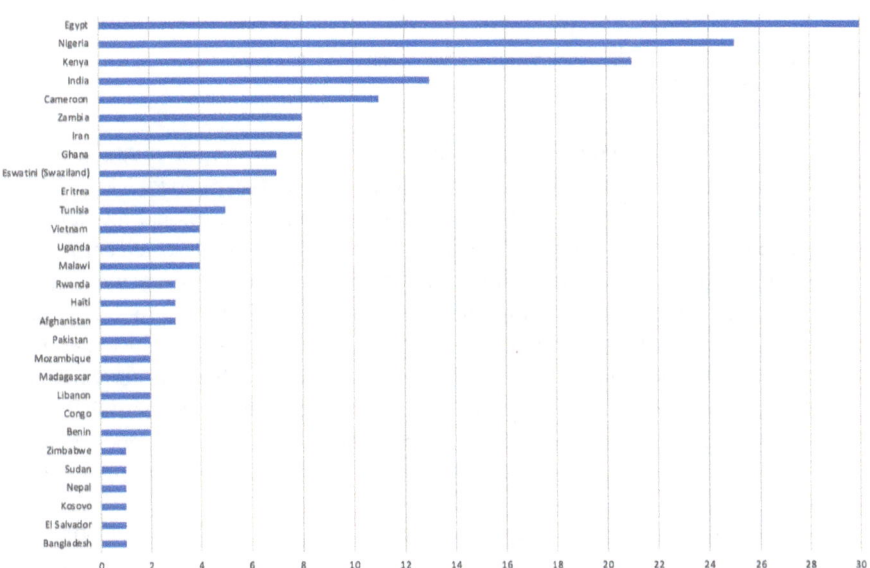

Fig. 16.3 Number of Eu2P trainees' registrants per Low- and Middle-income Country (2011–2022)

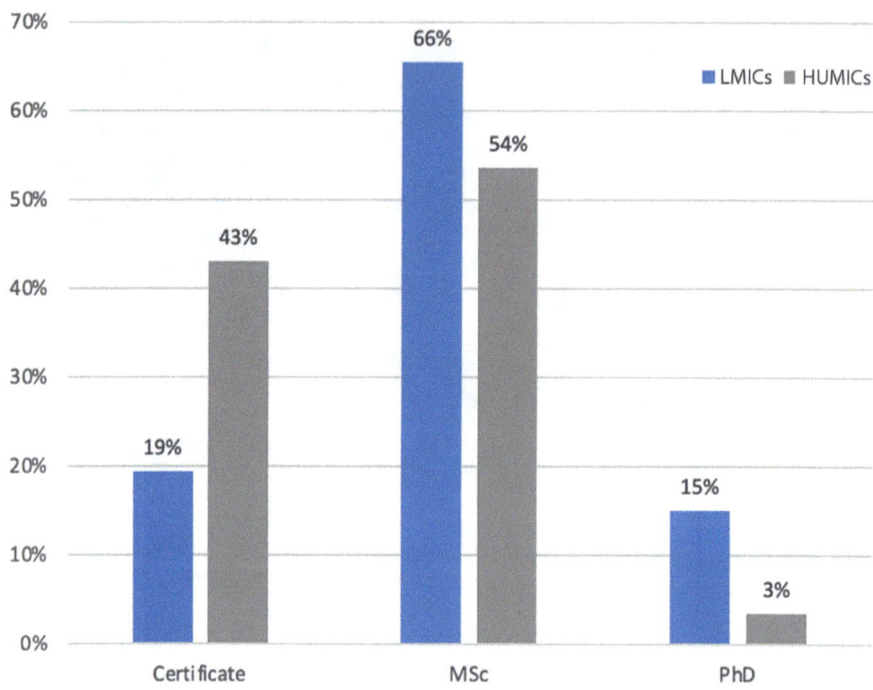

Fig. 16.4 Comparison of the proportions of LMICs and HUMICs groups according to the type of Eu2P diploma (2011–2022)

improvement or new competencies acquisition. It is interesting to note that all the Eu2P Master trainees living in LMICs conducted a project on regional LMICs problems such as the descriptive study of the pattern of use of traditional medicines in the area of Port-au-Prince; the adverse drug reactions caused by injected ceftriaxone sodium in Nepal; the assessment of prescribing practices for children attending the outpatient department of the children's hospital in Kabul; the factors associated with reduced efficacy of anti-malarial drugs: Kilifi District· Hospital experience. Besides, some of them have already published the results of their Master work conducted in LMICs such as the Pharmaceutical regulatory environment: challenges and opportunities in the Gulf Region [9] or the serious Adverse Events Reporting and Follow-Up Requirements in the European and Developing Countries Clinical Trials Partnership-Funded Clinical Trials: Current Practice [10].

The proportions of Eu2P course topics have been compared between LMICs and HUMICs groups depending on the offered specialties: basics in PV, benefit assessment, PV regulations, risk identification and quantification, benefit-risk assessment, public health and risk communication (cf. Fig. 16.5). Although before 2018, trainees from LMICs were mostly registered in Basics in PV (36%) compared to trainees living in HUMICs (19%), this figure now reflects similar PV training needs in LMICs as compared to HUMICs. This similarity may show that implementation of the PV systems in LMICs countries now requests and needs persons skilled in all

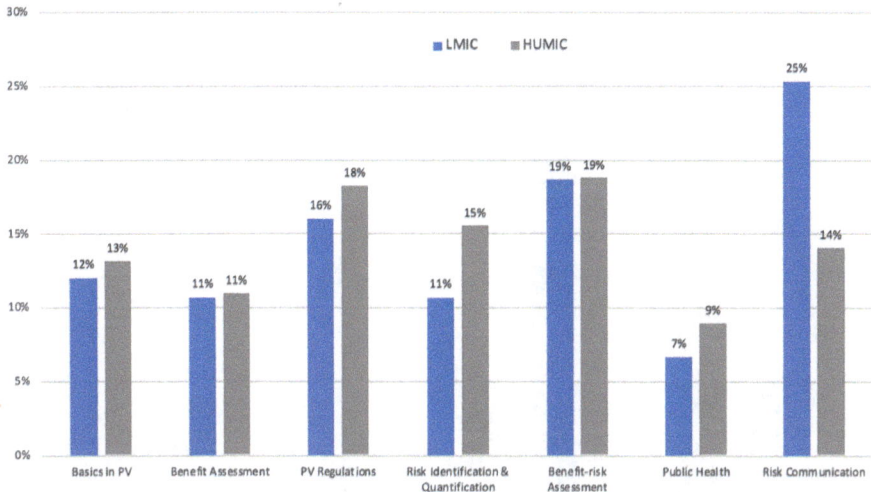

Fig. 16.5 Comparison of Eu2P course topics' interest between LMICs and HUMICs groups (2011–2022)

fields (PV, benefit assessment, PV regulations, risk identification and quantification, benefit-risk assessment, public health and risk communication) covered by Pharmacovigilance as well as in HUMICs.

16.3.3 Breakdown of the Trainee's Affiliation and Financial Support in Resource-Limited Countries

The proportions of Eu2P course registrations have been compared between LMICs and HUMICs groups depending on the type of the trainees' affiliation: private sector versus public academic and research organization versus regulatory agency versus none affiliation (cf. Fig. 16.6). Trainees from LMICs were mostly affiliated to a public academic and research organization, while trainees from HUMICs were mostly affiliated to the private sector. No difference could be observed in the proportions of LMICs and HUMICs trainees affiliated or not to a regulatory agency.

There is thus a room for improvement, particularly as regards the involvement of the private sector in the continuous training of its collaborators: this may ease the financial access to the training for such professional trainees and globally raise the quality level of the monitoring and enforcement of PV regulations in LMICs.

Indeed, the financial aspect remains a difficulty in the access to PV training in LMICs.

In this respect, the proportions of Eu2P trainees having received a grant between 2011 and 2022 to partially or fully cover their Eu2P course registrations fees have been compared between LMICs and HUMICs groups (cf. Fig. 16.7). Trainees from

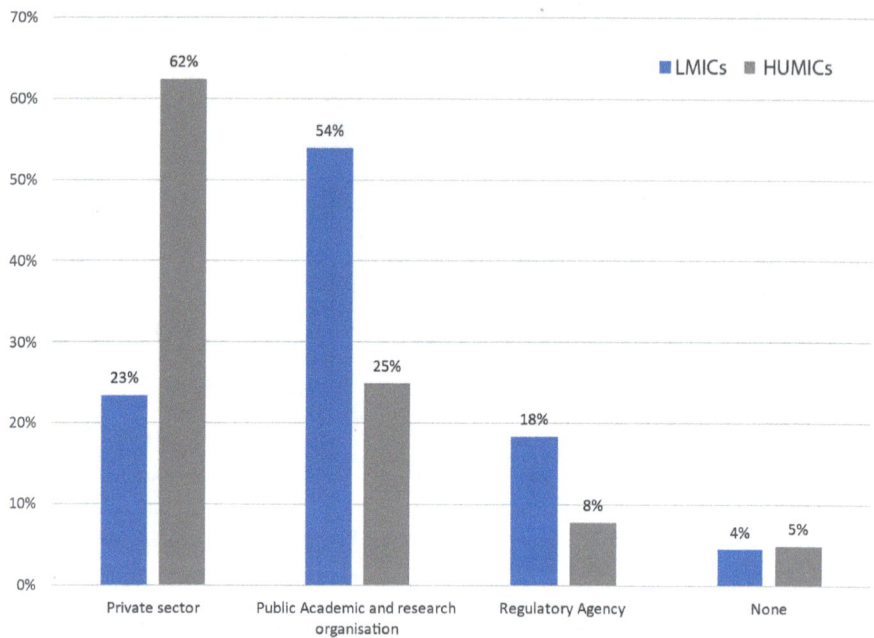

Fig. 16.6 Comparison of Eu2P trainees' affiliations between LMICs and HUMICs groups (2011–2022)

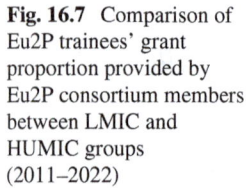

Fig. 16.7 Comparison of Eu2P trainees' grant proportion provided by Eu2P consortium members between LMIC and HUMIC groups (2011–2022)

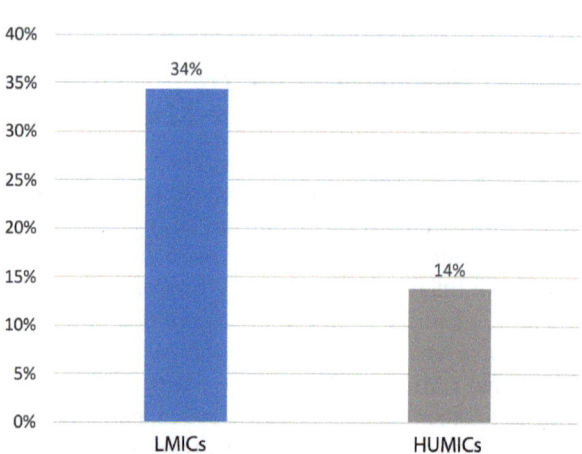

LMICs were more often awarded a grant (34%; $n = 62$ out of 180) than the trainees living in HUMICs (14%; $n = 121$ out 879). The grant represented from 20% up to 100% of the total fees amount; an average of 30% of grant amount was provided between 2011 and 2022 in both groups.

16.4 Conclusion

Thanks to the delivery of full-online courses and diplomas in English for the past 11 years, the Eu2P programme outputs that are mainly course contents and diverse professional expertise have rapidly and broadly spread within the scientific and industrial community of healthcare professionals. This is already demonstrated by the increasing number of student and professional trainees who registered and were awarded by the Eu2P consortium each academic year since 2011. The proportion of Eu2P trainees living in LMIC is significant in Africa countries where English is spoken, but also in Asia. E-learning facilities created by Eu2P consortium provide an equal chance of being trained in any country, without adding the cost of travels and accommodation. Furthermore, the savings offered by the Eu2P consortium is an effective opportunity to ease the registration and training of medicines-related stakeholders from LMIC.

The Eu2P programme strongly participates to the development of recognized post-graduate Education and Training of medicines-related stakeholders living in developing countries. The expected impact is to increase efficiency in the drug market surveillance within the developing countries as regards (i) enhanced quality through skilled and specifically trained persons, (ii) better understanding and knowledge of published papers, (iii) understanding of new needs and natural emergence of new job profiles, and (iv) facilitation of career development.

References

1. Olsson S, Pal SN, Dodoo A. Pharmacovigilance in resource-limited countries. Expert Rev Clin Pharmacol. 2015;8(4):449–60.
2. Cobert B. Organizations that deal with pharmacovigilance and drug safety – Part 2 Training & Education [Internet]. Bart's Corner: Expert PV Intelligence and Commentary (http://www.sentrx.com/). 2012 [cited 2013 Apr 22]. Available from: http://www.sentrx.com/2012/12/organizations-that-deal-with-pharmacovigilance-and-drug-safety-part-2-training-education/.
3. Beckmann J, Hagemann U, Bahri P, Bate A, Boyd IW, Pan GJD, et al. Teaching pharmacovigilance: the WHO-ISoP Core elements of a comprehensive modular curriculum. Drug Saf. 2014;30:1–17.
4. Hardman M. European initiatives for better training in medicines development. J Med Dev Sci [Internet]. 2015 [cited 2016 Mar 24];1(1). Available from: http://jmds.whioce.com/index.php/journal-of-medicines-development/article/view/01002.
5. Palin K, Bataille C, Liège S, Swain E, Fourrier-Reglat A, Schimmer R. Better comms in meds. Public Serv Rev Health Soc Care. 2013;34:71.
6. Klech H, Brooksbank C, Price S, Verpillat P, Bühler FR, Dubois D, et al. European initiative towards quality standards in education and training for discovery, development and use of medicines. Eur J Pharm Sci. 2012;45(5):515–20.
7. Goldman M. The innovative medicines initiative: a European response to the innovation challenge. Clin Pharmacol Ther. 2012;91(3):418–25.

8. Palin K, Bataille C, Liège S, Schimmer R, Fourrier-Réglat A. Eu2P: The First European Online Public–Private Joint Training Program in Pharmacovigilance and Pharmacoepidemiology. In: FISPE EBA MPH, FISPE NMM, FRCP(Edin), editors. Mann's Pharmacovigilance [Internet]. John Wiley & Sons, Ltd; 2014 [cited 2016 Mar 24]. p. 785–92. Available from: http://onlinelibrary.wiley.com/doi/10.1002/9781118820186.ch50/summary.

9. Al-Essa RK, Al-Rubaie M, Walker SR, Salek S. Pharmaceutical regulatory environment: challenges and opportunities in the Gulf Region [Internet]. 2015 [cited 2016 Mar 24]. Available from: http://search.ebscohost.com/login.aspx?direct=true&scope=site&db=nlebk&db=nlabk&AN=990730.

10. Habarugira JMV. Serious adverse events reporting and follow-up requirements in the European and Developing Countries Clinical Trials Partnership-funded clinical trials: current practice. J Pharmacovigil [Internet] 2014 [cited 2016 Mar 24];2(6). Available from: http://www.esciencecentral.org/journals/serious-adverse-events-reporting-and-followup-requirements-in-the-european-and-developing-countries-clinical-trials-current-practice-2329-6887-2-148.php?aid=32824.

Chapter 17
Pharmacy and Poisons Board: A Regional Centre of Regulatory Excellence (RCORE) in Africa on Pharmacovigilance

Christabel Khaemba, Pamela Nambwa, Martha Mandale, Edward Abwao, Karim Wanga, Kariuki Gachoki, and Fred M. Siyoi

Pharmacy and Poisons Board (PPB) was established in 1957 under the Pharmacy and Poisons Act of the laws of Kenya. The PPB is the National Medicines Regulatory Authority for Kenya whose mission is to protect the health of the public by regulating the profession of pharmacy and ensuring access to quality, safe, efficacious, and affordable health products and technologies (HPTs).[1] The mandate of PPB is achieved through implementing various regulatory functions such as pharmacovigilance and post-marketing surveillance.

As part of its mandate, the PPB has established and is implementing a pharmacovigilance (PV) system designed to monitor and respond to safety issues for HPTs circulating in the Kenyan market.

In May 2014, the Africa Union Development Agency-New Partnership for Africa's Development (AUDA-NEPAD) then NEPAD designated eleven (11) Regional Centres of Regulatory Excellence (RCOREs) in the Region as part of the African Medicines Regulatory Harmonization (AMRH) strategy for increasing human and institutional capacity in the regulation of HPTs on the African continent.[2]

The designation involved a number of processes including consultations with key stakeholders and experts in regulatory capacity building and a call for expression of interest for institutions interested to be selected as RCOREs in October 2013.[3] A selection criterion based on the infrastructure, governance, and manage-

---

[1] https://web.pharmacyboardkenya.org/about-us-2/

[2] https://www.nepad.org/publication/regional-centres-of-regulatory-excellence-rcores

[3] Report of Meeting of African Union and New Partnership for African Development's Regional Centres of Regulatory Excellence (RCOREs) in Pharmacovigilance, May 14–15 2015, Accra, Ghana. Submitted to the US Agency for International Development by the Systems for Improved Access to Pharmaceuticals and Services (SIAPS) Programme. Arlington, VA: Management Sciences for Health

---

C. Khaemba (✉) · P. Nambwa · M. Mandale · E. Abwao · K. Wanga · K. Gachoki · F. M. Siyoi
Pharmacy and Poisons Board, Nairobi, Kenya
e-mail: cnkhaemba@gmail.com

© Springer Nature Singapore Pte Ltd. 2025
S. R. Ahmad (ed.), *Special Issues in Pharmacovigilance in Resource-Limited Countries*, https://doi.org/10.1007/978-981-96-6154-1_17

ment systems alongside partnerships and collaborations was used. The criteria further looked at the training capacity and regulatory capabilities.[4]

The RCOREs were established to play a key role in regulatory capacity development in the region by providing academic and technical training in medicines regulatory sciences.[3]

Kenya's PPB was appointed by NEPAD as one of the two RCOREs in PV, the other one being the Collaborating Centre for Advocacy and Training in Pharmacovigilance at the University of Ghana which is a consortium comprising the World Health Organization–Collaborating Centre (WHO-CC), the National Pharmacovigilance Centres of Ghana, Nigeria, Tanzania, and Zimbabwe, Sante-Afrique International Limited of Ghana and Quintiles Clyndepharm of South Africa. The other RCOREs and their roles are described in the figure below.

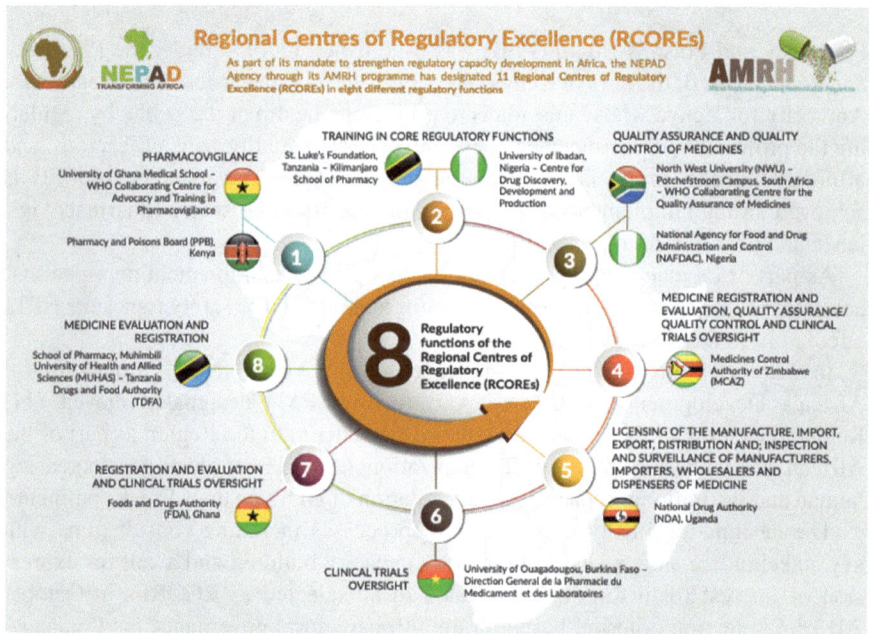

https://www.nepad.org/publication/regional-centres-of-regulatory-excellence-rcores#:~:text=As%20part%20of%20its%20mandate,RCOREs)%20in%20eight%20different%20functions.

In line with its mandate[1] through a systemic approach model of institutionalization, the PPB established the National Pharmacovigilance Centre (NPC) in 2004 as a department under the Product Registration Directorate. The Pharmacovigilance (PV) system was officially launched in June 2009 through the support of USAID's

---

[4] https://www.nepad.org/publication/guide-regional-centers-of-regulatory-excellence-rcores

Management Science for Health/Health Commodities and Services Management (MSH/HCSM) Programme.

The launch culminated in the roll-out of various activities including, capacity building of focal champions and regional trainers, the development and dissemination of guidelines, reporting tools and job aid, in-service training, and sensitization of healthcare workers.

The National Pharmacovigilance Centre (NPC) was able to collect and submit a total of 145 Individual Case Safety Reports (ICSRs) to the World Health Organization International Drug Monitoring Programme in 2010. Subsequently, the NPC became the 98th full official member of the Uppsala Monitoring Centre in May 2010.[5]

With the introduction of new medicines/regimens in the Kenyan market, the growth of the pharmaceutical sector, and an increase in the number of market complaints on substandard HPTs, there was the need to establish a robust post-marketing surveillance system for the detection and response to risks on quality of HPTs. The Pharmacovigilance department developed a Post-Marketing Surveillance (PMS) strategy to strengthen monitoring and response to quality issues of HPTs circulating in the Kenyan market.

To promote innovation, cost-effectiveness, and sustainability, the PPB with support from USAID through the HCSM Programme developed and implemented a Pharmacovigilance Electronic Reporting System (PvERS) in 2013, which was the first VigiFlow-compatible e-reporting system in Africa.

The PvERS system has undergone upgrades to make it responsive to emerging safety issues. Through stakeholder engagement, PPB identified gaps in the PVERs system, especially in the quality of reports submitted as well as the expanded scope of pharmacovigilance. This necessitated an upgrade of the system (v.1) to the current version II in 2021 (https://pv.pharmacyboardkenya.org/).

The Kenya Pharmacovigilance Electronic Reporting System II (PvERS II) is an electronic platform used for the collection and processing of information on individual case safety reports and suspected quality defects that occur with us of health products and technologies including adverse drug reactions, adverse events following immunization, medication errors, incidents related to medical devices and blood and blood product related reactions.

The PPB further enhanced the safety reporting platforms by developing and deploying a mobile phone application for safety reporting in 2022, dubbed the mobile pharmacovigilance electronic reporting systems (mPvERS)[6] which is available on both Android and iOS operating platforms. The platform enables reporting by both healthcare workers and members of the public. In addition, the PPB has established. Another reporting platform is based on USSD code that targets members of the public *271#.

The PPB in collaboration with development and technical partners has achieved several milestones since 2010 in strengthening the PV system in Kenya. They

---

[5] Uppsala Reports July 2010 https://who-umc.org/media/164023/ur50.pdf

[6] https://play.google.com/store/apps/details?id=com.ppb_app&hl=en_ZA&gl=US&pli=1

include the implementation of national PV guidelines and training packages, sensitization of healthcare providers on pharmacovigilance, and training and sensitization of undergraduate and graduate students on PV and Post Marketing Surveillance.

The PPB collaborated with the University of Nairobi, HCSM, University of Washington and SIAPS programme to implement a Post Graduate Masters' course in Pharmacoepidemiology and Pharmacovigilance (EPIVIGIL) in the year 2012. Almost 100 graduates of EPIVIGIL are currently implementing PV activities in public health programmes, PPB, at national, and county levels. The programme not only serves Kenyan students but also offers capacity building of regulatory and academia staff across the region among them Malawi, Rwanda, and Tanzania.

The achievements listed above contributed to the selection of Kenya as one of the Regional Centres of Regulatory Excellence (RCORES) in Africa for Pharmacovigilance in 2014. The Kenya PV-RCORE continues to strive for excellence and serve as a hub for good Pharmacovigilance practices in the continent and as the technical lead country for Pharmacovigilance and Post Marketing Surveillance in the East African Community and the Inter-Governmental Authority on Development (IGAD) under the Medicine Regulation Harmonization (MRH) initiative.

The strong pharmacovigilance system at PPB has attracted benchmarking visits by several countries including Afghanistan, Angola, Tanzania, Zimbabwe, Ethiopia, Somalia, Ghana, Bangladesh, and Mozambique.

In the year 2016, Kenya Spearheaded the development of East African Community Regional Economic Block harmonized PV indicators, which were used to perform a baseline assessment of the PV functions in the region. The results led to the development of the East Africa Community Pharmacovigilance Strategic Business Plan 2018–2023 for sourcing funds to oversee the strengthening of PV in the region. This led to the development of the EAC Harmonized Compendium on Safety and Vigilance of Medical Products and Health Technologies and SOPs that have been either adopted or domesticated in the partner countries.[7]

Some of the key activities that are under implementation include strengthening of pharmacovigilance activities in the Eastern Africa region through the PROFORMA Consortium, an EDCTP2-funded programme. The project is implemented by PPB in collaboration with other National Regulatory Authorities and training institutions in the region[8] (See Chap. 24).

Alongside Ethiopia, Nigeria, Ghana, and South, Kenya PV RCORE is also a part of the African Union's Smart Safety Surveillance (AU-3S) programme whose long-term goal is to strengthen the safety surveillance of priority medical products across the African continent.[9] The AU-3S team works closely with the medical products National Regulatory Authorities (NRAs) and Expanded Programmes on Immunisation (EPIs) from countries involved.

---

[7] https://www.eac.int/documents/category/pharmacovigilance

[8] https://proforma.ki.se/

[9] https://www.nepad.org/microsite/african-union-smart-safety-surveillance-au-3s

One of the key focuses of the AU-3S pilot is supporting the safety surveillance of COVID-19 vaccines, in the participating countries, and Kenya is currently undertaking an active surveillance of the vaccines through Cohort Event Monitoring (see Chap. 20).

The RCORE's functions and activities are currently funded through funds generated by PPB. Other financial or technical support comes from development and implementing partners as well as continued collaborations locally and globally.

There is a funding gap to support the RCORE activities, but with the continued support and collaboration with Regional Economic Communities (REC) MRH programs, the PPB RCORE will achieve its mandate of strengthening PV in Africa.

Chapter 18
KIDS-APEC Pharmacovigilance Center of Excellence Training

Euihwan Baek and E Na Song

To achieve regulatory harmonization in the Asia-Pacific Economic Cooperation (APEC) regions, Korea Institute of Drug Safety and Risk Management (KIDS)[1] provides pharmacovigilance training, namely 'KIDS-APEC Pharmacovigilance CoE Training' to the regulators.

18.1 What Is a CoE?

The establishment of a 'Training Center of Excellence for Regulatory Science (CoE)' was suggested by the Regulatory Harmonization Steering Committee (RHSC).[2] RHSC efforts have been guided by a Strategic Framework and Vision to

---

[1] Korea Institute of Drug Safety and Risk Management (KIDS) was established in January 2012 according to the regulation of Article 68-3 of Pharmaceutical Affairs Act. Its activities include collecting, analyzing, evaluating, and providing drug safety information, developing drug utilization review criteria, conducting causality assessments of adverse drug events, managing operation of Korea Adverse Drug Reaction (ADR) Relief programme, and Narcotics Information Management System for monitoring narcotics.

[2] The Regulatory Harmonization Steering Committee (RHSC) was formed in June 2009 under the auspices of the APEC Life Sciences Innovation Forum to promote a more strategic approach to regulatory harmonization by undertaking activities of greatest value to regulatory authorities and regulated industries.

E. Baek · E. N. Song (✉)
Korea Institute of Drug Safety and Risk Management,
Anyang-si, Gyeonggi-do, Republic of Korea
e-mail: kids_coe@drugsafe.or.kr

© Springer Nature Singapore Pte Ltd. 2025   341
S. R. Ahmad (ed.), *Special Issues in Pharmacovigilance in Resource-Limited Countries*, https://doi.org/10.1007/978-981-96-6154-1_18

promote greater regulatory convergence[3] by 2021. Roadmaps to analyze and address gaps have been developed for seven (7) priority work areas (PWAs),[4] which include pharmacovigilance.

The RHSC agreed in February 2013 to explore the establishment of CoEs in APEC, starting with a 3-day pilot workshop on Multi-Regional Clinical Trials (MRCT) and Good Clinical Practice Inspection at Duke-National University of Singapore in March 2014. After the successful pilot CoE workshop, the RHSC agreed in January 2015 to expand the CoE concept to other PWAs.

CoEs play a crucial role in sharing and disseminating knowledge and expertise, fostering advancements, and facilitating collaboration in their respective fields. The primary objectives of a CoE are to (1) build skilled human capacity in regulatory sciences to bring safe, effective, and quality medical products to patients and people as quickly as possible; (2) promote dialogue to share understanding in science and best practices; and (3) achieve a model of sustainable operation that includes periodic updates to maintain regulatory relevancy of materials and ensures continued value to all participating entities; and (4) avoid duplication of efforts and leverage work that already exists and has a level of convergence.

The key benefits expected from the implementation of CoEs include the following: CoEs will (1) deliver and/or support training by training experts and regulatory Subject Matter Experts as appropriate; (2) provide financial independence for sustainable training efforts, reduce reliance on funding; and (3) enable long-term, continuous training in the science and best practice(s) of a PWA.

KIDS was endorsed by members of the RHSC at the APEC RHSC meeting in February 2016 to host a pilot CoE in the PWA of pharmacovigilance. After the successful hosting of the APEC Pharmacovigilance CoE Pilot Programme in 2016, KIDS was endorsed as a formal CoE host institution in pharmacovigilance in 2017. Since then, with the guidance of a Strategic Framework and Vision aimed at fostering regulatory convergence, KIDS has been annually providing 'KIDS-APEC Pharmacovigilance CoE training' programmes to regulators (https://kidscoe.drugsafe.or.kr/).

---

[3] According to the RHSC's Operating Procedures (revised June 26, 2013), "regulatory convergence" represents a *voluntary process* whereby the regulatory requirements across economies become more similar or aligned over time as a result of the gradual adoption of internationally recognized technical guidance documents, standards, and scientific principles (harmonization) and common or similar practices and procedures. It *does not* represent the harmonization of laws and regulations, which is not necessary to allow for the alignment of technical requirements and for greater regulatory cooperation.

[4] Multi-Regional Clinical Trials (MRCT) and Good Clinical Practices (GCP) Inspection; Global Supply Chain Integrity; Biotherapeutics; Good Registration Management; Advanced Therapies; Medical Devices; and Pharmacovigilance.

18.2   Goals of the 'KIDS-APEC PV CoE Training' and the Programmes

The primary goals of the 'KIDS-APEC PV CoE Training' are to (1) provide a forum to facilitate understanding of the current pharmacovigilance activities in different APEC regions and beyond; (2) implement effective measures and system to promote global public health; and (3) strengthen the pharmacovigilance capacity of regulatory and public bodies and build capacity to improve the pharmacovigilance system (https://kidscoe.drugsafe.or.kr/).

Each year, the training programme is developed based on RHSC's core curriculum, survey results from the previous year, and relevant international standards via collaboration with the Pharmacovigilance Working Group—consisting of regulators and pharmacovigilance professionals from thirteen (13) economies (Chinese Taipei, Indonesia, Japan, Republic of Korea, Malaysia, Mexico, Peru, Philippines, Singapore, Sweden, Switzerland, Thailand, and USA) and sixteen (16) organizations (BIO, COFEPRIS, DIGEMID, FDA, FDA Thailand, HAS, JPMA, KIDS, MFDS, NADFC, NPRA, PFDA, PMDA, TFDA, UMC, and WHO).

The training programme focuses on the in-field capacity building of regulators, one of the essential requirements in achieving regulatory harmonization, and consists of lectures and hands-on exercises. The key topics taught cover the full life cycle of pharmacovigilance activities, which include adverse event reporting and collection; adverse event analysis and evaluation; decision making, safety measure, and risk communication. During the hands-on exercise sessions, participants are to apply the knowledge they have learned from the lectures through group discussions and voluntary presentations. The hands-on exercises from 2016 to 2024 covered topics such as writing individual case safety reports (ICSRs), learning methods for active AE collection, conducting causality assessments of ICSRs, signal detection, benefit-risk assessment, and decision making and communication in scenarios where a risk has been identified.

18.3   Participants of the 'KIDS-APEC PV CoE Training'

From 2016 to 2024, an average of 131 regulators from various economies per year have benefited from the 'KIDS-APEC Pharmacovigilance CoE training'. Among the participating economies, Korea had the highest number of total participants from 2016 to 2024, followed by Malaysia, Chinese Taipei, Azerbaijan, and Indonesia. Then came The Philippines, Thailand, Singapore, Mexico, and Peru. Papua New Guinea, Cambodia, and Chile, were next, followed by Hong Kong, China, Bangladesh, and Saudi Arabia. Lastly, Canada, Denmark, France, Germany, Ireland, Japan, New Zealand, Republic of Estonia, Sweden, The Czech Republic, The Netherlands, The United Kingdom, The United States, and Vietnam also had participants in the training.

Registration to attend the training is open to regulators only; however, all programs are recorded and made accessible on the KIDS-APEC official website (https://kidscoe.drugsafe.or.kr/) for anyone who may be interested, including non-regulators such as those from academia and industries.

18.4   Impact of the 'KIDS-APEC PV CoE Training'

Republic of Korea has emerged as the leading performing country in APEC PV CoE, a total of 1050 trainees with 30 economies attended the KIDS-APEC PV CoE workshops. Live hands-on exercise session programmes have helped participants share knowledge on the pharmacovigilance activities in their economies and strengthen networking relationships through discussions on the given cases and related issues. After the programmes ended, participants mentioned that their general understanding of pharmacovigilance has improved and they were able to grasp the trend of global pharmacovigilance. In addition, a need for cooperation among APEC regulators was reinforced, with an emphasis on continuous participation in global workshops and programmes where regulators can improve their professional capacity in drug safety and risk management. A forum where regulators from different economies and organizations could come together to discuss and exchange their ideas for international harmonization of pharmacovigilance and drug safety was highly valued.

Chapter 19
PMDA's Training and Capacity Building in Pharmacovigilance

Akiko Ogata

Pharmaceuticals and Medical Devices Agency (PMDA) is the regulatory authority for medical products in Japan. PMDA conducts scientific review of marketing authorization application of pharmaceuticals, medical devices and regenerative medical products and monitors their post-marketing safety in collaboration with the Ministry of Health, Labour and Welfare (MHLW).

19.1 Establishment of Asia Training Center (ATC) in PMDA

PMDA believes global cooperation is essential to accelerate clinical development of regulated medical products and to enhance benefit/risk balance in the post-marketing phase. On 1 April 2016, PMDA established the 'Asia Training Center for Pharmaceuticals and Medical Devices Regulatory Affairs' (PMDA-ATC) to contribute to enhancement of public health in Asia and universal health coverage (UHC) advocated by World Health Organization (WHO) through developing a foundation for international standards and regulatory harmonization, which will lead to faster and timely access to the advanced medical technologies for the patients especially in the Asian region. PMDA-ATC provides systematic trainings sharing the accumulated knowledge and experiences of PMDA. Since 2017, PMDA-ATC has been recognized as one of the Centers of Excellence (CoEs) in the area of pharmacovigilance by the Asia Pacific Economic Cooperation (APEC). Furthermore, in the joint statement of the Association of Southeast Asian Nations (ASEAN)-Japan Health Ministers' Meeting on Universal Health Coverage and Population Ageing in 2017,

A. Ogata (✉)
Division of Training Center Management, Office of International Programmes, Pharmaceuticals and Medical Devices Agency (PMDA), kasumigaseki, Chiyoda, Tokyo, Japan
e-mail: ogata-akiko@pmda.go.jp

© Springer Nature Singapore Pte Ltd. 2025
S. R. Ahmad (ed.), *Special Issues in Pharmacovigilance in Resource-Limited Countries*, https://doi.org/10.1007/978-981-96-6154-1_19

345

PMDA-ATC was specifically mentioned as the regulatory platform to improve the capabilities of ASEAN countries.

The PMDA-ATC Pharmacovigilance seminar provides latest comprehensive information and shares our experiences and knowledge. Its programme is typically 4 days long and consists of lectures and group works for case studies and offered in-person or virtual manner. The Seminar covers wide range of topics on pharmacovigilance area, such as global standards, global safety data collection, evaluation of accumulated adverse drug reaction (ADR) reports and other safety data, the risk management plan (RMP) including pharmacovigilance plan and risk minimization action plan, risk communication like labelling and dissemination of safety information.

In the PMDA-ATC seminar, participants are able to learn background information and practical case studies on different aspects of pharmacovigilance through lectures and group discussions. The purpose of the seminar is to provide global standards like International Conference on Harmonization (ICH) guidelines, not just Japanese regulations. However, knowing how the global standard is adopted by the US FDA, EMA or PMDA, as appropriately in each jurisdiction, and their backgrounds should help the participants to enhance the regulatory system in their own economies for pharmacovigilance.

The lectures are led not only by PMDA staff members from pharmacovigilance divisions but also by representatives from US FDA, academia and pharmaceutical industries. It allows participants to consider and discuss multiple perspectives on pharmacovigilance. In the group discussions, participants exchange their opinion and discuss safety specifications and risk minimization activities using the mock data for review reports or adverse reaction case reports. Through the interactive communication in the seminar programme, participants gain the chances to refer back to their work and to find any additional opportunity for enhancement of the regulatory system for pharmacovigilance in the post-marketing phase in their own countries and regions.

In the 7 years from 2017 to 2023, total 192 regulators from 34 countries and regions have participated in the PMDA-ATC pharmacovigilance seminars. About 80% of those participants are from Asian countries and regions (Bangladesh, Bhutan, Cambodia, China, Chinese Taipei, Hong Kong, India, Indonesia, Laos, Malaysia, Maldives, Myanmar, Nepal, Pakistan, Philippines, Singapore, South Korea, Sri Lanka, Thailand, and Vietnam), and the remaining 20% are from outside Asia (Azerbaijan, Brazil, Chile, Ethiopia, Nigeria, Papua New Guinea, Peru, Poland, Russia, Saudi Arabia, South Africa, Tanzania, Tunisia, and Uganda).

PMDA-ATC provides e-learning training materials as well. Learning videos are available in the 'Pmda Channel' of the YouTube for public. In the play list of 'Safety Measures', one can watch the several short videos introducing Safety Measures, E-labelling system in Japan, Pharmacovigilance activity utilizing Real world Data in Japan, etc., with the voice of a native English speaker. In addition, for only regulators, e-learning courses are also available that compiles several thematic contents into one course similar to PMDA-ATC seminars.

In Japan, all ICH guidelines are implemented and several unique systems are further included for pharmacovigilance, such as Early Post-marketing Phase Vigilance (EPPV), which provides updates of safety information and collects safety data intensively for 6 months immediately after marketing authorization, re-examination, re-evaluation and so on. These systems have been established based on our experiences that the real-world clinical settings are different from clinical trials in the development phase and that there is high possibility of occurrence of unforeseen risks just after the launch of new products. Risk Management Plan (RMP) is implemented in many countries/regions and the Japanese RMP, which was developed based on ICH-E2E and other relevant guidelines, was implemented in 2012. It is concise and easy to share comprehensive information on the product among stakeholders, regulators, marketing authorization holders (MAHs) and healthcare professionals.

PMDA publishes the information about revisions of label information (package inserts) for healthcare professionals as 'Safety Info', to be shared among regulatory authorities around the world. The information includes the list of the drugs that have come under review by PMDA/MHLW and are to proceed with revisions of precautions as recommended by PMDA based on safety concerns identified through analysis of a certain amount of information accumulated in the ADR reports, the data submitted as a part of EPPV or those from other sources.

As access to innovative medical products increases, post-marketing safety measures become more crucial. To provide appropriate drug therapies to the patients around the world, global data collection and aggregation, management and analysis of such data are vital for effective pharmacovigilance. Promoting public health is universal theme regardless of regions. PMDA is keen to contribute to build robust pharmacovigilance systems on a global basis for the patients through the PMDA-ATC Training Seminars.

Chapter 20
The UK MHRA's Collaboration to Improve Pharmacovigilance in Resource-Limited Settings

Mick Foy

A robust pharmacovigilance system is essential for the success of public health programmes. When new medicines or vaccines are used in large populations in a short timeframe, it is essential that safety information is gathered quickly to ensure the success of the product launch. New medicines and vaccines are much needed to treat and prevent disease, and this is particularly important in low- and middle-income countries (LMIC). Increasingly, such new medicines or vaccines are used for the first time in such settings, the uncertainties around their safety are greater, and the need for effective pharmacovigilance all the more compelling.

New medicines and vaccines, particularly in certain disease areas, such as malaria and HIV, may be introduced for the first time in LMICs where there are weak or no regulatory systems in place for effective pharmacovigilance. This can cause issues and a robust pharmacovigilance system is essential for the success of public health programs.

Without an effective pharmacovigilance system, public health programmes for the treatment of diseases such as malaria, HIV are at risk. Patients will be impacted as they may suffer from adverse drug reactions (ADRs), which are not promptly identified and treated. This can consequently undermine the programme as a loss of trust in the product or a vaccine will lead to lower uptake and the disease not being effectively treated. Furthermore, financial and reputational loss will be incurred by developers, manufacturers, and funders of the product(s) and programme(s).

These new treatments may have been developed with urgent public health needs in mind, and therefore, the need to gather and analyse information quickly on their safety and efficacy is important. The healthcare and regulatory systems in these settings may often lack the tools, training and capacity to operate a robust pharmacovigilance system. Whilst great progress has been made in the LMICs setting, with

M. Foy (✉)
Vigilance Intelligence and Research Group, Medicines and Healthcare Products Regulatory Agency (MHRA), London, UK
e-mail: mick@cimuna.co.uk

© Springer Nature Singapore Pte Ltd. 2025
S. R. Ahmad (ed.), *Special Issues in Pharmacovigilance in Resource-Limited Countries*, https://doi.org/10.1007/978-981-96-6154-1_20

many of the countries now involved as members of the World Health Organization Programme for International Drug Monitoring, the experience in collecting, assessing and acting on adverse reaction data, and risk management planning, is limited and the infrastructure in terms of data management and IT is also limited.

To address these issues, the Gates Foundation (GF) with the WHO created the Smart Safety Surveillance strategy or 3S for short. This identified products in critical disease areas, malaria, MDR-TB and rotavirus and countries where these products would be used to pilot programmes to improve pharmacovigilance capabilities. The concept is to target pharmacovigilance capacity building efforts around a drug or disease and then use the successes of that to build out to the rest of the safety system for all products.

The need for regulatory capacity building was seen as key to the success of the 3S programme and as such the Medicines and Healthcare products Regulatory Agency of the UK (MHRA) joined 3S as a regulatory partner in 2017.

The MHRA partnered with the WHO and the GF to strengthen the 3S initiative and to support ongoing work in Africa, Asia and the Americas. In particular work was carried out in Thailand, Armenia, Ethiopia and India.

The countries were selected for the 3S pilots by WHO together with the GF based on three factors: Being members of the WHO International Programme for Drug Monitoring, having a pharmacovigilance system rated as at least medium by WHO and having a high prevalence of the target disease being treated or going to be treated by the products.

The key problems to address were identified as:

- Potential risks of ADRs caused by new medicines/vaccines where the characteristics of the product and the ADR profile are not well established
- Under-reporting of ADRs from patients, healthcare professionals and pharmaceutical industry
- Limited capacity to effectively capture and analyse safety data
- Limited experience in risk management planning and the identification and assessment of signals
- Immature regulatory systems and limited capacity to support evidence based pharmacovigilance decisions

An example of the work carried out is the bedaquiline pilot in Armenia. This pilot was led by MHRA, a lead assessor was assigned, and additional MHRA support was brought in as required.

The pilot had the key objectives of:

- Enhance the National Regulatory Agency (NRA) capacity to collect and analyse safety data including reports of suspected ADRs through database development and availability of country-specific mobile application for reporting of ADRs (the Med Safety app). This mobile app has been made available via WHO and MHRA to a growing number of countries in LMICs. MHRA worked with the Armenia NRA to brand the App with the appropriate logos and translate the forms, which are in the ICH E2B format, into both Armenian and Russian.

- Increased healthcare professional and public awareness of the importance of ADR reporting was done using mainstream media and social media. This coincided with the launch of the App, and a press conference was arranged with the Health Minister and representatives of the WHO and the GF.
- Increased profile of the NRA; better public understanding of its role and knowledge of its activities relating to monitoring the safety of and risk management of medicines.
- Training and capacity building at the Armenian NRA in signal detection, risk benefit assessment and risk communication as well as the establishing of a safety committee to review newly identified risks. This was done through a series of site visits by the MHRA team to Armenia and study visits by the NRA to MHRA offices.
- Development of pharmacovigilance guidelines around PV responsibilities for the local pharmaceutical industry drafted by MHRA with Armenian counterparts.
- Studies were conducted to confirm that the safety profile of bedaquiline in clinical practice in Armenia is consistent with the current known safety profile and/or identify new signals, which may or may not be country specific.
- Improved Marketing Authorisation Holders' (MAHs) awareness and understanding of the NRAs expectations and requirements relating to submission of dossiers including Periodic Safety Update Reports, Risk Management Plans, and Post-Authorisation Safety Studies. Consequently, improved quality of regulatory submissions by MAHs enabling more efficient assessment by NRA and therefore better use of limited NRA resources.

Since 2019, the 3S initiative has had a greater focus on Africa, with the project being named AU3S (African Union Smart Safety Surveillance). Working with the African Union Development Agency (AUDA-NEPAD), there are extensive plans to take the learnings from the initial 3S pilots to improve pharmacovigilance across the African continent over a 10-year period. There will be a strong focus on technology and how Africa can implement international standards and methodologies for ADR collection and signal detection.

MHRA has again joined as partners to bring regulatory expertise to this programme, sharing insights from their extensive European experience on how a network of member states can effectively work together to share resources and establish standards, systems and processes for the benefit of all African citizens.

In the initial phase, the AU3S has concentrated on the surveillance of COVID-19 vaccines used in the African Union. Working with five countries initially, Ghana, Nigeria, South Africa, Ethiopia and Kenya, the AU3S project began looking at preparedness for collecting ADR reports and capacity strengthening for regulators and health care professionals involved in the immunisation programmes.

At the beginning of 2020, MHRA experts delivered a series of online training modules covering aspects of pharmacovigilance from data collection, case management, signal detection, risk benefit assessment and risk communication. These were all recorded and made available to stakeholders for future reference.

The Med Safety App was deployed in each country, and immunisation programmes and the regulatory authorities were given access to tools to manage follow-up. A specific AEFI (Adverse Event Following Immunisation) form was developed to improve data collection.

All data received was entered into the MHRA drug safety database and signal detection on the pooled African dataset was conducted each week. A "Joint Signal Management Group" (JSM) was convened with members from each country who meet each week to review potential signals of interest.

Over the 3 years since the introduction of the first COVID-19 vaccines in Africa, the AU3S project has facilitated over 85,000 new users of the Med Safety App. More than 38,000 AEFI reports have been submitted to the regulatory agencies representing a 15× increase in reporting. As a result the JSM group have analysed over 2.5 K vaccine/event combinations.

Following this successful period, the AU3S project will now expand to more countries and look at drugs and vaccines beyond those used for the COVID-19 pandemic.

More details on the results of AU3S will be subject of future publications and further information can be found at https://www.nepad.org/microsite/african-union-smart-safety-surveillance-au-3s.

Pharmacovigilance is a global concern, patients take the same medicines in LMICs as in Europe or other high income settings. Many treatments may be launched first in LMICs so it is now critical that all national regulators have the capacity to run effective pharmacovigilance systems not just for their citizens and patients but in the interests and for the benefit of all. Stringent regulators such as MHRA are well placed to join programmes like 3S and AU3S to share expertise and deliver training and tools for NRAs on pharmacovigilance techniques.

Chapter 21
Pragmatic Pharmacovigilance and Combatting Substandard and Falsified Medical Products (SFs)

Paul B. Huleatt

Over several decades, Australia, through the Therapeutic Goods Administration (TGA), has engaged in activities with counterpart regulatory authorities in the Indo-Pacific region, which come under the broad umbrella of 'regulatory systems strengthening and support'. In recent times, the WHO has effectively categorized regulatory functions through development and refinement of the Global Benchmarking Tool (GBT) and low- and middle-income countries (LMICs) often rely on the GBT methodology to inform and guide regulatory systems strengthening activities. Hence, it is a ubiquitous reference for technical assistance providers and National Regulatory Authorities (NRAs) alike.

Most GBT functions (e.g., Market Authorization (MA), Laboratory Testing (LT), Market Control (MC) etc.) fall primarily under the purview of the medical products regulatory authority and concern a limited group of external stakeholders (e.g. regulated industry). The Vigilance (VL) function is more complex in this regard, and strengthening Pharmacovigilance (PV) systems is particularly challenging as a result.

In LMICs settings, the majority of key stakeholders sit outside the National regulatory authority (NRA). The NRA typically, but not always, incorporates the National Pharmacovigilance Centre (the domestic entity which is linked to WHO's Programme on International Drug Monitoring (PIDM)) and in addition to regulated industry, an effective working relationship with a network of vertically integrated public health programmes (PHPs) and hospitals is an important foundation for a functional system. Organizational capacity, funding, staff turnover and competing priorities mean these important links are often difficult to build, harder to sustain and, therefore, should be the main target of Regulatory Systems Strengthening work aimed at developing PV systems.

P. B. Huleatt (✉)
Therapeutic Goods Administration (TGA), Woden, ACT, Australia
e-mail: paul.huleatt@dfat.gov.au

© Springer Nature Singapore Pte Ltd. 2025
S. R. Ahmad (ed.), *Special Issues in Pharmacovigilance in Resource-Limited Countries*, https://doi.org/10.1007/978-981-96-6154-1_21

Stringent Regulatory Authorities (SRAs) are well placed to deliver capacity building for staff in NRAs in LMICs guided by the GBT and leveraging Institutional Development Plans (IDPs) derived from GBT assessments wherever possible. However, this work mainly strengthens the Pharmacovigilance system at a single point, the regulator, and the potential value of these labours can only be realized with similar efforts at every touch point. Regulatory experts from SRAs whilst effective in training staff in NRAs are generally not equipped to deliver capacity building throughout the tiers of a PHP. Conversely, many non-government organisations lack the mandate, relationships and expertise required to train staff in NRAs but are optimally placed and well suited to working with PHPs (e.g. Medicines for Malaria Venture (MMV) and the Partnership for Vivax Elimination (PAVE) with National Malaria Control Programmes in the Greater Mekong Subregion). This is particularly important as information exchange relating to adverse events, any causality assessment and follow-ups may be unintentionally siloed within a PHP or duplicated at the NRA resulting in further strain on resource-limited organizations and may compromise the management of drug safety in these settings.

Therefore, with respect to NRA-PHP engagement, to truly strengthen the Pharmacovigilance system, a coordinated approach between all technical assistance providers is required. The strength of the working relationship between an NRA and the PHP will almost certainly reflect the effectiveness, cohesion and complementarity of the assistance provided by SRAs and NGOs. As important as it is, coordination and collaboration between relevant parties is often an ad hoc undertaking driven by individuals within concerned organizations. Fortunately, forums to systematize this type of engagement, such as WHOs long awaited Coalition of Interested Parties (of which TGA is a member), are moving from concept to reality at global, regional and national levels.

The PIDM has been running for over 50 years, and the PV systems in place in many high-income countries (HICs) have slowly matured over the course of many decades. It should therefore be apparent that building a strong PV system is a long-term undertaking. Technical assistance providers should ensure that initiatives undertaken to strengthen a nascent PV system are 'practical' in the sense of being readily implementable, sustainable and extensible rather than aiming for the HIC gold standard at the outset. In this regard, building a system which aims to help ensure medicine quality by inter alia effective identification of medicine quality problems rather than focusing on causality analysis and signal detection is a worthwhile consideration in many domestic contexts where prioritizing cost-effective procurement of essential medicines and vaccines and their sale through informal markets may introduce significant health risks. Substandard and Falsified Medical Products (SFs) are an ongoing scourge in the Indo-Pacific region and efforts to combat them employing Prevention, Detection and Response strategies continue to gain momentum. In the LMIC domestic setting, the PV system is an important piece of the 'Detection' pillar and reporting of medicine quality issues by consumers, health care professionals and industry should be enabled at every opportunity. SFs are an intercontinental, trans-national, cross-jurisdictional problem requiring a proportional multi-sectoral response. To facilitate such a response, it is important to rapidly communicate medicine quality issues linked to adverse events (including 'drug ineffective' cases or clusters) to the WHO via the Global Surveillance and Monitoring System (GSMS) for further investigation and subsequent publication of a Medical Product Alert in appropriate circumstances.

In LMICs, it is not uncommon for NRA staff in a National PV Centre to have responsibilities spanning multiple regulatory functions including market control and surveillance. To help balance competing priorities and capacity, it is important to augment technical assistance from SRAs like the Australian TGA, by leveraging other forums that allow the exchange of information and best practices. In this vein, NRA staff can work with counterparts through the WHO Member State Mechanism on Substandard and Falsified Medical Products (MSM). The Member State Mechanism was established by the World Health Assembly in 2012 to protect public health, promote access to affordable, safe, efficacious, and quality medical products and to promote the prevention and control of SF medical products and associated activities. MSM meetings, working groups and technical briefings cover a range of topics including risk communication, traceability and online sales, which are instructive and translate to pharmacovigilance activities in general. Greater engagement in the Member State Mechanism by countries in the Indo-Pacific will significantly enhance and reinforce this region's multi-pronged approach to securing medicine and vaccine quality and safety.

Chapter 22
Thirty Years of Safety and Vigilance Systems Strengthening in the WHO AFRO Region: From Buoyant Growth to Rigorous Protection of Public Health

Stanislav Kniazkov

22.1 Background

WHO Africa Region (AFRO) includes 47 Member States that have national medicines regulatory authorities (NMRAs) for medical products. These NMRAs vary a lot in their organizational models, the scope of regulation and maturity level. Medical product vigilance and safety is one of the core functions of these NMRAs. Over the past years substantial improvements have been recorded in pharmacovigilance implementation in Africa in quantitative and qualitative terms. However, the noticeable variance across the countries in Africa calls for continuation of technical support moving from the overall system strengthening to product/class-targeted assistance. A shift of focus from quantitative indicators to quality of the regulatory oversight introduced by the WHO AFRO (Regional Office for Africa) Regional Strategy for Medical Product Regulation in 2016 has yielded noticeable results. However, there is a need to change the approach and render technical assistance to the WHO Member States in the AFRO region in a more customer-tailored way through capacity building, reinforcement of legislative bases and emphasis on new medical products or products categories specifically developed to cater for the priority health needs in the countries.

S. Kniazkov (✉)
WHO Regional Office for Africa, AFRO, Brazzaville, Republic of the Congo

WHO Regional Office for Europe, Copenhagen, Denmark
e-mail: stansilav.kniazkov@gmail.com; kniazkovs@who.int

22.2 Growth of Pharmacovigilance

The vigilance and safety systems in Africa have witnessed an exponential growth from 1992 onwards when Morocco and South Africa became the first countries in the African continent to join the WHO Programme for International Drug Monitoring (PIDM) established in 1968 in response to the thalidomide crisis. United Republic of Tanzania and Tunisia became PIDM members in 1993 followed by Zimbabwe in 1998. By the end of 2015, there were already 35 countries with established pharmacovigilance programmes in the WHO AFRO region [1]. The portion of countries with vigilance and safety systems for medical products continues to grow.

During the 2017–2018 survey, a question NMRAs were asked to confirm was, if they have mandates for pharmacovigilance. It brought back 93% of positive answers. However, this was equally applicable to all product classes. When asked about the mandate for haemovigilance to ensure safety of blood and blood components, only 41% of responding authorities were able to confirm it. This unveiled a substantial gap that exists in the pharmacovigilance systems. Another example is safety and vigilance over medical devices, which returned 18% positive response for technovigilance and 23% cybervigilance. Although this survey did not aspire to analyse the root-causes, it emphasized the need for a greater focus on specific product classes and, thereby, justified a move from generic capacity building towards more targeted approaches [2].

22.3 Regional Strategy for Regulation of Medical Products

In August 2016, the WHO Regional Committee for Africa adopted Resolution 13/66/REG and endorsed the Regional Strategy for Regulation of Medical Products in the WHO Africa Region, 2016–2025. [https://www.afro.who.int/sites/default/files/2017-07/afrrc66-13-en-1011_0.pdf]. This strategy documented a remarkable change of approach towards regulatory strengthening shifting the emphasis from systems building to boosting regulation quality and scope. Progress evaluation was undertaken through surveys designed at the AFRO level and through the use of the WHO Global Benchmarking Tool (GBT). GBT incarnates an approach proposed by the International Organisation for Standardisation (ISO), which classifies systems into maturity levels to gauge their functionality and quality of processes they underpin. Maturity level 1 implies that some elements exist, whereas maturity level 4, currently the highest level for regulatory systems, is attributed to regulatory authorities with robust system capable to produce results of expected quality, which exercise the continuous improvement approach. The minimally recommended maturity level for regulatory systems is 3. At this level, regulatory systems enjoy stable functionality and exercise all critically important functions required to assure safety, efficacy and quality of medical products. In 2016–2020, WHO was invited by the national regulatory authorities to facilitate their self-assessment or to formally assess regulatory systems against GBT. Pharmacovigilance was one of the 8 common regulatory functions included into these assessments. Each function contributes to the overall maturity, which cannot surpass the least advanced of them, i.e., if 7 functions are assessed to be at maturity level 3 but one of them is at maturity level 2 with the implementation rate of less than 80%, the overall maturity cannot be higher than 2.

This strategic shift of focus from quantity to quality yielded results. This was formally confirmed in 2018 when the Tanzania Food and Drugs Authority (TFDA) became the first AFRO country with attained maturity level 3 [3]. In 2020, Ghana's Food and Drugs Authority also achieved maturity level 3 [4]. This demonstrates that the pharmacovigilance systems in these countries are also at maturity level 3 or above. These big achievements bear witness of the national commitment and investment, passion of the regulatory professional as well as results of many years of support delivered by the international community, including WHO. National regulatory systems across the continent continue gaining maturity. Although these remarkable achievements indicate that a lot has already been achieved, a survey conducted in 2017–2018 showed that a more specific focus is needed to ensure further growth and excellence of the national vigilance and safety systems for medical products.

Efficient reporting about substandard and falsified medical products (SF) serves as another, although indirect, evidence of the pharmacovigilance systems maturity in Africa. ADR reports signalling lack of therapeutic efficacy can be instrumental in SF identification. In the period from 2013 to 2017, the WHO AFRO was the leading region in WHO for SF reporting contributing 42% of the reports [5].

African countries with limited resources can no longer fully rely on the well-resourced nations in the aspects of safety and vigilance. Public Health Programmes for Neglected Tropical Diseases serve as a case in point. They use products developed specifically for Africa or other under-resourced countries. Due to the specificity of geographical spread of the diseases they treat, they cannot be used in the USA, Europe or other countries with well-established regulatory systems. Therefore, countries in Africa need to ensure that their pharmacovigilance systems are functional and this further emphasizes the necessity for product targeted technical support from international players. In line with this approach, the WHO conducted capacity building focused on pharmacovigilance for new TB treatments, new medicines for HIV and malaria in the AFRO region.

Pharmacovigilance is one of the regulatory functions that brings together clinicians, pharmacists and patients providing them with opportunities to make contributions to safeguarding public health. This unique quality of pharmacovigilance can be instrumental to implementing the vision of going away from vertical public health services towards integrated healthcare delivery. This will help shift the focus from diseases to patient, from medical procedures to ensuring health and wellbeing of people in Africa. But it cannot be achieved by regulators alone, this requires input of all the health system building blocks and goodwill and collaborative efforts of the key stakeholders. Consequently, this integrating role gives special importance to regulation and places it in the forefront of health systems.

22.4   Conclusions

Pharmacovigilance in the WHO AFRO region has been growing its maturity over the past 30 years. And there are substantial results the region can and should be proud of. The 2016 shift from quantity to quality was a strategic approach that has already yielded positive results. Technical support provided to the Member States in the AFRO region targets the overall strengthening of pharmacovigilance systems and requires building specialized expertise in the specific classes of medical products. This two-pronged approach aims at bringing pharmacovigilance in the region to the new level of excellence.

References

1. Ampadu HH, Hoekman J, de Bruin ML, Pal SN, Olsson S, Sartori D, Leufkens HG, Dodoo AN. Adverse drug reaction reporting in Africa and a comparison of individual case safety report characteristics between Africa and the Rest of the World: analyses of spontaneous reports in VigiBase®. Drug Saf. 2016;39(4):335–45. https://doi.org/10.1007/s40264-015-0387-4.
2. The state of health in the WHO African Region: an analysis of the status of health, health services and health systems in the context of the Sustainable Development Goals. Brazzaville: WHO Regional Office for Africa; 2018, p. 64.
3. https://www.afro.who.int/news/tanzania-food-and-drug-authority-becomes-first-reach-level-3-who-benchmarking-programme.
4. https://www.afro.who.int/news/ghana-foods-and-drugs-authority-fda-attains-maturity-level-3-regulatorystatus#:~:text=Level%203%20indicates%20that%20the,coverage%20and%20sustainable%20development%20goals.
5. WHO Global Surveillance and Monitoring System for substandard and falsified medical products. Geneva: World Health Organization; 2017, p. 11.

Chapter 23
Institutional and Individual Capacity Building in Pharmacovigilance

Tamara Hafner and Francis Aboagye-Nyame

The Medicines, Technologies and Pharmaceutical Services (MTaPS) programme (2018–2025) was the fifth iteration of a series of US Agency for International Development (USAID)-funded programmes implemented by Management Sciences for Health (MSH) that have worked since the early 1990s to strengthen pharmaceutical systems to improve access to and appropriate use of safe, effective, quality-assured medical products and pharmaceutical services. Pharmacovigilance (PV) has been one of the core technical areas in these programmes with MTaPS and its predecessors having contributed to building PV capacity at global, regional, national, sub-national, and health facility levels in the public and private sector using a comprehensive system building approach. Given that the Global Benchmarking Tool (GBT) developed by the World Health Organization (WHO) is now the accepted global standard for objectively assessing national regulatory capacity for medicines and vaccines, MTaPS has structured its PV capacity building efforts around the six critical elements defined in the tool's vigilance module. They include legal provisions, regulations, and guidelines required to define the PV regulatory framework; arrangements for effective organization and good governance; human resources; established and implemented procedures to effectively perform PV activities; mechanisms to monitor regulatory performance and outputs; and mechanisms to promote transparency, accountability, and communication [1]. MTaPS assisted five countries and three regional economic communities to strengthen their PV systems. MTaPS'

T. Hafner · F. Aboagye-Nyame (✉)
USAID Medicines, Technologies, and Pharmaceutical Services (MTaPS) Program,
Management Sciences for Health, Arlington, VA, USA
e-mail: kofinyame.pss@gmail.com

predecessor programme —the USAID Systems for Improved Access to Pharmaceuticals and Services (SIAPS) programme—supported PV capacity building in 12 countries.[1]

23.1 Key Achievements

At the global level, the programs collaborated with international organizations such as the WHO, Global Fund, World Bank, Gates Foundation; US government agencies such as the FDA and CDC; and USAID implementing partners to define the strategic direction for PV. For instance, SIAPS contributed to the development of several tuberculosis (TB) guidelines to guide PV centres and national TB programmes' staff in monitoring the safety of new or repurposed TB medicines (e.g., bedaquiline, linezolid) [2]. SIAPS also served as a member of the WHO-led working group that developed the framework for implementation of the active tuberculosis drug-safety monitoring and management (aDSM) [3]. MTaPS contributed to efforts to enhance and harmonize vaccine safety surveillance systems to guide processes for collecting, analyzing, and sharing safety data and information. As part of the WHO Global Advisory Committee on Vaccine Safety, MTaPS supported evidence-based programmatic decisions related to COVID-19 vaccines.

At the regional level, SIAPS and its predecessor programme—the Strengthening Pharmaceutical Systems (SPS) programme—conducted two multicountry PV assessments in nine sub-Saharan African countries and five Asian countries using a comparative regional perspective. These assessments benchmarked the performance of national PV systems, helped identify replicable and successful experiences, mapped out the contributions of donor agencies and global efforts toward PV, and recommended options for enhancing PV and post-market surveillance systems' capacity and performance [4, 5]. SIAPS also worked with the African Medicines Regulatory Harmonization Programme to establish the structures and mechanisms for coordination and governance of two PV Regional Centres of Regulatory Excellence (RCOREs). The programme also supported the East African Community (EAC) to launch its PV harmonization initiative in 2015. This initiative has led to the development of harmonized PV guidelines that have since been adopted and implemented by member countries.

Using the results of countries' Global Benchmarking Tool (GBT) assessments and building on the achievements of SIAPS, MTaPS supported the African Union Development Agency-New Partnership for Africa's Development (AUDA-NEPAD) by working with the EAC, Intergovernmental Authority on Development (IGAD), and Economic Communities of West African States (ECOWAS) to strengthen PV

---

[1] SIAPS supported Bangladesh, Burundi, Democratic Republic of the Congo (DRC), Ethiopia, Georgia, Kenya, Namibia, the Philippines, South Africa, Swaziland, Uganda, and Ukraine; and MTaPS is supporting Bangladesh, Mozambique, Nepal, the Philippines, Rwanda, East African Community, Intergovernmental Authority on Development, and Economic Communities of West African States.

systems in the regions. MTaPS supported the IGAD and EAC secretariats to fully operationalize their expert working groups on PV and facilitated the training of regional experts on the use of harmonized indicator-based assessment and monitoring tools. In the IGAD region, MTaPS worked with the secretariat to develop a harmonized IGAD PV training curriculum and a costed PV work plan. The programme also worked with the EAC secretariat and member states to develop and validate harmonized procedures for the EAC PV compendium implementation. Working with the West Africa Health Organization (WAHO) and the ECOWAS member states, MTaPS also developed a web-based platform for improving and harmonizing pharmacovigilance (PV) systems in ECOWAS. These regional networks and harmonization efforts have improved collaboration and reliance within the region and expanded safety surveillance and sharing of safety and quality information for better regulatory decision-making.

At the national level, the programmes supported NMRAs, departments and programs in ministries of health, drug and therapeutics committees, academic institutions, and professional associations as necessary to build institutional and individual PV capacity. Establishing a national PV system requires a strong legal framework that promotes an enabling environment with the development of appropriate legislations, regulations, and policies. In Eswatini, for example, SIAPS supported the development of the Medicines and Related Substances Control Bill, enacted into law in 2016, which provides for the establishment of Eswatini's first medicines regulatory authority. In Bangladesh, SIAPS supported the establishment of the adverse drug reaction advisory committee (ADRAC), and MTaPS continues to support and build the capacity of ADRAC members through training and provision of technical support. ADRAC in collaboration with the Adverse Drug Reaction Monitoring Cell provides technical guidance for implementing PV activities, evaluates adverse drug event (ADE) reports, and recommends regulatory decisions to the NMRA.

The procedures and tools used to implement PV activities contribute to the functional level of the system. MTaPS and its predecessor programmes worked with countries to develop or strengthen the procedures and tools—SOPs, reporting forms, information management systems, training—that support active and passive (spontaneous) surveillance. SIAPS, for example, supported the establishment of a national PV unit within the MOH in Eswatini through development of comprehensive PV tools, sensitization training, monthly support supervision of healthcare providers, and support for data analyses, causality assessment, and information dissemination. In the Democratic Republic of the Congo, SIAPS supported the establishment of a collaborative mechanism between key PV stakeholders, including the Drug Regulatory Authority, Drug and Therapeutics Committees, and the national PV centre, to ensure smooth implementation of PV activities at provincial and health facility levels. The programme developed the *Pharmacovigilance Monitoring System (PViMS)*, an electronic patient management system used at facility and central levels to monitor the safety and effectiveness of medicines [6]. PViMS enables the implementation of passive and active surveillance activities in countries by addressing the entire data collection, data analysis, and reporting process.

MTaPS supported PV system strengthening in Bangladesh, Jordan, Mozambique, Nepal, the Philippines, Rwanda, and Tanzania. For example, MTaPS supported Mozambique and the Philippines to use PViMS for their ongoing active surveillance programmes for HIV and TB, respectively, to facilitate identification of potential ADEs and decision making to improve patient safety. In Rwanda, MTaPS worked with the Food and Drugs Authority to develop a costed multi-year national PV implementation plan to guide patient safety monitoring. Generally, MTaPS support has led to the creation of, or the strengthening of PV units and active surveillance systems; development of PV strategies, guidelines, and SOPs; increased AE reporting and causality assessment through training; and the use of technologies such as PViMS for PV data management and decision-making.

Access to medicines is not only about ensuring product availability, but also ensuring they are safe, effective, quality-assured and being used appropriately. As MTaPS' experience has shown, PV capacity must be built at the global, regional, and national levels. At the national level, countries for the first time now have a valuable tool—the WHO GBT—which objectively defines national regulatory capacity for PV and other regulatory functions. The creation of an institutional development plan as part of the benchmarking process allows implementing partners like MTaPS to work with countries in a more streamlined process and an agreed upon framework in strengthening their regulatory capacity.

References

1. World Health Organization. WHO Global Benchmarking Tool (GBT) for evaluation of national regulatory system of medical products. Vigilance: indicators and fact sheets. Revision VI version 1 November 2018. https://www.who.int/medicines/regulation/03_GBT_VL_RevVI.pdf?ua=1. Accessed 20 July 2020.
2. SIAPS. Preventing and minimizing risks associated with Antituberculosis medicines to improve patient safety. Submitted to the US Agency for International Development by the Systems for Improved Access to Pharmaceuticals and Services (SIAPS) program. Arlington: Management Sciences for Health; 2013. https://www.msh.org/resources/preventing-and-minimizing-risks-associated-with-antituberculosis-medicines-to-improve. Accessed 23 July 2020.
3. World Health Organization. Active tuberculosis drug-safety monitoring and management (aDSM): framework for implementation; 2015. https://www.who.int/tb/publications/aDSM/en/. Accessed 23 July 2020.
4. SPS. Safety of medicines in Sub-Saharan Africa: assessment of pharmacovigilance systems and their performance. Submitted to the US Agency for International Development by the Strengthening Pharmaceutical Systems (SPS) Programme. Arlington: Management Sciences for Health; 2011. https://www.msh.org/sites/msh.org/files/Safety-of-Medicines-in-SSA.pdf. Accessed 5 Aug 2020.
5. SIAPS. Comparative analysis of pharmacovigilance Systems in Five Asian Countries. Submitted to the US Agency for international development by the Systems for Improved Access to Pharmaceuticals and Services (SIAPS) Programme. Arlington: Management Sciences for Health; 2013. http://siapsprogram.org/publication/comparative-analysis-of-pharmacovigilance-systems-in-five-asian-countries/. Accessed 5 Aug 2020.
6. USAID MTaPS. Pharmacovigilance monitoring system (PViMS). 2020. https://mtapsprogram.org/sites/default/files/PViMSbrochure-7-2-2020-2.pdf. Accessed 27 July 2020.

Chapter 24
PROFORMA Consortium to Strengthen Pharmacovigilance Capacity in Africa

Eleni Aklillu and Michelle Nderu

24.1 Background and Problem Statement

Access to medicine, particularly new treatments, vaccinations, and microbicides for the treatment of poverty-related illnesses (PRD), is on the rise in Sub-Saharan Africa. However, this effort falls short of National Medicines Regulatory Authorities' (NMRAs') capacity to oversee the quality and safety of new medications and interventions. The growing number of worldwide clinical trials being done in Africa highlights the need for a strong pharmacovigilance (PV) system that adheres to international standards and best practises. Pharmacovigilance is essential throughout clinical trials and beyond to monitor and update risk-benefit ratios and to avoid or minimise drug side effects.

Many African countries are currently deploying preventive chemotherapy through mass drug administrations and immunisation in various public health programmes to all eligible individuals. However, a significant gap in Sub-Saharan Africa is the lack of professional staff to lead and manage the regulatory pharmacovigilance process to monitor public safety, as well as the absence of a post-marketing surveillance system. In order to fill this void, the PROFORMA consortium was formed in 2018. PROFORMA is a 5-year international collaborative project funded by the European and Developing Countries Clinical Trials Partnership2 (EDCTP2)

This project is part of the EDCTP2 programme supported by the European Union (grant number CSA2016S-1618) and the Swedish International Development Cooperation Agency (SIDA). Project website: https://proforma.ki.se/

E. Aklillu (✉)
Department of Global Public Health, Karolinska Institutet,
Karolinska University Hospital, Stockholm, Sweden
e-mail: eleni.aklillu@ki.se

M. Nderu
EDCTP, The Hague, The Netherlands

to strengthen national pharmacovigilance and post-marketing surveillance capacity in Ethiopia, Kenya, Rwanda, and Tanzania.

PROFORMA is a collaboration between experts from academia, NMRAs, and WHO-collaborating pharmacovigilance centres, as well as Regional Centres of Regulatory Excellence (RCOREs), with the goal of developing a cohort of pharmacovigilance-trained personnel from all stakeholders, including patients, healthcare providers, and regulatory staffs, who are actively involved in pharmaco-vigilance data collection, analysis, interpretation, and data sharing. The primary focus is on pharmacovigilance implementation in clinical trial regulation and post-marketing surveillance in health initiatives involving national mass drug adminis-tration and immunisation campaigns.

24.2   Goals and Objectives

To strengthen the national pharmacovigilance infrastructure and post-marketing surveillance system involving mass drug administration and immunisation pro-grammes being deployed under public health programmes in four East African countries, namley, Ethiopia, Kenya, Rwanda, and Tanzania.

24.3   Specific Objectives

1. Using harmonised Pharmacovigilance Indicators methods, assess current phar-macovigilance policies, legislation, and infrastructures (in Ethiopia, Tanzania, Rwanda, and Kenya) to identify gaps, needs, and local priorities.
2. Implement comprehensive intervention programmes and Good Pharmacovigilance Practises to enhance pharmacovigilance capability in each country based on identified gaps, local priorities, and needs.
3. To develop a cohort of pharmacovigilance-trained people in NMRAs and medi-cal universities capable of leading and managing a sustainable national pharma-covigilance and regulatory process and training programmes.
4. To provide interregional training of trainers on pharmacovigilance and cohort event monitoring for patients, ADR collection and reporting, signal detection on mass drug administration (MDA), and immunisation programmes in East Africa.
5. To provide support for staff from regulatory agencies and higher education institutions to attend pharmacovigilance training and workshops both locally and globally. To ensure long-term viability, a total of 12 postgraduates (PhD/ MSc) in Pharmacovigilance and Pharmacoepidemiology will be taught and will help local medical universities in launching postgraduate PV programmes.

24.4 Project Activities

The research project began with an in-depth review of the current pharmacovigilance systems and practises in Ethiopia, Tanzania, Rwanda, and Kenya [1]. The goal was to identify the structures, strengths, shortcomings, and gaps in the missing pharmacovigilance systems. In each project participating country, a comprehensive baseline assessment of pharmacovigilance systems was conducted across the NMRAs, public health programmes, health facilities, and marketing authorization holders. This assessment revealed critical, country-specific deficiencies in areas such as policy and legislation, system infrastructure, stakeholder coordination, and core pharmacovigilance functions—including signal detection, risk assessment, and risk management. To address the gaps, the PROFORMA-Triangle Model - a trilateral partnership between academia, NMRAs, and public health programmes - was formed. Based on the identified deficiencies, each country developed and implemented a comprehensive national pharmacovigilance roadmap, strategies and intervention plans aligned with the local priorities and needs. Targeted interventions included policy and legislative reforms, workforce development, and sustainable capacity-building efforts. Pharmacovigilance was integrated into academic curricula, postgraduate training was provided for regulatory staff, and short courses and e-learning modules were introduced. Through a train-the-trainer cascade model, widespread capacity building was achieved, training more than 50,000 stakeholders, including staff from NMRAs, healthcare workers, personnel from public health programmes, and academic institutions.

PROFORMA has also formed collaborations with national public health programmes that use targeted mass drug administration (MDA) or immunisation programmes to monitor the safety of medicines and vaccines. Each country's partner NMRAs, medical universities, and neglected tropical diseases (NTD) programmes conducted active safety and efficacy surveillance of medications used in MDA. More than 45,000 people who received MDA as preventive chemotherapy for the treatment of NTDs have been regularly monitored for safety.

In 2019, the active safety and efficacy surveillance activities by PROFORMA included the following:

- Mass praziquantel and albendazole administration for the control of schistosomiasis and soil-transmitted helminths in 6000 school children from southern Ethiopia [2]
- A similar use of praziquantel and albendazole for the treatment and control of schistosomiasis and soil-transmitted helminths in 10,000 school children living near Lake Kivu in Rwanda [3]
- Targeted mass administration of ivermectin and albendazole for the control of lymphatic filariasis and onchocerciasis in 10,000 individuals from Tanga region, Tanzania [4]
- Targeted mass administration of ivermectin and albendazole and diethylcarbamazine for the control of lymphatic filariasis in 20,000 individuals from Mombasa, Kenya [5]

Key PROFORMA Project Achievements (2018–2024). Over six years, PROFORMA transformed pharmacovigilance systems and infrastructure in Ethiopia, Kenya, Tanzania, and Rwanda. These include:

- **Regulatory Strengthening:** Using WHO PV Indicators, baseline assessments identified gaps, leading to tailored five-year national PV roadmaps. Revised policies, guidelines, and regulations, including staff training, fortified pharmacovigilance frameworks. Outcomes included finalized pharmacovigilance regulations for Marketing Authorization Holders (MAHs), National pharmacovigilance Advisory Committees, electronic reporting systems, and decentralized PV centers in university hospitals
- **Capacity Building:** Trained 12 postgraduate experts (6 PhDs, 6 MScs) now leading pharmacovigilance efforts regionally and globally. Short-term training and a train-the-trainer model educated over 50,000 professionals, enhancing skills in risk management and safety monitoring.
- **Improved Education:** PV curricula were integrated into undergraduate and postgraduate programmes, supported by e-learning modules for continuous learning.
- **Scientific Impact**: Over 28 peer-reviewed original articles published and influenced national policies on PV, MDA, and immunization safety.
- **Adverse Event Reporting Surge:** Enhanced pharmacovigilance boosted ADR submissions to the WHO Programme for International Drug Monitoring. In 2024, Ethiopia ranked second in Africa for adverse event reporting, while Tanzania exceeded WHO targets with 11,904 ADRs and 1,200 AEFIs in 2023/24.
- **WHO Maturity Level:** Contributed to Rwanda FDA and Tanzania's TMDA achievement of WHO Maturity Level 3, with Ethiopia and Kenya nearing this benchmark, reflecting robust regulatory capacity.

PROFORMA has also developed networks with stakeholders in Sweden, notably the WHO Programme for International Drug Monitoring—Uppsala Monitoring Centre and the Swedish Medical Products Agency, to explore opportunities for future cooperation and knowledge sharing. In general, the project's results will improve the ability of national and regional health systems to establish capacity to assess the safety of innovative therapies for poverty-related disorders. The project has established a scalable and sustainable model for building resilient PV systems in resource-limited settings. Its integrated training frameworks, governance structures, and skilled workforce offer a practical blueprint for enhancing medicine safety across Sub-Saharan Africa and comparable regions globally. The legacy of the PROFORMA Project lies in its sustainable model—empowered professionals, strengthened pharmacovigilance systems and infrastructure, and a replicable Triangle Model. With trained postgraduates now leading pharmacovigilance initiatives at both national and regional levels, and countries actively contributing to global safety monitoring efforts, the project has established a solid foundation for safer medicines and healthier communities across East Africa and beyond.

The PROFORMA Consortium

Coordinator:

Karolinska Institutet, Sweden,
Professor Eleni Aklillu, PhD

Participants

1. Addis Ababa University (AAU), Ethiopia
2. Ethiopia Food and Drug (EFDA), Ethiopia
3. University of Nairobi, Kenya
4. Pharmacy and Poisons Board, Kenya
5. Tanzania Food and Drugs Authority (TFDA), Tanzania
6. Muhimbili University of Health & Allied Sciences (MUHAS), Tanzania
7. University of Rwanda, Rwanda
8. Ministry of Health, Rwanda
9. Stichting Lareb, The Netherlands

References

1. Barry A, et al. Comparative assessment of the National Pharmacovigilance Systems in East Africa: Ethiopia, Kenya, Rwanda and Tanzania. Drug Saf. 2020;43(4):339–50.
2. Gebreyesus TD, Makonnen E, Tadele T, Mekete K, Gashaw H, Gerba H, Aklillu E. Efficacy and safety of praziquantel preventive chemotherapy in Schistosoma mansoni infected school children in Southern Ethiopia: A prospective cohort study. Front Pharmacol. 20231;14:968106. https://doi.org/10.3389/fphar.2023.968106. PMID: 36937860; PMCID: PMC10014719.
3. Kabatende J, Barry A, Mugisha M, Ntirenganya L, Bergman U, Bienvenu E, Aklillu E. Safety of Praziquantel and Albendazole Coadministration for the Control and Elimination of Schistosomiasis and Soil-Transmitted Helminths Among Children in Rwanda: An Active Surveillance Study. Drug Saf. 2022;45(8):909-922. https://doi.org/10.1007/s40264-022-01201-3. Epub 2022 Jul 11. PMID: 35819751; PMCID: PMC9360141.
4. Fimbo AM, et al. Prevalence and correlates of lymphatic Filariasis infection and its morbidity following mass Ivermectin and Albendazole Administration in Mkinga District, North-Eastern Tanzania. J Clin Med. 2020;9(5):1550. https://doi.org/10.3390/jcm9051550.
5. Khaemba C, Njenga SM, Omondi WP, Kirui E, Oluka M, Guantai A, Aklillu E. Safety and effectiveness of triple-drug therapy with ivermectin, diethylcarbamazine, and albendazole in reducing lymphatic filariasis prevalence and clearing circulating filarial antigens in Mombasa, Kenya. Infect Dis Poverty. 2025;14(1):11. https://doi.org/10.1186/s40249-025-01282-z. PMID: 39994719; PMCID: PMC11849337.
6. Khaemba C, Njenga SM, Omondi WP, Kirui E, Oluka M, Guantai A, Aklillu E. Safety and Effectiveness of Triple-Drug Therapy with Ivermectin, Diethylcarbamazine, and Albendazole in Reducing Lymphatic Filariasis Prevalence and Clearing Circulating Filarial Antigens in Mombasa, Kenya. Infect Dis Poverty. 2025;14:11. https://doi.org/10.1186/s40249-025-01282-z.
7. Fimbo AM, Mnkugwe RH, Mlugu EM, Kumambi PP, Malishee A, Minzi OMS, Kamuhabwa AAR, Aklillu E. Efficacy of ivermectin and albendazole combination in suppressing transmission of lymphatic filariasis following mass administration in Tanzania: a prospective cohort study. Infect Dis Poverty. 2024;13:44. https://doi.org/10.1186/s40249-024-01214-3.
8. van Puijenbroek E, Barry A, Khaemba C, Ntirenganya L, Gebreyesus TD, Fimbo A, Minzi O, Makonnen E, Oluka M, Guantai A, Aklillu E. Short-term training, a useful approach for

sustainable pharmacovigilance knowledge development in Tanzania, Kenya, Ethiopia and Rwanda. Drug Saf. 2024;47(12):1193–202. https://doi.org/10.1007/s40264-024-01469-7.

9. Gebreyesus TD, Makonnen E, Tedele NF, Barry A, Mnkugwe RH, Gerba H, Dahl ML, Aklillu E. CYP2C19 and CYP2J2 genotypes predict praziquantel plasma exposure among Ethiopian school-aged children. Sci Rep. 2024;14:11730. https://doi.org/10.1038/s41598-024-62669-w.

10. Gebreyesus TD, Makonnen E, Tadele T, Mekete K, Gashaw H, Gerba H, Aklillu E. Reduced efficacy of single-dose albendazole against Ascaris lumbricoides, and Trichuris trichiura, and high reinfection rate after cure among school children in southern Ethiopia: a prospective cohort study. Infect Dis Poverty. 2024;13(1):8. https://doi.org/10.1186/s40249-024-01176-6.

11. Tadele T, Astatkie A, Tadesse BT, Makonnen E, Aklillu E, Abay SM. Efficacy and safety of praziquantel treatment against Schistosoma mansoni infection among pre-school age children in southern Ethiopia. Trop Med Health. 2023;51:72. https://doi.org/10.1186/s41182-023-00562-4.

12. Tadele T, Astatkie A, Abay SM, Tadesse BT, Makonnen E, Aklillu E. Prevalence and determinants of schistosoma mansoni infection among pre-school age children in southern ethiopia. Pathogens. 2023;12(7):858. https://doi.org/10.3390/pathogens12070858.

13. Khaemba C, Barry A, Omondi WP, Kirui E, Oluka M, Parthasarathi G, Njenga SM, Guantai A, Aklillu E. Comparative safety surveillance of triple (IDA) versus dual therapy (DA) in mass drug administration for elimination of lymphatic filariasis in kenya: a cohort event monitoring study. Drug Saf. 2023;46:961–74. https://doi.org/10.1007/s40264-023-01338-9.

14. Kabatende J, Ntirenganya L, Mugisha M, Barry A, Ruberanziza E, Bienvenu E, Bergman U, Aklillu E. Efficacy of Single-Dose Praziquantel for the Treatment of Schistosoma mansoni Infections among School Children in Rwanda. Pathogens. 2023;12(9):1170. https://doi.org/10.3390/pathogens12091170.

15. Kabatende J, Barry A, Mugisha M, Ntirenganya L, Bergman U, Bienvenu E, Aklillu E. Efficacy of single-dose albendazole for the treatment of soil-transmitted helminthic infections among school children in rwanda-a prospective cohort study. Pharmaceuticals (Basel). 2023;16:139. https://doi.org/10.3390/ph16020139.

16. Gebreyesus TD, Makonnen E, Tadele T, Mekete K, Gashaw H, Gerba H, Aklillu E. Efficacy and safety of praziquantel preventive chemotherapy in Schistosoma mansoni infected school children in Southern Ethiopia: A prospective cohort study. Front Pharmacol. 2023;14:968106. https://doi.org/10.3389/fphar.2023.968106.

17. Fimbo AM, Mlugu EM, Kitabi EN, Kulwa GS, Iwodyah MA, Mnkugwe RH, Kunambi PP, Malishee A, Kamuhabwa AAR, Minzi OM, Aklillu E. Population pharmacokinetics of ivermectin after mass drug administration in lymphatic filariasis endemic communities of Tanzania. CPT Pharmacometrics Syst Pharmacol. 2023;12:1884–96. https://doi.org/10.1002/psp4.13038.

18. Barry A, Kabatende J, Telele NF, Mnkugwe RH, Mugisha M, Ntirenganya L, Bienvenu E, Aklillu E. Effect of pharmacogenetic variations on praziquantel plasma concentration and safety outcomes among school children in Rwanda. Sci Rep. 2023;13:1446. https://doi.org/10.1038/s41598-023-28641-w.

19. Kabatende J, Barry A, Mugisha M, Ntirenganya L, Bergman U, Bienvenu E, Aklillu E. Safety of praziquantel and albendazole coadministration for the control and elimination of schistosomiasis and soil-transmitted helminths among children in rwanda: an active surveillance study. Drug Saf. 2022;45:909–22. https://doi.org/10.1007/s40264-022-01201-3.

20. Gebreyesus TD, Makonnen E, Tadele T, Gashaw H, Degefe W, Gerba H, Tadesse BT, Gurumurthy P, Aklillu E. Safety Surveillance of Mass Praziquantel and Albendazole Co-Administration in School Children from Southern Ethiopia: An Active Cohort Event Monitoring. J Clin Med. 2022;11(21):6300. https://doi.org/10.3390/jcm11216300.

21. Fimbo AM, Minzi OM, Mmbando BP, Gurumurthy P, Kamuhabwa AAR, Aklillu E. Safety and Tolerability of Ivermectin and Albendazole Mass Drug Administration in Lymphatic Filariasis Endemic Communities of Tanzania: A Cohort Event Monitoring Study. Pharmaceuticals (Basel). 2022;15(5):594. https://doi.org/10.3390/ph15050594.

22. Mnkugwe RH, Ngaimisi Kitabi E, Kinung'hi S, Kamuhabwa AAR, Minzi OM, Aklillu E. Optimal single sampling time-point for monitoring of praziquantel exposure in children. Sci Rep. 2021;11:17955. https://doi.org/10.1038/s41598-021-97409-x.

23. Mnkugwe RH, Minzi O, Kinung'hi S, Kamuhabwa A, Aklillu E. Effect of Pharmacogenetics Variations on Praziquantel Plasma Concentrations and Schistosomiasis Treatment Outcomes Among Infected School-Aged Children in Tanzania. Front Pharmacol. 2021;12:712084. https://doi.org/10.3389/fphar.2021.712084.

24. Minzi OM, Mnkugwe RH, Ngaimisi E, Kinung'hi S, Hansson A, Pohanka A, Kamuhabwa A, Aklillu E. Effect of Dihydroartemisinin-Piperaquine on the Pharmacokinetics of Praziquantel for Treatment of Schistosoma mansoni Infection. Pharmaceuticals (Basel). 2021;4(5):400. https://doi.org/10.3390/ph14050400.

25. Khaemba C, Barry A, Omondi WP, Bota K, Matendechero S, Wandera C, Siyoi F, Kirui E, Oluka M, Namibia P, Gurumurthy P, Njenga SM, Guantai A, Akilllu E. Safety and Tolerability of Mass Diethylcarbamazine and Albendazole Administration for the Elimination of Lymphatic Filariasis in Kenya: An Active Surveillance Study. Pharmaceuticals (Basel). 2021;14(3):264. https://doi.org/10.3390/ph14030264.

26. Barry A, Olsson S, Khaemba C, Kabatende J, Dires T, Fimbo A, Minzi O, Bienvenu E, Makonnen E, Kamuhabwa A, Oluka M, Guantai A, van Puijebroek E, Bergman U, Nkayamba A, Mugisha M, Gurumurthy P, Aklillu E. Comparative Assessment of the Pharmacovigilance Systems within the Neglected Tropical Diseases Programs in East Africa-Ethiopia, Kenya, Rwanda, and Tanzania. Int J Environ Res Public Health. 2021;18(4):1941. https://doi.org/10.3390/ijerph18041941.

27. Mnkugwe RH, Minzi OS, Kinung'hi SM, Kamuhabwa AA, Aklillu, E. Prevalence and correlates of intestinal schistosomiasis infection among school-aged children in North-Western Tanzania. PLoS One. 2020;15:e0228770. https://doi.org/10.1371/journal.pone.0228770.

28. Mnkugwe RH, Minzi O, Kinung'hi S, Kamuhabwa A, Aklillu E. Efficacy and safety of praziquantel and dihydroartemisinin piperaquine combination for treatment and control of intestinal schistosomiasis: A randomized, non-inferiority clinical trial. PLoS Negl Trop Dis. 2020;14:e0008619. https://doi.org/10.1371/journal.pntd.0008619.

29. Kabatende J, Mugisha M, Ntirenganya L, Barry A, Ruberanziza E, Mbonigaba JB, Bergman U, Bienvenu E, Aklillu E. Prevalence, Intensity, and Correlates of Soil-Transmitted Helminth Infections among School Children after a Decade of Preventive Chemotherapy in Western Rwanda. Pathogens. 2020;9(12):1076. https://doi.org/10.3390/pathogens9121076.

30. Gebreyesus TD, Tadele T, Mekete K, Barry A, Gashaw H, Degefe W, Tadesse BT, Gerba H, Gurumurthy P, Makonnen E, Aklillu E. Prevalence, Intensity, and Correlates of Schistosomiasis and Soil-Transmitted Helminth Infections after Five Rounds of Preventive Chemotherapy among School Children in Southern Ethiopia. Pathogens. 2020;9(11):920. https://doi.org/10.3390/pathogens9110920.

31. Fimbo AM, Minzi OMS, Mmbando BP, Barry A, Nkayamba AF, Mwamwitwa KW, Malishee A, Seth MD, Makunde WH, Gurumurthy P, Lusingu JPA, Kamuhabwa AAR, Aklillu E. Prevalence and Correlates of Lymphatic Filariasis Infection and Its Morbidity Following Mass Ivermectin and Albendazole Administration in Mkinga District, North-Eastern Tanzania. J Clin Med. 2020;9(5):1550. https://doi.org/10.3390/jcm9051550.

32. Barry A, Olsson S, Minzi O, Bienvenu E, Makonnen E, Kamuhabwa A, Oluka M, Guantai A, Bergman U, van Puijenbroek E, Gurumurthy P, Aklillu E. Comparative Assessment of the National Pharmacovigilance Systems in East Africa: Ethiopia, Kenya, Rwanda and Tanzania. Drug Saf. 2020;43:339–50. https://doi.org/10.1007/s40264-019-00898-z.

33. Mnkugwe RH, Minzi OS, Kinung'hi SM, Kamuhabwa AA, Aklillu E. Efficacy and Safety of Praziquantel for Treatment of Schistosoma mansoni Infection among School Children in Tanzania. Pathogens. 2019;9(1):28. https://doi.org/10.3390/pathogens9010028.

Chapter 25
Strengthening Pharmacovigilance in Africa: PhArmacoVigilance Africa (PAVIA)

Frank G. J. Cobelens and Michelle Nderu

PhArmacoVigilance Africa (PAVIA) is a project that was funded by the European Union under European and Developing Countries Clinical Trials Partnership (EDCTP2) program (grant number CSA2016S-1627-PAVIA). This was originally planned as a 4-year project to be executed from March 2018 until February 2022 but was granted a 1-year no-cost extension (ending February 2023) because activities could not be carried out as planned due to the COVID-19 pandemic. The project aimed to improve the ability of health systems in Sub-Saharan Africa (SSA) to deliver new medicinal products and monitor their post-market safety in an effective way. PAVIA's activities focused on strengthening collaboration between countries' regulatory authorities responsible for pharmacovigilance (PV) and public health control programs responsible for introduction of new drugs and vaccines for poverty-related infectious diseases. This is because new treatments for these diseases are introduced based on only limited safety data from clinical trials. The project aimed to ensure that introduction of these new or improved treatments is done in a unified manner and according to WHO's guidance by collecting safety data and acting upon safety signals.

This project is part of the EDCTP2 programme supported by the European Union (grant number CSA2016S-1627) and the United States Agency for International Development (United States of America).
Project website: https://pavia-project.net/
All public project documentation, including the Blueprint, is freely downloadable from The Global Health Network: https://globalpharmacovigilance.tghn.org/pavia/

F. G. J. Cobelens (✉)
Amsterdam Institute for Global Health and Development, Department of Global Health, Amsterdam University Medical Centers, Amsterdam, The Netherlands
e-mail: f.cobelens@aighd.org; https://www.aighd.org/

M. Nderu
EDCTP, The Hague, The Netherlands

© Springer Nature Singapore Pte Ltd. 2025
S. R. Ahmad (ed.), *Special Issues in Pharmacovigilance in Resource-Limited Countries*, https://doi.org/10.1007/978-981-96-6154-1_25

The PAVIA project was implemented in four African countries with different levels of maturity of their PV systems: Eswatini, Ethiopia, Nigeria, and Tanzania. The best practices learnt from these four countries were highlighted in a Blueprint document to be shared and cascaded to other African countries. To achieve its objectives, PAVIA harnessed the expertise from several African and European institutions.

25.1 Objectives and Strategy

These objectives were to strengthen the capacity for pharmacovigilance of new products for poverty-related diseases in these four countries by:

1. Improving PV governance by strengthening regulatory and organizational structures and defining clear roles and responsibilities for all stakeholders
2. Increasing the efficiency and effectiveness of national PV systems by strengthening the monitoring of adverse drug reactions and implementing tools and technologies for their detection, reporting, analysis, and dissemination
3. Enlarging the human capacity and building the skills to conduct effective safety surveillance throughout the country
4. Improving the readiness of the health systems for PV through performance assessment of PV systems and identifying, and acting upon, enablers and barriers for implementation

PAVIA's strategy was to forge effective collaborations around medicines safety surveillance between national medicines regulatory authorities and their associated pharmacovigilance agencies on the one hand, and public health programmes on the other hand. PAVIA's initial focus was on the introduction of new drugs and treatment regimens for multidrug-resistant tuberculosis (MDR-TB) by the national tuberculosis programmes (NTPs). The collaborative activities were aimed at increasing the quantity and quality of adverse event reports by NTPs to PV agencies in accordance with country policies by training health workers, improving reporting flows, and enhancing reporting through technological improvements. In addition, the capacity of the PV agencies to act upon these safety reports was improved by providing training and hands-on expert guidance on causality assessment, signal detection, and risk communication at the national and lower levels in the health system.

25.2 Triangle Model

In each of the participating countries, a uniquely designed "PAVIA Triangle" was established as a core coordinating mechanism for effective collaboration between the national medicine regulatory authority/national PV agency and the national public health program that was introducing a new drug or vaccine product. As a third key actor, the PAVIA Triangle also included one or more local medical research institutes that supported the PV process by providing medical expertise, training, and research.

Starting with PV for new drugs and treatment regimens for MDR-TB, the Triangle provided a channel for reporting and interpreting safety signals; served as a training ground for country PV staff and clinicians; and became a demonstration project for PV collaborations with other disease control programmes. During the course of the project, PAVIA expanded the Triangle Model to other public health programmes (e.g., HIV/AIDS, malaria, immunization), depending on country needs and preferences.

25.3 Stakeholder Engagement

The project partners included national medicine regulatory authorities, local medical research institutes, and NTPs (through KCNV Tuberculosis Foundation's country offices).

In addition, it included expert PV and TB centres: the University of Benin (Nigeria), the Netherlands Pharmacovigilance Centre LAREB (the Netherlands), KCNV Tuberculosis Foundation (the Netherlands), University of Verona (Italy), and the Amsterdam Institute for Global Health and Development (the Netherlands).

PAVIA engaged national and local stakeholders in the PV process in each of its project countries. In addition, the project strengthened collaborations with regional and global key stakeholders in the PV initiatives on the continent by aligning PV activities with AUDA/NEPAD, the Regional Economic Communities, the WHO Programme for International Drug Monitoring, and the Gates Foundation.

25.4 Project Activities and Achievements

The project started with baseline assessments of the PV situation in each of the project countries, both generic and with specific view to drug treatment of MDR-TB. Based on the results, country-specific PV Roadmaps were developed as a key step in the strategic planning process for activities aimed at strengthening country PV including, but not limited to, those supported by PAVIA. The Roadmaps were subsequently endorsed by the responsible national authorities.

Other activities included improvement of reporting flows, introduction of new reporting tools such as electronic reporting and strengthened supportive supervision of MDR-TB treatment sites. Trainings were held at various levels: PV agencies staff, MDR-TB nurses and clinicians, and general health care providers. For the latter, aimed at raising PV awareness among health care providers, a blended learning package consisting of e-learning and limited classroom teaching was developed, introduced, and implemented through step-down trainings.

PAVIA's activities have resulted in a surge of adverse drug reaction reports received at national PV agencies. In the final year, over 100 reports were received from MDR-TB patients in Nigeria and around 200 in Ethiopia. While the number of MDR-TB reports submitted was not separately counted for Tanzania and Eswatini, in both countries the total number of reports received has significantly increased: fivefold in Tanzania and fourfold in Eswatini.

Under the leadership of the University of Benin, Nigeria, PAVIA also advocated for PV policy strengthening at national levels in partner countries. After approval of the Ministry of Health, a Standalone PV Policy document in Eswatini was developed. The Nigerian PV Policy has been revised. The Tanzanian national medicines regulatory authority opted to use part of the PAVIA support to domesticate its Pharmacovigilance Regulations.

Furthermore, PAVIA conducted a continent-wide inventory of national approaches to funding for PV agencies and activities, and these have been published in a report on models for sustainable PV funding.

In its final project year, PAVIA conducted end-line assessments of the PV system in each of the countries. The findings were compiled in a Blueprint with the aim of guiding other countries wishing to strengthen their national PV system by improving the engagement of public health programs. The key output of the project, the Blueprint shows the lessons learnt and best practices from the project that are relevant and potentially applicable to other African countries. The Blueprint underscores the importance of a clear mandate provided by a set of laws, regulations, and policies, prioritized sustainable and sufficient funding for PV operations and maintenance of the requisite personnel with active support from national governments. These, well coupled with improved awareness and knowledge about PV through dedicated and focused trainings, are critical for a functional PV system in general and for drugs and vaccines for poverty-related diseases in particular.

25.5 Project Partners

1. Amsterdam Institute of Global Health and Development (AIGHD), Netherlands–Coordinator
2. Armauer Hansen Research Institute (AHRI), Ethiopia
3. Institute of Human Virology, Nigeria (IHVN), Nigeria
4. The Good Samaritan Foundation (Kilimanjaro Christian Medical Centre GSF KCMC), Tanzania
5. Stichting Lareb, Netherlands
6. University of Verona, Italy
7. KNCV Tuberculosis Foundation, Netherlands
8. University of Benin, Nigeria
9. National Agency for Food and Drug Administration and Control (NAFDAC)—Nigeria

10. Ministry of Health—Eswatini
11. Tanzania Food and Drug Administration (TFDA), Tanzania
12. Baylor College of Medicine Children's Foundation Swaziland (BIPAI), Eswatini
13. Ethiopia Food and Drug Administration (EFDA), Ethiopia

MIX

Papier | Fördert
gute Waldnutzung

FSC® C083411

Zeitfracht Medien GmbH
Ferdinand-Jühlke-Straße 7
99095 Erfurt, Deutschland
produktsicherheit@kolibri360.de